Rhinoplasty

Editors

SAM P. MOST
ALAN MATARASSO

CLINICS IN
PLASTIC SURGERY

www.plasticsurgery.theclinics.com

January 2022 • Volume 49 • Number 1

ELSEVIER

1600 John F. Kennedy Boulevard • Suite 1800 • Philadelphia, Pennsylvania, 19103-2899

http://www.theclinics.com

CLINICS IN PLASTIC SURGERY Volume 49, Number 1
January 2022 ISSN 0094-1298, ISBN-13: 978-0-323-83588-6

Editor: Stacy Eastman
Developmental Editor: Jessica Nicole B. Cañaberal

Clinics in Plastic Surgery (ISSN 0094-1298) is published quarterly by Elsevier Inc., 360 Park Avenue South, New York, NY 10010-1710. Months of issue are January, April, July, and October. Business and Editorial Offices: 1600 John F. Kennedy Blvd., Suite 1800, Philadelphia, PA 19103-2899. Periodicals postage paid at New York, NY and additional mailing offices. Subscription prices are $548.00 per year for US individuals, $1234.00 per year for US institutions, $100.00 per year for US students and residents, $613.00 per year for Canadian individuals, $1,259.00 per year for Canadian institutions, $682.00 per year for international individuals, $1,259.00 per year for international institutions, $100.00 per year for Canadian and $305.00 per year for international students/residents. To receive student/resident rate, orders must be accompanied by name of affiliated institution, date of term, and the *signature* of program/residency coordinator on institution letterhead. Orders will be billed at individual rate until proof of status is received. Foreign air speed delivery is included in all *Clinics* subscription prices. All prices are subject to change without notice. **POSTMASTER:** Send address changes to *Clinics in Plastic Surgery*, Elsevier Health Sciences Division, Subscription Customer Service, 3251 Riverport Lane, Maryland Heights, MO 63043. **Customer Service: 1-800-654-2452 (US and Canada). From outside of the United States and Canada, call 314-447-8871. Fax: 314-447-8029. E-mail: JournalsCustomerService-usa@elsevier.com (for print support); JournalsOnline-Support-usa@elsevier.com (for online support).**

Reprints. For copies of 100 or more of articles in this publication, please contact the Commercial Reprints Department, Elsevier Inc., 360 Park Avenue South, New York, New York 10010-1710. Tel.: +1-212-633-3874; Fax: +1-212-633-3820; E-mail: reprints@elsevier.com.

Clinics in Plastic Surgery is covered in *Current Contents, EMBASE/Excerpta Medica, Science Citation Index, MEDLINE/ PubMed (Index Medicus), ASCA, and ISI/BIOMED.*

Contributors

EDITORS

SAM P. MOST, MD, FACS
Chief, Division of Facial Plastic and
Reconstructive Surgery, Director, Fellowship in
Facial Plastic and Reconstructive Surgery,
Professor, Departments of Otolaryngology–
Head and Neck Surgery and Surgery (Plastic),
Professor, Division of Facial Plastic and
Reconstructive Surgery, Stanford University
School of Medicine, Stanford, California, USA

ALAN MATARASSO, MD, FACS
Clinical Professor of Surgery, Hofstra-
Northwell Health System, New York, New York,
USA

AUTHORS

SARAH R. AKKINA, MD, MS
Department of Otolaryngology–Head and Neck
Surgery, University of Washington, Seattle,
Washington, USA; Division of Facial Plastic
and Reconstructive Surgery, Department of
Otolaryngology–Head and Neck Surgery,
Stanford University School of Medicine, Palo
Alto, California, USA

BRENDAN ALLEYNE, MD
Renaissance Plastic Surgery and Medical Spa,
Saint Peters, Missouri, USA

ANDREW N. ATIA, MD
Division of Plastic, Maxillofacial, and Oral
Surgery, Duke University Hospital, Durham,
North Carolina, USA

JUSTIN BELLAMY, MD
Dallas Plastic Surgery Institute, Dallas, Texas,
USA

MATTHEW A. BRIDGES, MD, FACS
Private Practice, Facial Plastic Surgery
(Commonwealth Facial Plastic Surgery),
Assistant Clinical Professor, Department
of Otolaryngology–Head and Neck Surgery,
Virginia Commonwealth University School of
Medicine, Richmond, Virginia, USA

JAY W. CALVERT, MD
Aesthetic Surgery Fellowship Director, Division
of Plastic and Reconstructive Surgery,
University of Southern California, Beverly Hills,
California, USA

NAZIM CERKES, MD
Private Practice, Istanbul, Turkey

EDWARD CHAMATA, MD
Dallas Plastic Surgery Institute, Division of
Plastic Surgery, Baylor College of Medicine,
Houston, Texas, USA

MONA CLAPPIER, BA
Division of Plastic and Reconstructive Surgery,
Northwell Health, Great Neck, New York, USA;
Division of Plastic and Reconstructive Surgery,
Donald and Barbara Zucker School of
Medicine at Hofstra/Northwell, Hempstead,
New York, USA

ROXANA COBO, MD
Private Practice Facial Plastic Surgery, Chief, Department of Otolaryngology, Clinica Imbanaco, Grupo Quiron Salud, Cali, Colombia

MARK B. CONSTANTIAN, MD, FACS
Private Practice, Plastic Surgery, Traveling Professor, American Society for Aesthetic Plastic Surgery, Clinical Adjunct Professor of Surgery, (Plastic Surgery), University of Wisconsin-Madison, Clinical Professor, Department of Surgery, Division of Plastic and Reconstructive Surgery, University of Wisconsin-Madison School of Medicine and Public Health, Madison, Wisconsin, USA; Visiting Professor, Department of Plastic Surgery, University of Virginia Medical School, Charlottesville, Virginia, USA

DANIELLE F. EYTAN, MD
Assistant Professor, Division of Facial Plastic and Reconstructive Surgery, Department of Otolaryngology–Head and Neck Surgery, New York University School of Medicine, New York, New York, USA

GRACE J. GRAW, MD
Private Practice, Graw Beauty | Dr. Grace, Palo Alto, California, USA

BAHMAN GUYURON, MD
Zeeba Clinic, Lyndhurst, Ohio, USA; Professor Emeritus, Case Western Reserve University, Cleveland, Ohio, USA

ANDREA HANICK, MD
Department of Otolaryngology–Head and Neck Surgery, Washington University School of Medicine, Missouri, USA

CHERINE H. KIM, MD, PhD
Division of Facial Plastic and Reconstructive Surgery, Department of Otolaryngology–Head and Neck Surgery, Loma Linda University School of Medicine, Loma Linda, California, USA

JEFFREY R. MARCUS, MD
Division of Plastic, Maxillofacial, and Oral Surgery, Duke University Hospital, Durham, North Carolina, USA

SAM P. MOST, MD, FACS
Chief, Division of Facial Plastic and Reconstructive Surgery, Director, Fellowship in Facial Plastic and Reconstructive Surgery, Professor, Departments of Otolaryngology–Head and Neck Surgery and Surgery (Plastic), Professor, Division of Facial Plastic and Reconstructive Surgery, Stanford University School of Medicine, Stanford, California, USA

SAMI P. MOUBAYED, MD
Assistant Professor of Surgery, University of Montreal, Montreal, Canada

MATTHEW NOVAK, MD
Dallas Plastic Surgery Institute, Dallas, Texas, USA

CRISTEN E. OLDS, MD
Roxbury Institute, Beverly Hills, California, USA

PRIYESH N. PATEL, MD
Assistant Professor, Division of Facial Plastic and Reconstructive Surgery, Department of Otolaryngology, Vanderbilt University Medical Center, Nashville, Tennessee, USA

BRYAN J. PYFER, MD, MBA
Division of Plastic, Maxillofacial, and Oral Surgery, Duke University Hospital, Durham, North Carolina, USA

ARIEL N. RAD, MD, PhD
Private Practice, Plastic Surgery (SHERBER+RAD), Clinical Assistant Professor, Department of Plastic Surgery, The Johns Hopkins Hospital, Baltimore, Maryland, USA

ROD ROHRICH, MD
Dallas Plastic Surgery Institute, Dallas, Texas, USA; Division of Plastic Surgery, Baylor College of Medicine, Houston, Texas, USA

SEBASTIAN SCIEGIENKA, MD
Department of Otolaryngology–Head and Neck Surgery, Washington University School of Medicine, Missouri, USA

EMILY SPATARO, MD
Department of Otolaryngology–Head and Neck Surgery, Washington University School of Medicine, Missouri, USA

JONATHAN M. SYKES, MD
Roxbury Institute, Beverly Hills, California, USA; Facial Plastic and Reconstructive

Surgery, UC Davis Medical Center, Sacramento, California, USA

NEIL TANNA, MD, MBA
Associate Program Director of Plastic Surgery, Division of Plastic and Reconstructive Surgery, Northwell Health, Great Neck, New York, USA; Professor of Surgery, Division of Plastic and Reconstructive Surgery, Donald and Barbara Zucker School of Medicine at Hofstra/ Northwell, Hempstead, New York, USA

ALI TOTONCHI, MD
Associate Professor, Case Western Reserve University, MetroHealth Hospital, Medical Director, Craniofacial Deformity Clinic, Cleveland, Ohio, USA

TOM D. WANG, MD
Professor, Division of Facial Plastic and Reconstructive Surgery, Department of Otolaryngology–Head and Neck Surgery, Oregon Health & Sciences University, Portland, Oregon, USA

Surgery, UC Davis Medical Center, Sacramento, California, USA

NEIL TANNA, MD, MBA
Associate Program Director of Plastic Surgery, Division of Plastic and Reconstructive Surgery, Northwell Health, New York, USA; Professor of Surgery, Division of Plastic and Reconstructive Surgery, Donald and Barbara Zucker School of Medicine at Hofstra/ Northwell, Hempstead, New York, USA

ALI TOTONCHI, MD
Associate Professor, Case Western Reserve University, MetroHealth Hospital; Medical Director, Cranial Deformity Clinic, Cleveland, Ohio, USA

TOM D. WANG, MD
Professor, Division of Facial Plastic and Reconstructive Surgery, Department of Otolaryngology/Head and neck Surgery, Oregon Health & Sciences University, Portland, Oregon, USA

Contents

Requiring both high-level technical skills and artistic sense, rhinoplasty continues to be one of the most challenging procedures in plastic surgery despite its popularity. A thorough preoperative consultation of the rhinoplasty patient forms the foundation of a successful case. During the consultation, the physician should obtain a detailed medical and nasal history, understand the patient's areas of concern, conduct a nasal analysis, and evaluate the patient's candidacy for surgery. This article reviews the key functional, esthetic, and psychosocial considerations that should be taken into account during a preoperative consultation for a rhinoplasty patient.

Photodocumentation is an essential part of a rhinoplasty surgeon's practice. Preoperative photographs are an indispensable device for patient counseling and surgical planning. Comparison of preoperative and postoperative photographs allow for outcome evaluation, which has a variety of applications—clinical, research, teaching, medicolegal. The ever-evolving technology of photography may seem daunting, but developing a basic understanding of this tool is imperative for a successful rhinoplasty practice. This article reviews the basic photographic principles, equipment, and techniques that are essential to produce high-quality and standardized patient photographs.

Nasal airway obstruction is a very common phenomenon that can significantly decrease patients' quality of life. This review article summarizes in an evidence-based fashion the diagnosis and treatment of nasal airway obstruction. The nasal airway may be obstructed at the level of the nasal valve, septum, nasal turbinates, sinonasal mucosa, or nasopharynx. Nasal valve obstruction and septal deviations are usually treated surgically depending on the level of valve obstruction. Isolated turbinate hypertrophy is usually managed medically as part of the treatment of rhinitis, with surgery reserved for cases refractory to medical care. Sinonasal and nasopharyngeal conditions are treated according to the diagnosis.

Endonasal rhinoplasty is a minimally invasive approach in which esthetic and functional improvements are made solely through intranasal, without transcolumellar, incisions and with limited soft tissue and skeletal disruption. In addition to intentionally limiting surgical dissection, the rhinoplasty surgeon must preoperatively recognize and surgically correct 4 common anatomic variants which predictably create all 3 patterns of secondary deformity. In combination, respecting these principles gives the surgeon greater predictability in achieving esthetic and functional improvements, and the ability to limit the adverse effects of skin contractility and postoperative scar contracture, thus reducing the risk of secondary deformity, patient dissatisfaction, and reoperation.

The nose is a complex three-dimensional structure with critical structural and functional roles; its relationship to surrounding structures is, in part, responsible for a harmonious, pleasing visage as a whole. There are many variables and dimensions that can be adjusted to alter the esthetic appearance, structural components, and functional role of the nose and many tools and maneuvers available to the rhinoplasty surgeon to adjust these numerous variables. Although every rhinoplasty operation should be individualized, a systematic order and algorithm may be helpful in operative planning as well as establishing a logical progression of steps and maintaining stability. While each adjustment may have a primary anticipated effect, it will invariably have a secondary impact.

Controlling the nasal tip to achieve excellent structural and cosmetic outcomes is challenging in rhinoplasty surgery. A strong foundation and understanding of the nasal tripod complex and the various methods for restoring tip support mechanisms when disrupted either from surgery or other means is critical. The columellar strut graft, septal extension graft, and tongue-in-groove suture technique are well-described methods to control and support the nasal tip. There are advantages and disadvantages to each method, but one should be comfortable with the nuances of each to master nasal tip surgery.

Tip reduction and refinement require a thorough understanding of the contributing anatomy, the impact of deprojection on tip stability, and how to control these variables. This article reviews the anatomy, the steps of analysis, and the essential components of the surgical approach. The surgical approach utilized emphasizes open reductive techniques combined with strong and stable central support using the batten-type septal extension graft. This approach allows robust tip-shaping techniques in the setting of an inherently destabilizing tip reduction procedure, effectuating significant tip change while maintaining long-term tip stability.

Dorsal hump reduction is one of the most common techniques used in modern rhinoplasty, yet it carries a high propensity for untoward aesthetic and functional sequelae, as evidenced by a nontrivial revision rate. Component dorsal hump reduction with stepwise deconstruction and manipulation of component parts allows for an adaptable and precise approach to variances in anatomy and in desired aesthetic result. Secondary changes must be anticipated and addressed at the index operation to avoid negative results and prevent the need for revision. Adequate reconstruction of the midvault is paramount to achieving optimal aesthetic and functional outcomes.

Combining Open Structural and Dorsal Preservation Rhinoplasty

Priyesh N. Patel and Sam P. Most

There has been a resurgence in dorsal preservation rhinoplasty (DPR) caused by theoretic aesthetic and functional advantages compared with conventional hump takedown rhinoplasty. Classically, the push-down and let-down maneuvers have been described for management of the bony nasal vault. There have been a variety of modifications in the septal resection that is a requisite for dorsal lowering in DPR. Partial dorsal preservation techniques, including cartilage-only preservation, have also been described. Although several studies have reported aesthetic and functional success with a variety of techniques, few have used objective or patient-centered subjective measures.

Treatment of the Crooked Nose

Sarah R. Akkina and Sam P. Most

The crooked nose is a challenging esthetic and functional problem. The surgeon must carefully evaluate baseline facial asymmetry as well as whether deviation stems from the upper third, middle third, or lower third of the nose. Surgical intervention should be tailored accordingly, with techniques geared toward addressing each deviated section. Modified dorsal preservation techniques represent a newer means to address deviations. Operative results must be measured, ideally through patient-reported outcomes measures, to quantify overall success.

Cleft Rhinoplasty

Cristen E. Olds and Jonathan M. Sykes

An understanding of anatomy and pathophysiology of the cleft nasal deformity is crucial to its management, including selection of correct surgical techniques for repair. Timing of intermediate and definitive rhinoplasty should be considered carefully, with definitive rhinoplasty occurring after management of facial skeletal deformities. At the time of definitive rhinoplasty, the septum, external and internal nasal valves, alar base malposition (and corresponding bony deficiency), and position and shape of the lower lateral cartilage and the columella all must be individually considered. Thorough knowledge of rhinoplasty techniques is crucial to address the cleft nasal deformity with optimal functional and aesthetic outcomes.

Dorsal Augmentation

Grace J. Graw and Jay W. Calvert

 Video content accompanies this article at http://www.plasticsurgery.theclinics.com.

To manage the deficient nasal dorsum, a thorough knowledge of dorsal augmentation techniques should be mastered by the rhinoplasty specialist. Indications for dorsal augmentation may arise in both primary and revision rhinoplasty presentations. To direct operative planning, a complete facial analysis, noting the importance of maintaining overall nasofacial balance, is essential. An array of techniques, including autologous and nonautologous (ie, allogeneic and synthetic) sources, have been used globally—each carrying its own advantages and disadvantages. The authors believe autologous grafts to be the optimal source for dorsal augmentation because of their biocompatibility and ability to produce natural and long-lasting outcomes.

Today non-Caucasian patients comprise an important group of patients seeking rhinoplasty. The term non-Caucasian is used interchangeably to speak about patients of ethnic origin. It becomes important to understand the interplay of culture, race, and ethnicity when evaluating patients and defining what their aesthetic ideals are and what will be needed for surgery. An integrated approach and management of the non-Caucasian patient is presented in which medical and surgical options are explored. The final goal when treating non-Caucasian patients should be trying to help patients achieve their aesthetic ideal in the best possible fashion.

Treatment of nasal base deformities is critical for a successful rhinoplasty. Several anatomic variations are seen on nasal base. Alar base deformities can be horizontal excess or deficiency, vertical excess or deficiency, cephalic malposition or caudal malposition of alar base, wide or narrow nostril sills, and columellar base deformities. Columellar base should be addressed before alar base resections. Correction of columellar base deformities and positioning of medial crural footplates should be the primary step of nasal base surgery to attain aesthetic ideals of the columellar base and improve external nasal valve function. The most common deformities requiring alar base modification include wide nasal base, alar flaring, large nostril size, and asymmetries of nostrils or alae. There are 3 basic types of excision on alar base surgery. (1) Alar wedge excision, (2) nostril sill excision, and (3) combined alar wedge and nostril sill excision. The alar wedge excision is an elliptical excision placed in the alar crease that is used to reduce the size and shorten the vertical length of alar lobule and correct the excessive flaring on the frontal view. Nostril sill excision is the technique which is used to decrease interalar distance and nostril sill length, and reduce the size of nostril. The combined alar wedge and nostril sill excision is used in cases with wide alar base and additionally, there is excessive flaring and large alar lobule.

Rhinoplasty is widely regarded as one of the more technically challenging surgeries, owing in part to the many possible short- and long-term complications that can arise. Although severe complications are uncommon, unforeseen complications can lead to esthetic and functional compromise, patient dissatisfaction, and need for revision surgery. The rhinoplasty surgeon must be prepared to counsel patients and identify and manage the range of complications that may result from this procedure. This article reviews some of the most frequently encountered complications related to rhinoplasty and their management approaches.

Nonsurgical Rhinoplasty   191

Rod Rohrich, Brendan Alleyne, Matthew Novak, Justin Bellamy, and Edward Chamata

 Video content accompanies this article at http://www.plasticsurgery.theclinics.com.

Nonsurgical rhinoplasty is increasing in popularity, and when used appropriately, can be less costly and have less downtime than surgical rhinoplasty. It can offer patients a means of seeing how they would feel about a surgical rhinoplasty later. Injection can be safe but patients should still be counseled regarding the rare, possible risks of tissue loss and potentially irreversible tissue ischemia and irreversible blindness. Treatment with hyaluronidase can be partially effective when signs and symptoms are caught early; however, avoidance is still the best medicine along with seeking an experienced, qualified rhinoplasty plastic surgeon.

CLINICS IN PLASTIC SURGERY

ISSUE OF RELATED INTEREST

Facial Plastic Surgery Clinics
https://www.facialplastic.theclinics.com/
Otolaryngologic Clinics
https://www.oto.theclinics.com/

THE CLINICS ARE AVAILABLE ONLINE!
Access your subscription at:
www.theclinics.com

Preface
Rhinoplasty: A Complex, Four-Dimensional Procedure

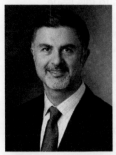 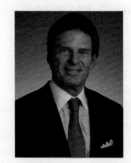

Sam P. Most, MD, FACS   Alan Matarasso, MD, FACS

Editors

Rhinoplasty is widely accepted as one of the most, if not the most, challenging procedures in plastic surgery, comprising numerous interconnected maneuvers that have immediate and long-term consequences on aesthetics and function. Rhinoplasty requires mastering reshaping a three-dimensional bony and cartilaginous structure that projects from the face, taking into account the effect of the skin–soft tissue envelope on results. Finally, the fourth dimension of rhinoplasty surgery, the changes that occur over time, requires the long view in determining success or failure in our results. The results are scrutinized, "front and center," for patients' entire lives. As such, it is fair to say that rhinoplasty impacts appearance perhaps more than any procedure we do.

While John Orlando Roe, an otolaryngologist in Michigan, was the first to publish an article describing this operation in 1887, it was Jacques Joseph, an orthopedic surgeon by training and considered a father of plastic surgery, who pioneered and popularized many of the techniques and instruments used in rhinoplasty in the early twentieth century. Indeed, most common dorsal hump reduction methods are derived from his concepts. In the mid-twentieth century, Maurice Cottle championed concepts of the central importance of nasal physiology and popularized another method for dorsal hump reduction, involving impaction of the dorsum into the maxilla. Many of the leaders in the field of rhinoplasty, plastic surgeons, otolaryngologists, and facial plastic surgeons, continued to develop and teach methods of rhinoplasty from these early pioneers. Over the past century and more, countless articles and textbooks have been published on the art and science of this operation.

So, why the need for yet another compilation on this well-described procedure? Simply put, the bar for measuring success of our results in the procedure is constantly rising. As masters of this operation have shared their experience, our

Clin Plastic Surg 49 (2022) xiii–xiv
https://doi.org/10.1016/j.cps.2021.08.006
0094-1298/22/© 2021 Published by Elsevier Inc.

understanding of associated complications and corrective measures has increased. One obvious example would be Jack Sheen's understanding of the importance of midvault reconstruction after dorsal hump resection. Another example: the idea that one could use the excess upper lateral cartilages as spreader grafts was first described by Fomon in the 1950s but was not popularized for another 50 years.

In the past decade, new ideas have been added to our armamentarium. The use of powered instrumentation has gained acceptance. We are moving from minimizing removal of alar cartilages to complete alar preservation during tip plasty. And, of course, the concept of dorsal preservation, over 100 years old, is now making a comeback.

Countless other examples exist and are constantly being added to our literature. We are constantly evolving our practice to improve outcomes for our patients. As such, we have attempted in this issue to update our readers on some of the advances in rhinoplasty concepts and practice. This issue of *Clinics in Plastic Surgery* has

something for rhinoplasty surgeons of all levels of interest and experience. We hope this brings all readers another step closer to improving our rhinoplasty outcomes and patient satisfaction. We would like to thank our authors, all esteemed members of the community of rhinoplasty surgeons, for their contributions to this issue.

Sam P. Most, MD, FACS
Division of Facial Plastic and Reconstructive Surgery
Stanford University School of Medicine
801 Welch Road
Stanford, CA 94304, USA

Alan Matarasso, MD, FACS
Hofstra-Northwell Health System
New York, NY 10028, USA

E-mail addresses:
Smost@stanford.edu (S.P. Most)
amatarasso@drmatarasso.com (A. Matarasso)

Preoperative Evaluation of the Rhinoplasty Patient

Mona Clappier, BA[a,b], Neil Tanna, MD, MBA[a,b],*

KEYWORDS

• Rhinoplasty • Rhinoplasty consultation • Preoperative evaluation • Facial proportions
• Nasal surgery • Cosmetic surgery

KEY POINTS

- The goals of the preoperative consultation for rhinoplasty are to obtain a medical and nasal history, understand the patient's areas of concern, conduct a nasal analysis, and evaluate patient candidacy for surgery.
- The nasal analysis is conducted from the frontal, lateral, and basal views, and should also include dynamic assessments.
- Overall facial proportions and facial features surrounding the nose should be taken into account when conducting a nasal analysis to ensure that the nose is well-balanced and suits the patient.
- Ideal nasal characteristics and proportions may differ substantially depending on the patient's ethnicity, gender, and age.
- An ideal patient is emotionally stable, well-informed, secure, and understanding of the limitations of rhinoplasty surgery. Physicians are cautioned against operating on patients who hold unrealistic expectations, severe insecurities, and excessive concerns about minor deformities, as they are likely to be unsatisfied with the outcome of the surgery.

INTRODUCTION

According to the American Society of Plastic Surgeons, more than 200,000 rhinoplasties are performed each year in the United States.[1] Requiring both high-level technical skills and artistic sense, rhinoplasty continues to be one of the most challenging procedures in plastic surgery despite its popularity. Ensuring the best possible functional and esthetic outcome for this challenging procedure begins with conducting a thorough preoperative evaluation of the patient.[2] The goals of the preoperative assessment are to (1) obtain a medical and nasal history, (2) understand the patient's areas of concern, (3) conduct a nasal analysis, and (4) evaluate patient candidacy for rhinoplasty surgery. This article will review the key functional, esthetic, and psychological considerations to take into account during the preoperative consultation.

PREOPERATIVE CONSULTATION
Nasal History

The preoperative assessment is an important opportunity for the surgeon to learn about the patient's concerns and motivations for undergoing rhinoplasty and to conduct a thorough nasal examination that will inform subsequent surgical planning. First, a comprehensive nasal history is obtained, in addition to a standard medical history. The surgeon should seek to understand the esthetic and functional concerns that a patient has regarding their nose and note the associated duration, frequency, laterality, and timing (ie, only occurs at work or seasonally) of any symptoms

[a] Division of Plastic & Reconstructive Surgery, Northwell Health, 600 Northern Boulevard, Suite 310, Great Neck, NY 11021, USA; [b] Division of Plastic & Reconstructive Surgery, Zucker School of Medicine at Hofstra/Northwell, Hempstead, NY, USA
* Corresponding author. Division of Plastic & Reconstructive Surgery, Northwell Health, 600 Northern Blvd. Suite 310, Great Neck, NY 11021.
E-mail address: ntanna@northwell.edu

Clin Plastic Surg 49 (2022) 1–11
https://doi.org/10.1016/j.cps.2021.07.002

mentioned.[3] Any allergies, prior nasal trauma, previous nasal surgery, medications, and use of dietary supplements should be documented.[4,5] Factors that are associated with poor wound healing such as metabolic disorders, smoking, alcohol, and illicit drug use should also be recorded.[6]

Nasal Airway Examination

Nasal airway obstruction is a common symptom presented by rhinoplasty patients. Nasal airway examination is conducted with the patient seated in a chair with his or her head at eye level with the examiner. It involves an evaluation of the external and internal nasal valves, the inferior turbinate, and the septum.[3,7,8]

A collapse of the external nasal valves on deep inspiration can indicate inadequate airway. In addition, the Cottle maneuver can be used to examine the integrity of the internal nasal valves. If the patient's breathing is improved upon retraction of the cheek, the nasal valves may be compromised.[9,10]

The physician conducts anterior rhinoscopy using a nasal speculum and bright light to reveal abnormal narrowing or collapse of internal valves with inspiration. If mucosal edema is present, one can use oxymetazoline nasal spray to alleviate mucosal constriction. In addition, the septum is examined for deformities (ie, deviation, tilt, spurs, and perforations). Any signs of septal deviation are noted along with inferior turbinate hypertrophy on the side opposite of the septum deviation.[10] The septal cartilage is also assessed for the availability of cartilage to assess its candidacy as a source of graft material.[3,10] If nasal polyps or tumors are discovered, further investigation may be necessary. (Readers may refer to Sami P. Moubayed and Sam P. Most's article, "Evaluation and Management of the Nasal Airway," in this issue for a full discussion on the topic of nasal airway examination.)

Dynamic View Assessment

The nasal examination should also include a dynamic view assessment. Often, actions such as smiling or breathing can reveal features involving the collapse of the nasal valves, nasal tip ptosis, and shortening of the upper lip that are not evident when the patient is still.[10,11] In cases involving nasal airway obstruction, the surgeon should also differentiate whether it occurs during quiet and/or heavy inspiration; obstruction that only occurs during heavy inspiration may signal an incompetent valve rather than a fixed obstruction like a septal deviation or mass.[3,12]

Paying attention to these subtleties will help ensure the best functional and esthetic outcomes.

Photographs

Photographs of the patient should be taken during the preoperative examination. Frontal, lateral, oblique, and basal views should be captured, in addition to animated and inspiratory views that expose features only evident upon muscle activation.[11,13] These photographs can be used as a visual tool for the patient and surgeon to communicate concerns and determine the surgical plan. They can also be morphed using modern digital imaging tools to aid surgical planning and to discuss surgical goals with the patient.[14–16] The patient should understand, however, that the edited images are not representative of the guaranteed outcome.[13]

Nasal Analysis

The nasal analysis is one of the most important parts of the preoperative assessment and must be conducted from several angles. Here, we describe the general principles of facial and nasal esthetics that may serve as a starting point for the nasal analysis. The surgeon must recognize, however, that there is no universal standard that applies to every patient. We cannot understate the importance of taking an individualized approach to understanding each patient's unique anatomy and goals for rhinoplasty surgery. **Fig. 1** summarizes the nasal analysis.

Frontal View Assessment

The frontal view is crucial for assessing the patient's nose within the context of overall facial proportions.[9] The nose is the central feature of the face so it must be balanced with the surrounding facial features as well as the stature of the patient.

The face is divided into horizontal thirds by 4 lines that cross the mentum, subnasale, brow at the supraorbital notch, and hairline (**Fig. 2**).[17] The bottom third is further divided into an upper third and lower two-third section by a horizontal line that goes across the oral commissures.[17] Vertically, the face is divided into 5 planes by lines crossing the most lateral portion of the head, the lateral canthi, and the medial canthi (**Fig. 3**).[18] Although there are significant individual differences and variations in facial harmony, this principle of dividing the face into sections can help identify areas of the face that deviate from ideal proportions and may influence the outcome of the surgery. Areas of incongruence should be discussed with the patient before surgery when considering the possibilities and limitations of the operation—often, patients are unaware of existing subtle deviations that may influence their perception of the outcome of the surgery.[10] If a patient

Nasal Analysis Worksheet

FRONTAL VIEW

Skin Type:

    Fitzpatrick Skin Type: ☐I ☐II ☐III ☐IV ☐V ☐VI

    Thickness: ☐Thick ☐Normal ☐Thin

    Sebaceous: ☐Yes ☐No

Nasal Symmetry:

    Symmetric Bony Vault: ☐Yes ☐No

    Mid-Vault Symmetry: ☐Yes ☐No

    Symmetric Dorsal Aesthetic Lines (DAL): ☐Yes ☐No

    Septal Deviation:

        Type: ☐C-Shaped ☐Reverse C-Shaped ☐S-Shaped

    Notes:

Nasal Length:

    ☐Normal (Equal to distance from stomion to menton)

    ☐Short

    ☐Long

Nasal Width

    ☐Alar base width equal to intercanthal distance

    ☐Bony base width equal to 75%–80% of alar base width

    Notes:

Nasal Tip:

    Alar Rims in shape of seagull wings: ☐Yes ☐No

    Shape: ☐Boxy ☐Bulbous ☐Pinched

    Length of Upper Lip:

        ☐Adequate (11 mm–13 mm)

        ☐Excessive (>13 mm)

        ☐Insufficient

LATERAL VIEW

Dorsal Profile: ☐Smooth ☐Concave ☐Convex ☐Saddle Nose Deformity ☐Pollybeak Deformity

Nasofrontal Angle: ☐Adequate (115°–130°) ☐Small(<115°) ☐Large (>130°)

Radix Height: ☐Normal ☐High ☐Low

Tip Projection : ☐Adequate (50%–60% of in front of upper lip)
             ☐Over-projected (>60% of in front of upper lip)
             ☐Under-projected(<50% of in front of upper lip)

Tip Rotation
    Nasolabial Angle:
        ☐Adequate (90°–120°)
        ☐Small (<90°)
        ☐Large (>120°)

Columellar Show: ☐Adequate (2-4 mm) ☐Excessive (>4 mm) ☐Lacking (<2 mm)

Lip-Chin Relationship: _____

Notes:

BASAL / INTERNAL VIEW

☐Symmetry of Alar Base

☐Symmetry of Nostrils

Lobule to Columella Ratio: ☐Appropriate (1:2) ☐Excessive Columella ☐Excessive Lobule

Note Signs of Buckling: _____

Angle of Divergence ☐Appropriate (30°) ☐Small(<30°) ☐Large (>30°)

If increased alar base width is observed, it is caused by:
    ☐Alar flaring
    ☐Horizontal Position of Alar Insertions

Fig. 1. Nasal analysis worksheet for use during the preoperative rhinoplasty consultation.

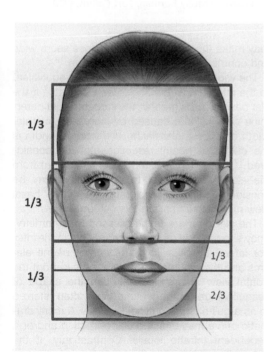

Fig. 2. Ideal facial proportions demonstrated from a frontal view. Lines crossing the mentum, subnasale, brow at the supraorbital notch, and hairline divide the face into horizontal thirds. The bottom third is further divided into an upper third and lower two-third section by a line that goes through the oral commissures. (*Courtesy of* Molly Borman, Fort Collins, CO.)

presents proportions that dramatically differ from the average range, orthodontics, and orthognathic interventions may also be necessary.[17]

During the facial analysis, the surgeon should also note the thickness and quality of the skin and underlying subcutaneous tissue.[19] These factors can influence surgical plans and pose limitations on the outcome of the procedure; patients with thicker skin have a higher risk for prolonged postoperative edema and scar formation and may require a longer recovery. In addition, patients with thicker skin may require greater intraoperative manipulations compared to patients with thinner skin, as subtle changes may be less visible.[9,20]

After a broad facial analysis is conducted, the surgeon may focus on subtleties involving the nose. The nasal length, defined as the distance from the nasal root to tip, should be equal to the vertical distance from the stomion to the menton.[9]

The nasal dorsum should be contoured by 2 slightly curved lines referred to as the dorsal esthetic lines (DALs), which extend from the medial superciliary ridges, travel down the radix, and terminate at the tip-defining points (**Fig. 4**).[17] The DALs should be smooth, symmetric, and continuous. Any asymmetries and deformities on the bony vault and the midvault should be documented and further investigated.[6] Patients seeking revision rhinoplasty sometimes present an inverted-V deformity, where a visible and palpable indentation between the nasal bones and the start

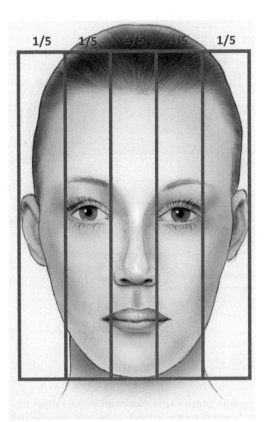

Fig. 3. Ideal facial proportions demonstrated using vertical fifths from a frontal view. Vertical lines cross the most lateral portion of the head, the lateral canthi, and the medial canthi. (*Courtesy of* Molly Borman, Fort Collins, CO.)

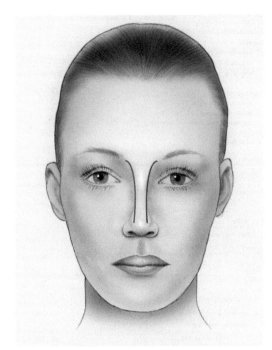

Fig. 4. DALs extend from medial superciliary ridges, travel down the radix, and terminate at the tip-defining points. DALs are smooth and symmetric. (*Courtesy of* Molly Borman, Fort Collins, CO.)

of the upper lateral cartilages disrupts the DALs.[21] The inverted-V deformity is often a result of a previous hump removal procedure and can also affect the patient's airway by narrowing the internal nasal valves.[21]

A vertical line drawn from the midglabellar area to the menton can also be used to determine any form of septal deviation and to assess overall symmetry (**Fig. 5**). This line should pass through the nasal ridge, upper lip, and Cupid's bow, and the nasal bones and septum should be symmetric. A C-shaped, reversed-C-shaped, or S-shaped curvature may indicate a deviated septum.[4,9]

The width of the bony base should be 75% to 80% of the alar base width (**Fig. 6**).[17] If the bony base is wider, mobilization of the bones may be required to narrow the dorsum. It should be noted that a dorsal hump may give the illusion of a narrow dorsum and decreased projection, while the presence of a saddle deformity in the bony or cartilaginous dorsum can cause the dorsum to appear wide in the frontal view.[19] Likewise, a bony dorsum

may make the upper third of the nose seem wide and contribute to pseudohypertelorism.[19]

The width of the alar base should be equivalent to the intercanthal distance (see **Fig. 6**).[9,17] If the alar base width is greater, the surgeon must determine whether it is caused by increased interalar width or excess alar flaring.[17] If interalar width is the culprit, a nostril resection may be considered.[17] If the flaring extends beyond 2 mm from the alar base, an alar base resection may be considered. Further exploration from the basal view may help in making this determination.[17]

The alar rims are then assessed for symmetry. They should have a slight outward flare in the inferior lateral direction.[18,19] The outline of the alar rims and the columella is also assessed from the frontal view and should take on the shape of seagull wings with a gentle curve—often referred to as a gull-shaped outline (**Fig. 7**).[18] A more dramatic curve may indicate alar retraction and/or a dependent infratip lobule. Contrastingly, if the columella is not visible, this may be an indication of a hidden or retracted columella.[19] The surgeon should also make note of alar rims and bases that are boxy, bulbous, pinched, or drooping.[11]

From the frontal view, the tip of the nose can be outlined using 4 landmarks: 1 at the supratip break, 1 at the columellar-lobule angle, and

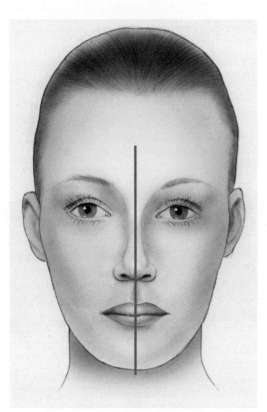

Fig. 5. Vertical line drawn from the midglabellar area to the menton to assess symmetry. (*Courtesy of* Molly Borman, Fort Collins, CO.)

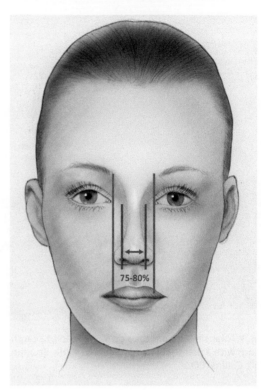

75-80%

Fig. 6. The width of the alar base should be equivalent to the intercanthal distance. The width of the bony base should be 75% to 80% the width of the alar base. (*Courtesy of* Molly Borman, Fort Collins, CO.)

2 on either side of the tip (**Fig. 8**).[17] Straight lines that connect these 4 points should resemble 2 equilateral triangles that face opposite directions. Distortion of these triangles should be further investigated. The tip is also assessed for bulbosity. In cases where an increased distance between the domes is causing the bulbosity, the surgeon may consider bringing them in closer together, while in cases where thick skin is the cause of bulbosity, debulking may help. Otherwise, a bulbous tip may need to be addressed by modifying the lower cartilages.[19] Cephalically oriented (vertically malpositioned) lateral crura results in a parenthesis-shaped tip deformity. Furthermore, the cranial and caudal edges of the lateral crus should be level with each other; a higher cephalic edge can lead to supratip fullness. As such, the lower lateral cartilage should have the cephalic margin down and the caudal margin up.[19]

The upper lip should be assessed to ensure that it adequately counterbalances the nose. Some patients may present insufficient or excessive length of the upper lip.[9] The surgeon should also make sure to conduct a dynamic view assessment;

activation of the depressor septi nasi muscle, which runs from the upper lip to the inserts on the septum and alae, can distort the appearance of the nasal tip, columella, and alae and reveal key insights.[9,10,14]

Lateral View Assessment

The lateral view provides the opportunity to focus on the nasal profile and to investigate features such as the nasofrontal angle, tip projection, nasal length, dorsal profile, and the alar-columellar relationship.

First, the position and depth of the nasofrontal angle are determined. This angle is defined as the juncture where the line from the glabella to the nasion intersects with a line drawn from the nasion to the tip (**Fig. 9**).[19] The deepest portion of the nasofrontal angle should lie between the upper eyelash line and the supratarsal fold when the eyes are in a relaxed horizontal gaze.[17] The ideal esthetic nasal dorsum is characterized by a nasofrontal angle between 115° and 130° and is greater in women than in men.[19] The nasal length can be assessed from the lateral view as well, with the

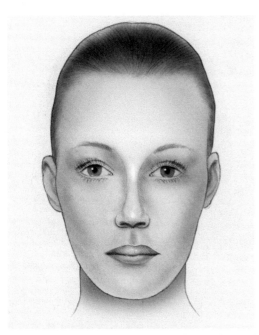

Fig. 7. Alar rims should take on the shape of seagull wings with a gentle curve. (*Courtesy of* Molly Borman, Fort Collins, CO.)

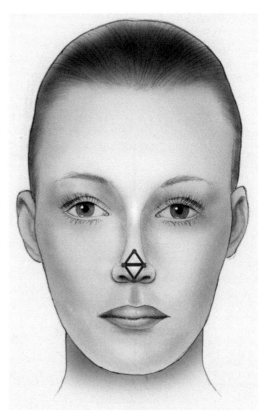

Fig. 8. The tip of the nose can be outlined using 4 points—1 at the supratip break, 1 at the columellar-lobule angle, and 2 on either side of the tip. When connected, the lines should form 2 equilateral triangles oriented in opposite directions. (*Courtesy of* Molly Borman, Fort Collins, CO.)

ideal length being equal to the vertical distance from the stomion to the menton. It is important to realize that a large nasofrontal angle can give an illusion of a long nose, whereas a small nasofrontal angle may create the illusion of a short nose.[19]

The dorsal profile should be described as smooth, convex, or concave.[9] Cases involving a saddle-nose deformity may implicate inadequate bony and cartilaginous support of the nasal vault caused by previous nasal surgery, trauma, vascular compromise, neoplasms, or systemic abnormalities.[9,22] In addition, in women, a slight concavity at the rhinion is often preferred, whereas in men, a minor dorsal hump may be acceptable or even desirable. When considering a dorsal hump reduction or dorsal augmentation, it is important to remember that the skin at the rhinion is typically thinner than the skin at the nasion, making it particularly susceptible to even the slightest visible and palpable irregularities.[19]

The ideal nasal starting point for the dorsum is at the level of the superior palpebral fold, and the ideal position for the nasion is between the supratarsal fold and the lash line of the upper eyelid.[20] It should be noted, however, that the average radix height differs substantially with the ethnicity of the patient.[9]

The degree of supratip break should also be assessed. A slight supratip break enhances nasal definition and distinguishes the dorsum from the tip and is preferred in women but not in men.[9,17]

To assess nasal tip projection, a line is drawn from the alar-cheek junction to the tip of the nose (**Fig. 10**). Tip projection is considered adequate when 50% to 60% of the nasal projection is in front of the most projected part of the upper lip.[9] If it is greater than 50% to 60%, the tip may be over-projected and require reduction. Some patients may also present a Pollybeak deformity, in which the nasal tip hangs over excessively, resembling a parrot's beak.[23] This deformity can be caused by excessive dorsal prominence, scar tissue in the supratip region, lack of tip support, and/or excess of soft tissue in the region (periapical hypoplasia).[14,21,23] If the nose has less than 50% of the tip in front of the upper lip, augmentation may be necessary. According to Byrd and Burt's analysis, the ideal nasal length can also be described as a ratio of nasal length to tip projection of 1:0.67.[24]

The nasolabial angle is measured at the juncture between the columella and the upper lip and can be used to assess tip rotation (**Fig. 11**).[19] The ideal nasolabial angle is between 90° and 120°. A more

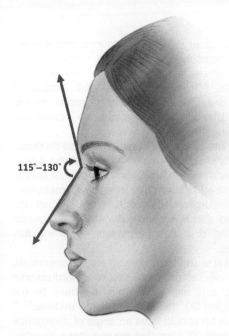

115°–130°

Fig. 9. The nasofrontal angle is defined as the juncture where the line from the glabella to the nasion intersects a line drawn from the nasion to the tip. (*Courtesy of* Molly Borman, Fort Collins, CO.)

obtuse angle within this range is preferred in women, whereas an angle closer to 90° is preferred in men.[19] Similar to the nasofrontal angle, the nasolabial angle can influence the perception of nasal length; a more obtuse

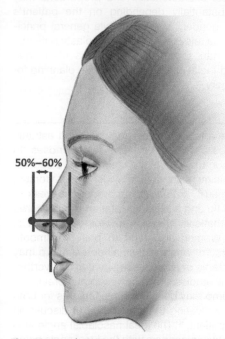

50%–60%

Fig. 10. Nasal tip projection is considered adequate when 50% to 60% of nasal projection is in front of the most projected part of the upper lip. (*Courtesy of* Molly Borman, Fort Collins, CO.)

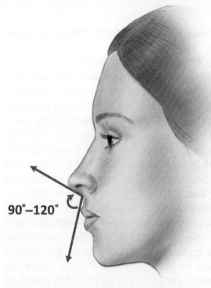

90°–120°

Fig. 11. The ideal nasolabial angle is 90° to 120° and is used to assess tip rotation. A larger angle within this range is preferred in women, whereas a smaller angle within this range is preferred in men. (*Courtesy of* Molly Borman, Fort Collins, CO.)

nasolabial angle can create the illusion of a short nose, whereas a more acute angle can create the illusion of a long nose.[19] A prominent caudal septum can cause increased fullness in this area and contribute to greater tip rotation, even when the nasolabial angle is in the ideal range.[17]

The columellar-lobular angle, which is formed at the juncture between the columella and the infratip lobule, is considered normal at 45° (**Fig. 12**).[17] An

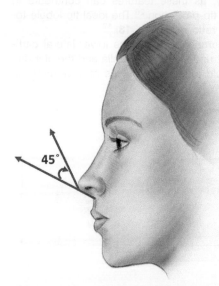

45°

Fig. 12. The columellar-lobule angle is formed at the juncture between the columella and the infratip lobule and is considered normal at 45°. (*Courtesy of* Molly Borman, Fort Collins, CO.)

acute columellar-lobule angle is often associated with a long upper lip.[25]

The insertion of the alae on the face should be 2 to 3 mm above the columella plane. The outline of the alar rim from the lateral view should resemble a lazy-S shape and should be described if this contour is exaggerated or not present.[19] The alar-lobule size should also be documented. The alae should be at a similar height as the columella, with about 2 to 4 mm of columellar show and any retraction, notching, or collapse of the alae should be documented.[9,26] When viewed laterally, the ideal nostril to tip ratio is 55:45.[27]

Finally, it is important to assess the esthetic relationship of the chin and lips with the nose; retrognathia or micrognathia may create the illusion that a nose is over-projected.[28] The upper lip should project about 2 mm beyond the lower lip and in most women, the chin will be slightly posterior to the lower lip (2-3 mm). In men, the chin may be slightly longer.[17]

Basal and Internal View Assessment

The basal and internal view assessment allows the surgeon to further investigate the lobule-to-columella ratio and the shape, symmetry, width, and insertion of the alar base. The outline of the nasal base should form a triangle with a slightly tapered apex or infratip lobule that is not boxy or bulbous. A lack of a triangular shape or a trapezoidal configuration can indicate a diverged intermediate crura.[19] In addition, the surgeon should pay attention to the length of the columella and its rigidity, as these features can contribute to the nasal tip projection.[26] The ideal tip lobule-to-columella ratio is 1:2 (**Fig. 13**).[17]

If the surgeon can see the lower lateral cartilages that underly the columella and the alar rim, they should look for any signs of asymmetry or

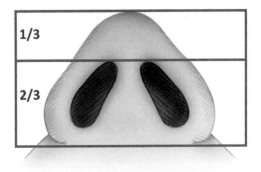

1/3

2/3

Fig. 13. Basal view of the nose. Ideal lobule-to-columella ratio is 1:2. (*Courtesy of* Molly Borman, Fort Collins, CO.)

buckling. Other details to note include the presence of excessively long or short medial crura, a wide columella, and flaring of the medial crural footplates.[19] Uneven nostrils and protruding medial crural footplates may signal a caudal septum that is protruding into the nostril and obstructing the patient's airway.[19]

The width of the alar base should also be documented and should ideally lie between the 2 lines that extend downwards from the medial canthi. As described in the frontal view assessment section, the surgeon must determine whether the increased alar base width is caused by excess alar flaring or horizontal positioning of the alar insertions.[17]

Nostril size and shape should also be described, with the ideal shape being that of a teardrop with the long axis extending from the base to the apex angled 30° to 45° toward the midline.[17,19] The nasal tip should have an angle of divergence smaller than 30°; tips that exceed these parameters are likely to be bulbous or boxy.[29]

The thickness of the alar walls, as well as the orientation of the base insertions, are also described—with the 2 extremes being straight insertions that run directly into the face and horizontal insertions that run directly into the columella.[19]

Variation with Gender, Race, and Age

Ideal nasal characteristics and proportions may differ substantially depending on the patient's ethnicity, gender, and age. While general principles may be relevant to most rhinoplasty patients, it is important to consider each person's unique nasal and facial characteristics when planning for their surgery.

Gender

There are a few common anatomic and esthetic differences between male and female noses. In comparison to women, men tend to have squarer faces, thicker skin, and a wider nasal dorsum than women.[13,30] In addition, a supratip break of the nasal tip and a slight tip rotation is considered to be esthetically pleasing in women but not in men.[9,13] Women also tend to prefer a smooth linear dorsum, whereas a small dorsal hump may be acceptable or even desired in men.[9] Nevertheless, some studies show that a supratip break and dorsal hump may be undesirable features for both genders, indicating the importance of discussion with the patient.[30] The ideal nasolabial angle also differs between genders with the ideal angle being 110° and 90° to 100° for women and men, respectively.[9,30] Men also tend to have broader nasal tips and weaker medial crura than women. While they often have wider bony vaults than women, with age, the bony vaults can narrow due to weakening and interfere with the proper functioning of the internal nasal valves.[13]

Age

Aging is associated with weaker lower lateral crura and external nasal valves that are caused by the weakening of the underlying cartilage.[13] Aging-associated changes in skin laxity and resorption of septal cartilage can also lead to nasal tip ptosis and columellar retraction.[13] Furthermore, as a person ages, dorsal skin thins while the nasal tip skin thickens and develops large pores.[13] These factors should be taken into account when evaluating older patients and determining the goals and limitations of rhinoplasty surgery.

Ethnicity

There are several well-documented differences across patients of various ethnicities that can influence surgical goals and planning.[31] The surgeon needs to understand these differences so that they can modify a patient's nose while maintaining facial harmony and respect for cultural differences in esthetics.[32]

First, Caucasians generally have a more prominent and a higher radix compared with patients of Asian or African ethnicities.[9,33,34] Asian skin also tends to be thick with abundant fibrofatty tissue, particularly at the nasal tip which is commonly bulbous and less defined.[33] Thicker skin, however, offers the advantage of being more tolerable to alloplastic or autogenous material than thin skin.[33] In addition, Asian noses often have an overall weak cartilaginous structure and a lack of septal cartilage. These features can present a challenge to the surgeon if the patient desires dorsal augmentation, which is a common concern reported by Asian patients.[20,33]

Middle Eastern patients also commonly have thick, sebaceous skin.[35] However, this patient population often present concerns related to a wide and high nasal dorsum, a pronounced dorsal hump, over-projected tip, and/or nostril-tip imbalance.[31,35,36] African American patients commonly present a wide nasal base, low nasal dorsum, and deepened nasofrontal angle.[31,37] Alar base abnormalities such as increase interalar space and excessive alar flaring are often reported.[31,37]

These variations across age, gender, and ethnicity emphasize the importance of the preoperative evaluation. The success of rhinoplasty rests not only on creating an esthetically pleasing nose, but one that will harmonize with the rest of the patient's appearance and take into account an individual's natural skin quality, cartilage structure, and facial composition.[37] Surgeons must engage in a clear and candid discussion with the patient to prevent postoperative dissatisfaction and unrealistic expectations.

Psychosocial Assessment of the Rhinoplasty Patient

The preoperative consultation is an important opportunity for the surgeon to evaluate patient candidacy for rhinoplasty surgery. An ideal patient is emotionally stable, well-informed, secure, and understanding of the limitations of rhinoplasty surgery.[10,38,39] They are also able to articulate their major concerns and rank them in order of importance when they have multiple points they would like to address.[9,10,17,38,39]

However, physicians are cautioned against operating on patients who hold unrealistic expectations, severe insecurities, and excessive concerns about minor deformities, as they will likely be unsatisfied regardless of the outcome of the surgery.[17,38,40] These characteristics can signal underlying psychiatric conditions as well, such as body dysmorphic disorder in which a patient has an intense preoccupation with a physical trait that is hardly noticeable to others.[9,10,39] Motivation for surgery in these patients stems from a strong sense of flawed self-image and a disturbed state of mind. Surgeons are also cautioned against operating on "surgiholics" or patients who have had multiple rhinoplasties and other esthetic surgeries; not only are these patients likely to be unsatisfied with the postoperative result, operating on a nose that has been subjected to multiple surgeries can make a case extremely difficult and carry a high risk of complications.[17,39] Surgeons may also benefit from using a patient-reported outcome measure to evaluate function, esthetics, and psychosocial parameters as they have been shown to be predictive of outcomes.[40–42]

Other warning signs include patients who have unrealistic expectations that their lives will be drastically changed because of rhinoplasty surgery, who are currently going through a deeply emotional period in their lives (ie, grieving loss of loved one, divorce, etc.) and patients who are manipulative or hostile toward the surgeon and medical staff.[10,13,39,43]

Historically, surgeons have been warned against operating on patients who are described by the acronym SIMON: single, immature, male, overly expectant, and narcissistic and to choose patients who fit the acronym SYLVIA: secure, young, listens, verbal, intelligent, and attractive.[17,38] Although these acronyms may serve as a reminder of some common signs to look out for, they are at most generalizations—many male patients, for example, make for great rhinoplasty candidates.[13] This point highlights the importance of taking an individualized approach with each patient and to focus on determining their main goals and motivations for surgery. Although techniques and skill level are important from rhinoplasties, bidirectional communication between the physician and the patient is crucial to achieve a postoperative outcome that satisfies both parties.

CLINICS CARE POINTS: EVALUATING PATIENT CANDIDACY

- An ideal rhinoplasty patient is emotionally stable, well-informed, secure, and understanding of the limitations of surgery. They should also be able to articulate and rank their major concerns.
- Patients with unrealistic expectations, severe insecurities, and excessive concerns about minor deformities are likely to be unsatisfied regardless of the outcome of the surgery.
- Operating on a patient who has had multiple rhinoplasties in the past can be difficult and additional surgery may be associated with a high risk of complications.

SUMMARY

In this article, we have highlighted the key components of the preoperative evaluation for rhinoplasty patients. The preoperative consultation should always include a thorough medical and nasal history and nasal analysis conducted from the frontal, lateral, and basal views. The surgeon must also take the time to understand the patient's primary areas of concern, while also assessing the patient's candidacy for rhinoplasty. The ideal facial and nasal proportions presented here should be used as a rough guideline, with the understanding that each individual must be assessed independently and analyzed based on their age, ethnicity, and gender. Doing so will ensure that both the surgeon and the patient are satisfied with the outcome of the operation.

DISCLOSURE

The authors have nothing to disclose.

REFERENCES

1. 2019 national plastic surgery statistics report. Availble at: https://www.plasticsurgery.org/documents/News/Statistics/2019/plastic-surgery-statistics-report-2019.pdf. Accessed February 15, 2021.
2. Lu SM, Hsu DT, Perry AD, et al. The public face of rhinoplasty: impact on perceived attractiveness and personality. Plast Reconstr Surg 2018;142(4):881–7.
3. Howard BK, Rohrich RJ. Understanding the nasal airway: principles and practice. Plast Reconstr Surg 2002;109(3):1128–46. Available at: https://journals.lww.com/plasreconsurg/Fulltext/2002/03000/Understanding_the_Nasal_Airway__Principles_and.54.aspx.
4. Ahmad J, Rohrich RJ. The crooked nose. Clin Plast Surg 2016;43(1):99–113.
5. Teichgraeber JF, Gruber RP, Tanna N. Surgical management of nasal airway obstruction. Clin Plast Surg 2016;43(1):41–6.
6. Beck DO, Kenkel JM. Evidence-based medicine: rhinoplasty. Plast Reconstr Surg 2014;134(6):1356–71.
7. Tanna N, Im DD, Azhar H, et al. Inferior turbinoplasty during cosmetic rhinoplasty: techniques and trends. Ann Plast Surg 2014;72(1):5–8.
8. Tanna N, Lesavoy MA, Abou-Sayed HA, et al. Septoturbinotomy. Aesthet Surg J 2013;33(8):1199–205.
9. Tanna N, Nguyen KT, Ghavami A, et al. Evidence-based medicine: current practices in rhinoplasty. Plast Reconstr Surg 2018;141(1):137e–51e.
10. Rohrich RJ, Ahmad J. A practical approach to rhinoplasty. Plast Reconstr Surg 2016;137(4):725e–46e.
11. Dhir K, Ghavami A. Reshaping of the broad and bulbous nasal tip. Clin Plast Surg 2016;43(1):115–26.
12. Tanna N, Smith BD, Zapanta PE, et al. Surgical management of obstructive sleep apnea. Plast Reconstr Surg 2016;137(4):1263–72.
13. Rohrich RJ, Mohan R. Male rhinoplasty: update. Plast Reconstr Surg 2020;145(4):744e–53e.
14. Rohrich RJ, Ahmad J. Rhinoplasty. Plast Reconstr Surg 2011;128(2):49e–73e.
15. Mühlbauer W, Holm C. Computer imaging and surgical reality in aesthetic rhinoplasty. Plast Reconstr Surg 2005;115(7):2098–104.
16. Mahajan A, Shefiei M, Marcus BC. Analysis of patient-determined preoperative computer imaging. Arch Facial Plast Surg 2009;11:290–5.
17. Rohrich RJ, Potter jason K, Landecker A. Preoperative concepts for rhinoplasty. In: Rohrich RJ, editor. Dallas rhinoplasty: nasal surgery by the masters. 2nd edition. St Louis, (MO): Quality Medical Publishing; 2007. p. 59–79.
18. Gunter JP, Hackney FL. Clinical assessment and facial analysis. In: Rohrich RJ, editor. Dallas rhinoplasty: nasal surgery by the masters. 2nd edition. St Louis, (MO): Quality Medical Publishing; 2007. p. 106–23.
19. Toriumi DM, Becker DG. Rhinoplasty analysis. In: Toriumi DM, editor. Rhinoplasty dissection manual. Philadelphia: Lippincott Williams & Wilkins; 1999. p. 9–23.

20. Suhk J, Park J, Nguyen AH. Nasal analysis and anatomy: anthropometric proportional assessment in asians—aesthetic balance from Forehead to chin, Part I. Semin Plast Surg 2015;29(04):219–25.
21. Hamilton G. Dorsal Failures: from saddle deformity to Pollybeak. Facial Plast Surg 2018;34(03):261–9.
22. Pribitkin EA, Ezzat WH. Classification and treatment of the saddle nose deformity. Otolaryngol Clin North Am 2009;42(3):437–61.
23. Rohrich RJ, Shanmugakrishnan RR, Mohan R. Rhinoplasty refinements: addressing the Pollybeak deformity. Plast Reconstr Surg 2020;145(3):696–9.
24. Byrd H, Burt J, El-Musa K, et al. Dimensional approach to rhinoplasty: perfecting the aesthetic balance between the nose and chin. In: Rohrich RJ, editor. Dallas rhinoplasty: nasal surgery by the masters, vol. 1. St Louis, (MO): Quality Medical Publishing; 2002. p. 135.
25. Filho DH, Alonso N, Oksman D, et al. Surgical treatment of the acute columellar-labial angle. Aesthet Surg J 2008;28(6):627–30. https://doi.org/10.1016/j.asj.2008.10.003.
26. Hamilton GS. Form and function of the nasal tip: re-orienting and reshaping the lateral crus. Facial Plast Surg 2016;32(01):049–58.
27. Daniel R. Rhinoplasty: large nostril/small tip disproportion. Plast Reconstr Surg 2001;107(7):1874–81 [discussion: 1882–3].
28. Ahmed J, Patil S, Jayaraj S. Assessment of the chin in patients undergoing rhinoplasty: what proportion may benefit from chin augmentation? Otolaryngol Neck Surg 2010;142(2):164–8.
29. Berger CAS, Mocelin M, Soares CMC, et al. Lateral intercrural suture in the caucasian nose: decreased domal divergence angle in endonasal rhinoplasty without delivery. Int Arch Otorhinolaryngol 2012;16(2):232–5.
30. Springer IN, Zernial O, Nölke F, et al. Gender and nasal shape: measures for rhinoplasty. Plast Reconstr Surg 2008;121(2):629–37.
31. Rohrich RJ, Bolden K. Ethnic rhinoplasty. Clin Plast Surg 2010;37(2):353–70.
32. Broer PN, Buonocore S, Morillas A, et al. Nasal aesthetics: a cross-cultural analysis. Plast Reconstr Surg 2012;130(6):843e–50e.
33. Jin HR, Won T-B. Rhinoplasty in the asian patient. Clin Plast Surg 2016;43(1):265–79.
34. Naini FB, Cobourne MT, Garagiola U, et al. Nasofacial angle and nasal prominence: a quantitative investigation of idealized and normative values. J Craniomaxillofac Surg 2016;44(4):446–52.
35. Sajjadian A. Rhinoplasty in middle Eastern patients. Clin Plast Surg 2016;43(1):281–94.
36. Rohrich RJ, Ghavami A. Rhinoplasty for middle Eastern noses. Plast Reconstr Surg 2009;123(4):1343–54.
37. Peng GL, Nassif PS. Rhinoplasty in the african American patient. Clin Plast Surg 2016;43(1):255–64.
38. Gorney M, Martello J. Patient selection criteria. Clin Plast Surg 1999;26(1):37–40.
39. Tasman A-J. The psychological aspects of rhinoplasty. Curr Opin Otolaryngol Neck Surg 2010;18:290–4.
40. Kandathil CK, Patel PN, Spataro EA, et al. Examining preoperative expectations and postoperative satisfaction in rhinoplasty patients: a single-center study. Facial Plast Surg Aesthet Med 2020. https://doi.org/10.1089/fpsam.2020.0406. fpsam.2020.0406.
41. Spataro EA, Kandathil CK, Saltychev M, et al. Correlation of the standardized cosmesis and health nasal outcomes survey with psychiatric screening tools. Aesthet Surg J 2020;40(12):1373–80.
42. Okland TS, Patel P, Liu GS, et al. Using nasal self-Esteem to predict revision in cosmetic rhinoplasty. Aesthet Surg J 2021;41(6):652–6.
43. Spataro EA, Olds CE, Kandathil CK, et al. Comparison of reconstructive plastic surgery rates and 30-day postoperative complications between patients with and without psychiatric diagnoses. Aesthet Surg J 2021;41(6):NP684–94.

Photography and Photodocumentation for the Rhinoplasty Patient

Cherine H. Kim, MD, PhD[a],*, Sam P. Most, MD[b]

KEYWORDS

• Rhinoplasty • Photography • Digital single-lens reflex camera • Mirrorless camera

KEY POINTS

- Understanding basic photography equipment and principles is crucial for developing a technique to produce high-quality and accurate images of the rhinoplasty patient.
- Careful patient preparation and positioning is critical for consistent, standardized images.
- Digital single-lens-reflex (DSLR) cameras are the gold standard for facial plastic photography; however, digital mirrorless camera technology has quickly evolved and is a viable alternative to DSLR.
- The emergence of 3-dimensional photography has exciting implications for the future of medical photography but has yet to be adopted as a standard for the facial plastic surgery practice.

INTRODUCTION/HISTORY/DEFINITIONS/BACKGROUND

Photodocumentation is an essential part of a rhinoplasty surgeon's practice. Preoperative photographs are an indispensable device for patient counseling and surgical planning.[1,2] Comparison of preoperative and postoperative photographs allow for outcome evaluation, which has a variety of applications—clinical, research, teaching, medicolegal.[3] The ever-evolving technology of photography may be daunting; yet developing a basic understanding of this tool is imperative for a successful rhinoplasty practice. This article reviews the basic photographic principles, equipment, and techniques that are essential to produce high-quality and standardized patient photographs.

EQUIPMENT
Camera

The single-lens reflex 35-mm camera was historically the gold standard for patient photodocumentation in facial plastic surgery[1] but has been replaced by digital photography.[4] Digital photography offers immediate viewing and use during consultation, ability to serve in computer imaging simulations, decreased production cost, and easy storage and organization. Although digital point-and-shoot cameras are smaller, lighter, and more affordable, they lack the resolution and versatility that digital single-lens reflex (DSLR) cameras provide. DSLR cameras offer the ability to change lenses and allow manipulation of exposure, aperture size, and shutter speed.

Digital cameras capture images using a light sensitive sensor. Currently there are 2 types of image sensors: charged coupled devices and complementary metal-oxide-semiconductors. The mechanical differences and ensuing advantages and disadvantages of each type of sensor are beyond the scope of this review; however, the working principle of these sensors is that they capture and convert light into an electrical pattern that is then converted and stored as a digital image. The sensor is composed of millions of capacitors, each of which accounts for one pixel of the

[a] Division of Facial Plastic and Reconstructive Surgery, Department of Otolaryngology - Head and Neck Surgery, Loma Linda University School of Medicine, 11234 Anderson Street, Room 2586A, Loma Linda, CA 92354, USA; [b] Division of Facial Plastic and Reconstructive Surgery, Department of Otolaryngology - Head and Neck Surgery, Stanford University School of Medicine, 801 Welch Road, Stanford, CA 94305, USA
* Corresponding author.
E-mail address: chekim@llu.edu

Clin Plastic Surg 49 (2022) 13–22
https://doi.org/10.1016/j.cps.2021.07.003

image.[5] Pixel density is related to resolution, a factor in image quality. A resolution of 1.5 megapixels was once considered acceptable for medical photography.[6] At the advent of digital photography, adequate resolution was a topic of frequent discussion. Considerations include how much a given image will be enlarged. For viewing on a typical computer screen (eg, blowing up to 11 × 14 inches), 5 megapixels should be adequate and would likely be considered the minimum. To enlarge specific areas of the image, or to view on a projected screen, higher resolution may be required. Currently, with the rapid improvement of digital photography technology, even entry-level DSLR cameras boast a 24-megapixel sensor.

Typical digital image sensors are smaller than the traditional 35-mm film frame. In an identical photographic setting, the smaller image sensor captures a smaller central area of an image when compared with that of a full 35-mm frame. This effectively crops the image and decreases the field of view, mimicking the characteristics of a lens with a longer focal length. The effective lengthening of focal length is designated the focal length multiplier (FLM), which corrects for the size of the sensor in relationship to the traditional 35-mm frame. The FLM is calculated by dividing the diagonal of a 35-mm film frame by the diagonal of the sensor. For example, a DSLR with an FLM of 1.5 and a lens with a 70 mm focal length will produce an image comparable to a 35-mm film SLR with a focal length of 105 mm (70 mm x 1.5).[7–9] Full-frame digital sensors are available and have the advantage of eliminating the need for FLM calculations, but they are significantly more costly (**Fig. 1**).

Lens

Interchangeability of lenses is one of the many advantages of a DSLR camera. The lens directs the path of captured light onto the film medium or image sensor. Each lens has a set focal length, which measures the distance from the optical center of the lens to the focal point located on the image sensor or film. Proper lens selection is critical for producing accurate images that provide fine details of the face with minimal distortion. In facial plastic surgery, the ideal focal length is between 90 and 105 mm.[6,10] These lenses are known as

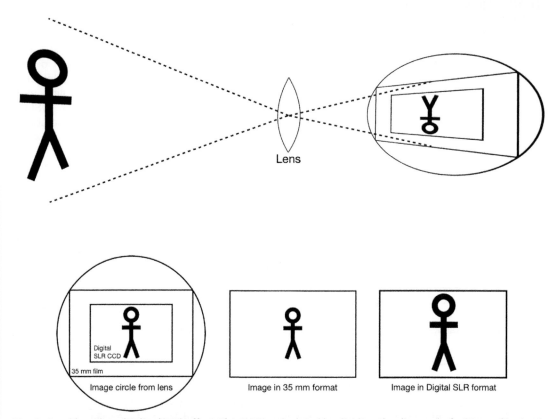

Fig. 1. Focal length multiplier (FLM) effect. The FLM is calculated by dividing the diagonal of a 35-mm film by the diagonal of the CCD sensor size used by the DSLR camera. The multiplier provides the effective increase in the focal length propagated by the use of the DSLR. The subject appears larger in the image captured by the DSLR, which is effectively the equivalent of using a lens with a longer focal length. CCD, charged coupled device.

"macro" or "portrait" lenses and are made for near focusing. Lenses with shorter focal lengths have a wider angle of view and produce a central-bulging "fish-eye" appearance when used to photograph the face (**Fig. 2**).[6,9]

In addition to focal length, several other factors influence image characteristics. Depth of field (DOF) refers to the distance range in which all portions of a photograph appear in focus. For the purposes of rhinoplasty, the DOF should include the entire face with the nose at the focal point and with the greatest definition. DOF may be manipulated by altering 3 factors—focal length of lens, distance between photographer and subject, and aperture size. Yet in the facial plastic clinic, focal length and photographer-to-subject distance are difficult to adjust. As discussed earlier, the ideal focal length is between 90 and 105 mm because this produces minimal distortion. Considering the space restrictions of the clinic, photographer-to-subject distance may also be difficult to alter.[9] Thus, aperture setting is the simplest way to adjust the DOF.

The lens aperture is made up of an adjustable diaphragm that controls the passage of light through the lens. Aperture size is measured as f-stops, calculated based on the ratio of the focal length to the aperture diameter. Therefore, f-stop values have an inverse relationship to aperture size; larger f-stop values correspond to a smaller aperture size. Decreasing aperture size will increase the DOF; f-stop values of f11 to 22 will typically ensure that the entire subject will be in focus (**Fig. 3**).[6] Yet a smaller aperture size decreases the amount of light that enters the camera, potentially resulting in an underexposed photograph. To counteract the small aperture, decrease the shutter speed and lengthen the amount of time the film or image sensor is exposed to light.

Manually fine-tuning DSLR settings to obtain the correct DOF while ensuring proper exposure may be cumbersome for the novice photographer. Fortunately, most DSLR cameras provide automated modes that adjust these settings based on photographer preference. The aperture-priority mode allows the photographer to manually set the aperture size, whereas the camera automatically adjusts the shutter speed using through-the-lens light metering to ensure adequate exposure.[6,9]

Lighting

Lighting is a critical component of obtaining high-quality images. It is especially important in extracting the fine anatomic details and contours of the nose that are crucial for rhinoplasty evaluation.

The arrangements of light sources may vary widely, having dramatic effects on the captured images.

The simplest and economic arrangement is the single camera-mounted flash. This approach will produce harsh lighting as well as undesirable shadowing effects.[9,11] Shadowing may be mitigated by a ring flash, a circular flash that emit light around the circumference of the lens; however, these tend to produce a flat, washed out image that causes loss of DOF and detail.[3]

Preferably, lighting consists of studio-grade electronic flash units, which provide diffuse, indirect light to produce shadowless images while allowing for the aperture settings of f11 to 22 and adequate DOF. The distance between the lights, termed the horizontal angle of incidence, has a significant effect on the appearance of the nasal tip; the ideal angle is 45°.[12] If the angle is increased, the tip defining points may seem wider, and vice versa. Maintaining the light sources at a fixed angle to the subject for all photos over time ensures that changes in the horizontal angle of incidence are not responsible for narrowing of the nasal tip, termed a "photographic tip rhinoplasty."[12]

Two types of studio lighting arrangements have been described—the key light system and the quarter light system. In portrait photography, the key light system uses one light as the major light source (key light); a less-intense second fill light is then positioned to light the area of the shadow on the face made by the key light. The downside of this is asymmetrical lighting that may give the illusion of anatomic asymmetry. Although this may be tolerated in nonmedical portraiture, it is problematic for the purposes of rhinoplasty photography, which relies on nasal tip light reflexes to evaluate for deformity and deviation. Consequently, medical photography has largely adopted the quarter light system.

The quarter light system includes 2 equal intensity lights positioned 45° from the subject-camera axis and 36 inches from the patient, as well as 2 additional backlights at 45° and 36 inches from the background to eliminate background shadows (**Fig. 4**). An alternative option to the 2 backlights is a single top light placed above the patient and directed at the background.[12] Although this setup produces excellent lighting, it requires a large space and budget. The senior author uses a modified version of the quarter light system that consists of only 2 synchronized studio flashes of equal intensity positioned 45° from the subject-camera axis with the patient placed 12 to 18 inches from the background, which minimizes the background shadows and eliminates the need for backlights (**Fig. 5**).[9,13]

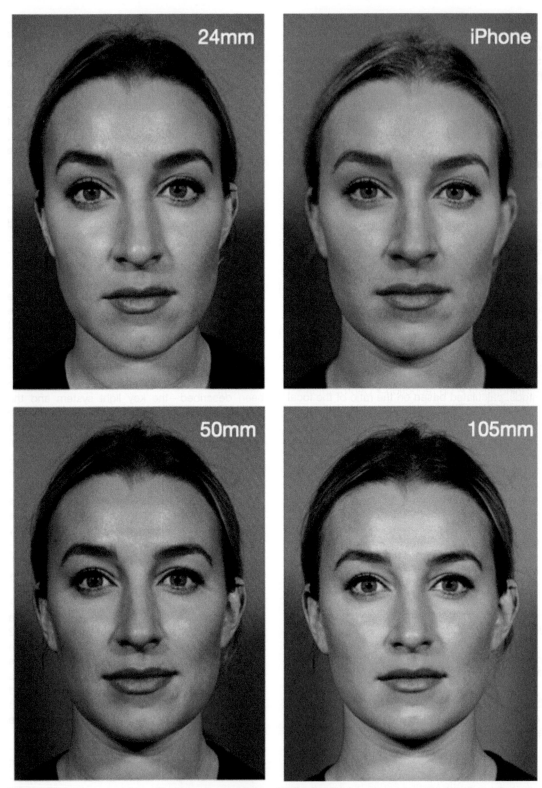

Fig. 2. Effect of lens focal length on facial proportions. With a 24-mm lens, there is noticeable facial distortion with a central-bulging or "fish-eye" effect. The image captured with a smartphone shows a similar result. The image obtained with a 50-mm lens shows less facial distortion. More realistic facial proportions are achieved with a 105-mm lens. The subject was photographed in the same sitting in a dual flash studio with a DSLR camera.

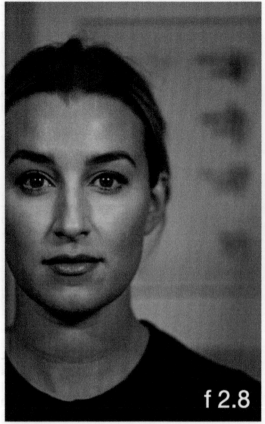 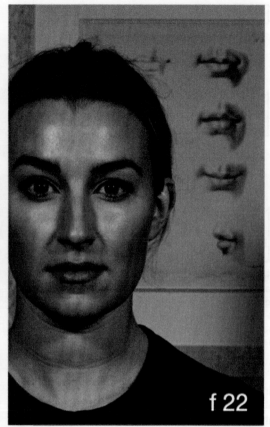

Fig. 3. Effect of aperture on depth of field (DOF). The left panel exhibits the limited DOF of an image taken with a larger aperture (f 2.8). The plane of focus is limited to the nasal tip, whereas the ears, hair, and background are out of focus. In the right panel, the image taken with a smaller aperture (f 22), the DOF is increased to include the nasal tip, ears, hair, and background in clear focus. The smaller aperture required additional lighting to maintain appropriate exposure.

Background

The photographic background should be a solid uniform color to eliminate distractions and place focus on the patient. A white background will produce harsh shadows; a black background can hide these shadows but is suboptimal for subjects with dark skin color and provides less contrast. A blue background is often used, as it provides adequate contrast and temper shadows.[3,6,14]

Digital Imaging Software/Storage

A key advantage of digital photography is the ability to immediately use imaging to facilitate communication with the patient during consultation. Computing imaging software may be used to create simulations of anticipated postoperative results and better understand the patient's expectations from rhinoplasty. It is an invaluable tool to communicate aesthetic changes that may be more difficult to convey verbally.

There are 2 types of imaging software systems. All-in-one systems, such as the Canfield Mirror imaging system (Canfield Scientific Inc., Parsippany, NJ), use an integrated program for both storage and image simulation and may be compatible with electronic medical record systems. The other system uses a separate program for storage and simulations. Adobe Photoshop (Adobe Systems Inc.) is a commonly used imaging editing program that can perform all editing functions that the all-in-one programs offer. The all-in-one system is expensive and may store images in a proprietary format but streamlines work flow. In contrast, using a stand-alone image editing program, such as Adobe Photoshop, is more cost-effective but the learning curve is steeper.[15,16] Another consideration is storage and organization. Patient images are protected health information and must be handled in a way that is compliant with the Health Insurance Portability and Accountability Act (HIPAA). All-in-one system images are encrypted

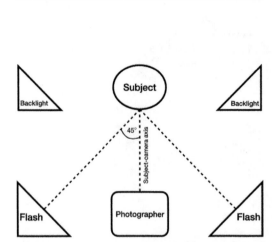

Fig. 4. The ideal quarter light photography setup for facial plastic surgery. Two equal-intensity flashes are set up at 45° to the subject-camera axis. The patient is placed 36 inches in front of the background. Two backlights are placed facing the background to eliminate background shadows.

and stored in a proprietary format and are organized within its system. Stand-alone programs allow for flexibility in selection of storage system, as long as it is appropriately encrypted according to HIPAA guidelines. Ultimately, both systems are viable options, and it is up to the surgeon to choose according to their needs.

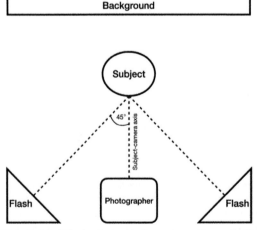

Fig. 5. Modified photography setup. Two studio flashes of equal intensity are positioned 45° from the subject-camera axis. The patient is placed 12 to 18 inches from the background, which minimizes the background shadows and eliminates the need for backlights.

Computer imaging software is a powerful device that allows both surgeon and patient to visualize the effects of a proposed rhinoplasty. Yet showing computer simulations with outcomes that are not surgically feasible will most certainly result in a dissatisfied patient postoperatively. It is imperative that the surgeon tempers the image editing to what is anatomically achievable. If used judiciously, imaging software can be an effective tool for patient communication and preoperative planning.

TECHNIQUE
Patient Preparation

Standardized patient preparation is crucial to obtaining consistent preoperative and postoperative images that depict accurate structural details of the rhinoplasty patient. Distracting accessories, such as eyeglasses, necklaces, and large earrings, should be removed. Clips or bands should be used to pull back the patient's hair to expose the ears and forehead.

Consent

Patients must understand how their photographs will be incorporated into their medical record and used as a tool for surgical planning. If the surgeon anticipates using the images for nonmedical purposes—such as publications, education, or marketing—a consent detailing intended uses of the photographs should be obtained.[3]

Patient Positioning

Identical positioning should be used preoperatively and postoperatively. The camera should be positioned at the eye level of the patient. The Frankfort horizontal line, an imaginary line from the infraorbital rim to the top of the tragus, should be used as a reference (**Fig. 6**). Proper head positioning places this line in a parallel plane to the ground.[17,18]

Standard Photographic Views

Standardized views for rhinoplasty photography have been previously described in detail.[18] These views include the anteroposterior view, right lateral view, right oblique view, left oblique view, left lateral view, and the basal view (**Fig. 7**). Additional views that may be beneficial for rhinoplasty are the cephalic view and a smiling lateral view (**Fig. 8**). The cephalic view allows evaluations of subtle deviations of the nasal dorsum. The smiling lateral view captures the dynamic changes of the nasal tip with the action of the depressor septi muscle.[13]

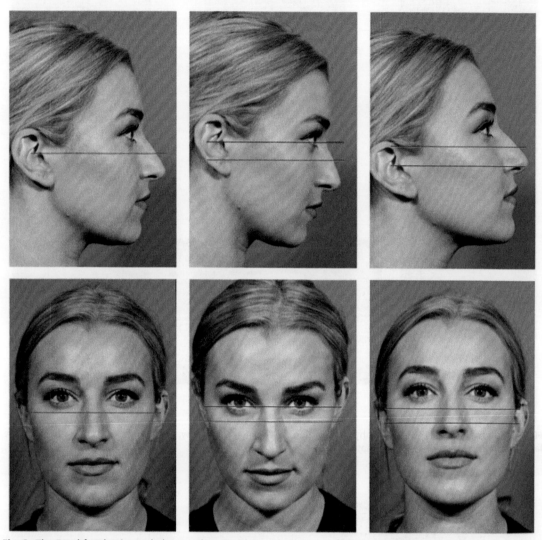

Fig. 6. The Frankfort horizontal plane and positioning. In both rows of photos, the left photograph demonstrates the proper position with the Frankfort horizontal plane, with the green line passing through the infraorbital rim and the external auditory canal. In the middle and right photos, the green line passes through the infraorbital rim and parallel to the floor, and the redline passes through the external auditory canal and parallel to the floor. Improper positioning leads to apparent changes in tip rotation.

DISCUSSION

In the past 2 decades, technological advancements brought about the transition in photography from film to digital media, and the 35-mm film SLR was largely replaced by DSLR cameras by professional and amateur photographers alike. As photography continues to evolve, emerging technology may again replace the current gold standard in facial plastic surgery—the DSLR.

Digital mirrorless camera technology has made great strides in the past decade. DSLR cameras contain a mirror that reflects light into the optical viewfinder, allowing the photographer to see precisely what the lens is capturing, and the mirror moves to expose the image sense when the image is captured. In mirrorless cameras, the light passes through the lens and directly onto the image sensor. The image is displayed on a monitor or the electronic viewfinder. Initially, mirrorless cameras had lagged behind DSLR in resolution and autofocusing features but recent advancements have placed mirrorless technology on par with that of DSLRs. The main advantage of the mirrorless system is that it is mechanically simpler and therefore smaller and lighter.[19] Native macro lenses for mirrorless cameras are now available in the 90 to 105 mm focal point range, making them a viable option for the facial plastic surgery setting. Lens adaptors are also available to allow

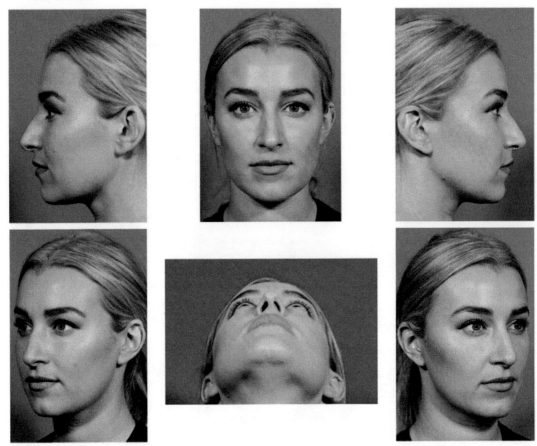

Fig. 7. Standard views for photography of the rhinoplasty patient. Top row: right lateral, anterior-posterior, left lateral. Bottom row: right oblique, basal view, left oblique.

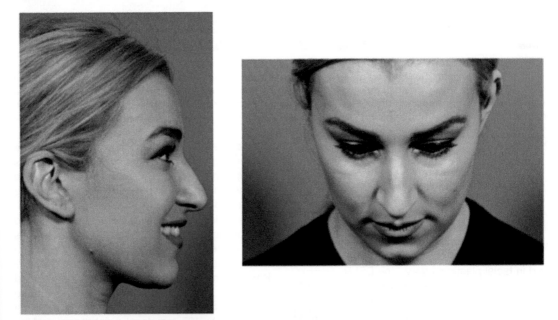

Fig. 8. Additional views for photography of the rhinoplasty patient. The left photo is the smiling lateral view; in some patients, smiling may cause downward tip movement. The right photo is a cephalic view, which may show dorsum additional irregularities not appreciated on the standard anterior-posterior view.

use of existing lenses for DSLR systems. Furthermore, the development of full-frame sensors in mirrorless cameras obviate the correction of crop factor with an FLM calculation.

Another emerging technology is 3-dimensional (3D) photography. There are many techniques that have been used to measure the 3D complexities of the face. These include stereophotogrammetry, image subtraction, moiré topography, liquid crystal scanning, light luminance scanning, laser scanning, and stereolithography; discussion of available 3D photography commercial systems and the techniques they use is beyond the scope of this discussion but have been previously discussed in detail.[20–22] Most current systems use stereophotogrammetry, in a process that use multiple 2-dimensional (2D) images taken by one or more cameras arranged around the subject. The 2D images are then integrated to produce a 3D image that is a result of thousands of points in space.[23,24] As discussed earlier, even slight discrepancies in 2D photograph lighting or angles may have significant ramifications for structural and aesthetic interpretation. 3D imaging has the potential to eliminate this problem. It may also enhance communications between surgeon and patient. Lekakis and colleagues examined whether rhinoplasty patients found that 3D morphing provided added benefit over 2D morphing during preoperative consultations; of the 172 study participants, 95% considered 3D simulation an added value over 2D.[25] A major disadvantage of 3D imaging is that most systems require a multicamera, multiangle setup that require a large, dedicated space. Another disadvantage is that these systems are significantly more expensive than a standard DSLR camera system. In its current state, 3D photography is physically burdensome and costly, rendering it largely impractical for the standard rhinoplasty practice. However, as technological progress allows for standardization of 3D image format as well as produces smaller and cheaper systems, 3D photography will provide a powerful tool for the facial plastic surgeon and may someday serve as a superior instrument for patient communication and surgical planning.

SUMMARY

Photography is a fundamental tool for the facial plastic surgeon. It is an invaluable resource for patient communication and education, surgical planning, medical record keeping, and for scholarly communication. Understanding the basic principles of photography equipment and technique is critical for obtaining high-quality, consistent, and accurate images.

CLINICS CARE POINTS

- Understanding basic photography equipment and principles is crucial for developing a technique to produce high-quality and accurate images of the rhinoplasty patient.

- Careful patient preparation and positioning is critical for consistent, standardized images.

- DSLR cameras are the gold standard for facial plastic photography; however, digital mirrorless camera technology has quickly evolved and is a viable alternative to DSLR.

- The emergence of 3D photography has exciting implications for the future of medical photography but has yet to be adopted as a standard for the facial plastic surgery practice.

DISCLOSURE

The authors have nothing to disclose.

REFERENCES

1. JENNES ML. Photography in rhinoplasty: an office technique. AMA Arch Otolaryngol 1954;60(6):695–701.
2. Karlan MS. Photographic documentation techniques. Ear Nose Throat J 1979;58(6):246–51.
3. Yavuzer R, Smirnes S, Jackson IT. Guidelines for standard photography in plastic surgery. Ann Plast Surg 2001;46(3):293–300.
4. Persichetti P, Simone P, Langella M, et al. Digital photography in plastic surgery: how to achieve reasonable standardization outside a photographic studio. Aesthet Plast Surg 2007;31(2):194–200.
5. Riley RS, Ben-Ezra JM, Massey D, et al. Digital photography: a primer for pathologists. J Clin Lab Anal 2004;18(2):91–128.
6. Galdino GM, DaSilva And D, Gunter JP. Digital photography for rhinoplasty. Plast Reconstr Surg 2002;109(4):1421–34.
7. Young S. Maintaining standard scales of reproduction in patient photography using digital cameras. J Audiov Media Med 2001;24(4):162–5.
8. Young S, Lake A. Calibrating lenses for standard scales of reproduction with digital SLR cameras. J Vis Commun Med 2008;31(1):11–5.
9. Swamy RS, Sykes JM, Most SP. Principles of photography in rhinoplasty for the digital photographer. Clin Plast Surg 2010;37(2):213–21.
10. Thomas JR, Tardy ME, Przekop H. Uniform photographic documentation in facial plastic surgery. Otolaryngol Clin North Am 1980;13(2):367–81.

11. Becker DG, Tardy ME. Standardized photography in facial plastic surgery: pearls and pitfalls. Facial Plast Surg 1999;15(2):93–9.

12. Daniel RK, Hodgson J, Lambros VS. Rhinoplasty: the light reflexes. Plast Reconstr Surg 1990;85(6): 859–66 [discussion: 867–8].

13. Swamy RS, Most SP. Pre- and postoperative portrait photography: standardized photos for various procedures. Facial Plast Surg Clin North Am 2010; 18(2):245–52. Table of Contents.

14. Zarem HA. Standards of photography. Plast Reconstr Surg 1984;74(1):137–46.

15. Hamilton GS. Morphing images to demonstrate potential surgical outcomes. Facial Plast Surg Clin North Am 2010;18(2):267–82. Table of Contents.

16. Ewart CJ, Leonard CJ, Harper JG, et al. A simple and inexpensive method of preoperative computer imaging for rhinoplasty. Ann Plast Surg 2006;56(1): 46–9.

17. DiBernardo BE, Adams RL, Krause J, et al. Photographic standards in plastic surgery. Plast Reconstr Surg 1998;102(2):559–68.

18. Henderson JL, Larrabee WF, Krieger BD. Photographic standards for facial plastic surgery. Arch Facial Plast Surg 2005;7(5):331–3.

19. Zoltie T. Mirrorless cameras for medical photography - time to switch? J Vis Commun Med 2018; 41(3):103–8.

20. Tzou CH, Frey M. Evolution of 3D surface imaging systems in facial plastic surgery. Facial Plast Surg Clin North Am 2011;19(4):591–602, vii.

21. Tzou CH, Artner NM, Pona I, et al. Comparison of three-dimensional surface-imaging systems. J Plast Reconstr Aesthet Surg 2014;67(4):489–97.

22. Lekakis G, Claes P, Hamilton GS, et al. Three-dimensional surface imaging and the continuous evolution of preoperative and postoperative assessment in rhinoplasty. Facial Plast Surg 2016;32(1):88–94.

23. Matthews HS, Burge JA, Verhelst PR, et al. Pitfalls and promise of 3-dimensional image Comparison for craniofacial surgical assessment. Plast Reconstr Surg Glob Open 2020;8(5):e2847.

24. Lee S. Three-dimensional photography and its application to facial plastic surgery. Arch Facial Plast Surg 2004;6(6):410–4.

25. Lekakis G, Hens G, Claes P, et al. Three-dimensional morphing and its added value in the rhinoplasty consult. Plast Reconstr Surg Glob Open 2019;7(1): e2063.

Evaluation and Management of the Nasal Airway

Sami P. Moubayed, MD[a],*, Sam P. Most, MD[b]

KEYWORDS

- Rhinoplasty • Airway obstruction • Septorhinoplasty • Functional rhinoplasty • Septoplasty
- Nasal valve collapse • Lateral wall insufficiency • Turbinate reduction

KEY POINTS

- The nasal airway may be obstructed at the level of the nasal valve, septum, nasal turbinates, sinonasal mucosa or nasopharynx.
- Nasal valve obstruction and septal deviations are usually treated surgically depending on the level of valve obstruction.
- Isolated turbinate hypertrophy is usually managed medically as part of the treatment of rhinitis, with surgery reserved for cases refractory to medical care.
- Sinonasal and nasopharyngeal conditions are treated according to the diagnosis.

INTRODUCTION

The nasal airway starts at the nasal vestibule and ends at the nasopharynx. *Nasal airway obstruction* is defined as the sensation of insufficient airflow or difficulty breathing through the nose.[1] Nasal obstruction is frequently encountered in primary care, otolaryngology, facial plastic surgery, and allergy, and is the major symptom of a broad spectrum of conditions.[2] Although data sources vary, the overwhelming conclusion from several studies is that nasal obstruction is very common, affecting up to half of the population depending on how it is evaluated.[2] It results in significantly decreased quality of life, with hundreds of thousands of patients in the United States seeking treatment for nasal obstruction annually.[3] Every year, about 5 billion dollars are spent to treat nasal obstruction and around 60 million dollars are spent on surgical treatment of nasal airway obstruction.[4]

CLASSIFICATION

There are multiple classification systems to categorize nasal obstruction, but we prefer a classification system that is, anatomically based (**Table 1**).

The external nasal valve (ENV) is the entry point (vestibule) of the nasal airway. It is formed by the caudal septum, medial crura of the alar cartilages, alar rim, and nasal sill.[5] Deviations in the caudal septum, post-traumatic or iatrogenic stenosis or synechiae, and neoplastic conditions may arise in this area. There are no studies of the exact prevalence of obstruction at the ENV, but caudal septal deviations produce a much greater symptomatic nasal obstruction than posterior septal deviations.[6] Caudal septal deviation is defined as deviation in the anteriormost portion of the nasal septum, as represents 5% to 8% of all septal deviations.[7,8] Moreover, dynamic collapse due to contralateral caudal septal deviation due to the

The authors have nothing to disclose.
[a] University of Montreal, Montreal, Canada; [b] Stanford University, Stanford
* Corresponding author. 245 Victoria, Suite 10, Westmount, Quebec H3Z 2M5, Canada.
E-mail address: sp.moubayed@umontreal.ca

Clin Plastic Surg 49 (2022) 23–31
https://doi.org/10.1016/j.cps.2021.08.001
0094-1298/22/© 2021 Elsevier Inc. All rights reserved.

Table 1
Etiologies of nasal airway obstruction according to obstruction level

Nasal valve	Static external nasal valve collapse (congenital, caudal septal deviation, synechiae, nostril stenosis)
	Dynamic external nasal valve collapse (iatrogenic, congenical)
	Static internal nasal valve collapse (hump takedown during rhinoplasty without midvault reconstruction, synechiaie, congenital)
	Dynamic internal nasal valve collapse (iatrogenic, congenital)
Nasal septum	Nasal septal deviations (congenital, traumatic, iatrogenic)
	Synechiae (traumatic or iatrogenic)
Turbinates	Inferior turbinate hypertrophy
Sinonasal mucosa	Rhinitis (allergic and nonallergic)
	Rhinosinusitis with or without polyposis
	Benign or malignant neoplasms
	Vascular malformations
Nasopharynx	Choanal atresia
	Adenoid hypertrophy
	Benign or malignant neoplasms

Bernoulli effect is a condition that is, usually corrected with caudal septoplasty.[9] Dynamic collapse may also occur iatrogenically after weakened of the sidewall following rhinoplasty with lower lateral cartilage resection or a congenitally weak lateral nasal wall. This is termed lateral wall insufficiency (LWI).[10] A severely ptotic nasal tip is also a recognized cause of external valve collapse.[5]

The internal nasal valve (INV) is bound by the septum medially, the nasal sidewall, and inferior turbinate laterally, and the upper lateral cartilages (ULCs) and nasal floor laterally.[11] It represents the cross sectional segment of the nasal airway most resistive to air flow, and as such it plays a central role in the pathophysiology of nasal obstruction. Congenital narrowing or iatrogenic synechiae or narrowing may affect this condition. Of significant clinical importance, dorsal hump reduction procedures in the primary rhinoplasty setting can result in destabilization of the nasal midvault and subsequent static compromise of the INV.[12] The INV may also be affected by dynamic collapse, either due to congenital or iatrogenic reasons, and is also termed LWI.[10] We categorize LWI as occurring in two distinct zones divided roughly at the level of the upper LLC and scroll region, as shown in **Fig. 1** (MOST, Trends in Functional Rhinoplasty). Zone 1 LWI occurs superior to this, and zone 2 LWI occurs caudal to this. Note that zone 2 LWI is analogous to classical "external valve collapse", whereas zone 1 LWI was not previously categorized as a dynamic issue.

Septal deviations are an extremely common occurrence in the general population, although not all will result in nasal obstruction. Nasal septal deviations may be congenital or acquired, most commonly during trauma, whether accidental or iatrogenic.[13] In patients with no clear history of trauma, a common overlooked trauma is vaginal birth. Studies have shown prevalence of septal deviations in children to be of up to 60%.[13] In adults, a wide variety of prevalences has been reported,

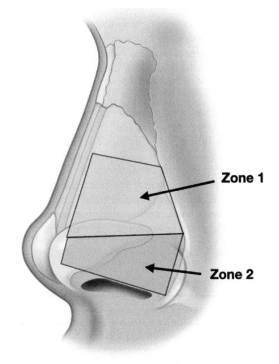

Zone 1

Zone 2

Fig. 1. Zones of lateral wall insuffiency.

with certain studies reporting a prevalence of up to 90%.[13] An interesting Turkish study of 9835 young men aged 20 to 29 years showed a prevalence of septal deviation of 47% in this population.[14] All of these patients were examined by otolaryngologists as part of a routine mandatory examination before undergoing physical activity.[14] However, 30% of the patients with septal deviations did not complain of nasal obstruction.[14] In nasal obstruction patients, a large study by Clark and colleagues[15] in 1906 patients has shown that nasal obstruction is a contributor, in isolation or in conjuction with other conditions in 80% of cases.

Inferior turbinate hypertrophy may be congenital or due to rhinitis. One of the largest studies of prevalence of nasal obstruction showed that inferior turbinate hypertrophy is a component of nasal obstruction in 72% of cases.[15]

Rhinitis is defined as inflammation of the nasal mucosa. The most common cause of rhinitis is allergic rhinitis, which affects up to 40% of the population, and with a higher occurrence in children.[16] The most common symptom of allergic rhinitis is nasal obstruction.[3] Allergic rhinitis may be seasonal (due to pollens, most commonly) or perennial (due to dust mites, molds, insects, and animal dander). Other common causes of rhinitis, that are nonallergic, are infectious, hormonally induced, drug-induced, rhinitis medicamentosa, occupational rhinitis, smoke-induced, food-induced, alcohol-induced, vasomotor rhinitis, atrophic rhinitis, autoimmune rhinitis, vasculitis rhinitis, NARES syndrome, and many others.[16]

Rhinosinusitis is defined as inflammation in the sinonasal mucosa and is classified as rhinosinusitis with or without nasal polyps.[17] Rhinosinusitis may be acute or chronic.[17] Chronic rhinosinusitis (CRS) affects around 5% of the population and is responsible for significant health expenditures every year.[17] Nasal obstruction is reported in 70% of rhinosinusitis patients.[3] Other symptoms include congestion, facial pain/pressure, discharge, and smell alterations.[17] Patients with CRS have a health status similar to patients with cancer, arthritis, asthma, and inflammatory bowel disease.[17]

Intranasal masses may be benign or malignant and may be of epithelial and nonepithelial in origin.[18] More than 70 benign and malignant sinonasal neoplastic conditions have been described, and malignant sinonasal tumors comprise 3% of all head and neck malignancy.[19] Nasal obstruction can be a cardinal feature in these conditions. The most common benign conditions are osteoma, fibrous dysplasia, juvenile nasal angiofibroma, schwannoma, and nasal papilloma.[19] The most common malignant conditions are squamous cell

carcinoma, adenocarcinoma, sinonasal undifferentiated carcinoma, lymphoma, chondrosarcoma, salivary tumors, neuroendocrine carcinoma, and melanoma.[19]

Nasopharyngeal conditions such as adenoid hypertrophy, nasopharyngeal tumors, or choanal atresia are also responsible for nasal obstruction. For this reason, it is important to examine the nasopharynx in patients complaining of nasal obstruction.

Finally, recumbency has been shown to increase nasal resistance and nasal obstruction in both normal patients and patients suffering from rhinitis.[20] The pathophysiology includes local factors (congestion of capacitance vessels of inferior concha mucosa) and systemic ones (increase in venous pressure by the affection of hydrostatic pressure), and both are related to cutaneous and vascular reflexes.[21]

HISTORY AND PHYSICAL EXAMINATION

The basis of proper treatment involves proper diagnosis. Appropriate diagnosis can be made in most cases using thorough history and physical examination. As nasal obstruction is present in a variety of conditions, focused medical history should include the following:

- Onset: long-standing since childhood, post-traumatic or postsurgical, or following changes in a patient's life such as acquiring a pet or moving to a new city may help narrow down the cause[2]
- Laterality: unilateral obstruction suggest anatomic causes although bilateral obstruction does not exclude anatomic conditions[2]
- Duration of symptoms: intermittent duration suggest inflammatory conditions such as rhinitis[2]
- Specific triggers: exposure to allergens, foods, medications, smoke, medications or pregnancy may alert the physician to the presence of a certain type of rhinitis.
- Alleviating factors: nasal dilator cones or strips may suggest nasal valve compromise or caudal septal deviations, alleviation with nasal steroids may suggest the presence of underlying rhinitis
- Associated rhinitis or rhinosinusitis symptoms
- Associated epistaxis or pain, which would elicit possibilty of malignancy
- Drugs and substance abuse, such as nasal decongestant or intranasal illicit drugs
- Comorbidities and personal history:

Physical examination is of utmost importance and should include the following:

- Inspection of the nasal vestibule: a columellar deviation may suggest the presence of an underlying caudal septal deviation, and stenotic nostrils may be congenital or following accidental trauma, surgical trauma or trauma following nasal packing,
- Inspection of the nasal septum using a headlight: posterior (noncaudal) nasal septal deviations
- Inspection of the nasal turbinates using a headlight: enlarged turbinates must be identified. To optimize the evaluation of resulting medical or surgical treatment, we recommend documenting the size of the turbinates using a classification system. One validated classification system that has been described is the 25% (grades 1–4) inferior turbinate classification system[22]
- Inspection for dynamic collapse: as previously described[23] and validated[10] by most, dynamic LWI must be evaluated by looking into the nasal valve area using a light in zone 1 (INV) and zone 2 (external nasal) valve and classified as 0-1-2-3 depending on the distance the lateral nasal wall moves into the nasal septum (0%, 0%–33%, 33%–66%, more than 66%)
- The modified Cottle maneuver for static or dynamic valve collapse: the modified Cottle maneuver can be alternately performed by manual intranasal lateralization or stabilization of the lateral nasal wall using an ear curette or the wooden end of a cotton-tipped applicator.[24] In cases of dynamic collapse, we test for suitability for surgery by noting improvement in obstruction resulting from simple stabilization (vs lateralization) of the nasal wall at the level of collapse. In cases of static collapse, improvement in obstruction on the obstructed side with lateralization, with an identifiable area of narrowing such as a deviated caudal septum, may indicate suitability for surgery, if the surgeon feels this outcome is achievable.
- The original Cottle maneuver (lateral distraction of the cheek) should not be used as it demonstrates low construct validity[25]
- Decongestion of the turbinates with resulting improvement in obstruction can help diagnose rhinitis, although is not diagnostic
- Nasal endoscopy is helpful in identifying benign or malignant masses, polyps, very posterior septal deviations, or nasopharyngeal conditions such as adenoid hypertrophy

Ancillary testing such as computed tomography of the sinuses and allergy testing can help diagnose rhinosinusitis and allergic rhinitis when clinical suspicion is present after history and physical examination.

EVALUATION OF OBJECTIVE OUTCOMES

Nasal obstruction is often multifactorial and may be due to a variety of conditions.[26] For this reason, measurement of outcomes has historically been difficult and a variety of recommendations[5] exist in published consensus statements, and sometimes there is even an absence of recommendations in this regard.[27]

Several objective anatomic and physiologic measures of the nasal airway exist, such as acoustic rhinometry, sinonasal imaging, rhinomanometry, nasal peak inspiratory flow, and computational fluid dynamics.[26] Most studies do not find a significant correlation between these measures and a patient's subjective complaint of nasal obstruction.[28–32] Currently, there is a lack of a "gold standard" objective test for nasal airway obstruction.[5]

Patient-reported outcome measures (PROMs) evaluate the subjective experience of the patient and the patient's self reported assessment of the efficacy of a treatment without interpretation from the physician.[26] Thus, PROMs seem to provide a measurable assessment of otherwise subjective results. Both the nasal valve compromise and rhinoplasty clinical practice guidelines recommend the routine use of PROMs in nasal surgical patients.[5,33] Unfortunately, only 14% of published functional rhinoplasty outcome studies involve the use of validated PROMs.[11]

With regards to nasal obstruction, the most commonly used PROM to evaluate nasal obstruction is the Nasal Obstruction Symptom Evaluation (NOSE) score.[26] The NOSE score is a disease-specific questionnaire to assess nasal obstruction and was shown to be valid, reliable, and sensitive in evaluation of nasal obstruction.[34] The questionnaire has 5 questions based on a 4-point scale, with scores reported on a scale of 0 to 100 (raw score multiplied by 5). It was initially validated with patients undergoing septoplasty but is now used in many studies of functional rhinoplasty as well.[26]

As nasal obstruction is often a component of other conditions, such as nasal valve collapse or rhinosinusitis, several other questionnaires exist that assess the outcomes of interventions that impact other symptoms that are specific to each particular disease. For functional rhinoplasty, intervention at the level of the nasal valve may modify nasal appearance, and a combined functional and cosmetic PROM should be administered both before and after surgery to evaluate the change in both components. An extensively validated PROM that adheres to international development guidelines is the Standardized Cosmesis and Health Nasal Outcomes Survey (SCHNOS, **Fig. 2**).[35] This outcome measure has been translated into multiple languages, characterized temporally, correlated with psychiatric disease, as well as used to predict likelihood of revision.[36–38] As such, it is our preferred outcome measure and has been recommended for wide adoption by a multispecialty rhinoplasty work group.[39] Other combined functional and cosmetic PROMs include the Rhinoplasty Outcomes Evaluation, Functional Rhinoplasty Outcomes Inventory (FROI-17), RHINO scale, and Evaluation of Esthetic Rhinoplasty Scale, but none have been validated or characterized as extensively.[26]

Other validated measures focus on inflammatory nasal disease such as the Rhinosinusitis Disability Index and SNOT-22.[26] However, as their primary goal of these PROMs is to evaluate inflammatory nasal disease, nasal obstruction measured by these instruments is more often secondary to inflammatory disease, rather than a structural abnormality.

TREATMENTS

Nasal obstruction is multifactorial. Proper diagnosis enables appropriate treatment to be tailored to each specific anatomic area of obstruction.

Nasal Valve

In 2010, the American Academy of Otolaryngology-Head and Neck Surgery released a clinical

Over the past **month**, how much of a **problem** was the following:

	No problem					Extreme problem
1. Having a blocked or obstructed nose	0	1	2	3	4	5
2. Getting air through my nose during exercise	0	1	2	3	4	5
3. Having a congested nose	0	1	2	3	4	5
4. Breathing through my nose during sleep	0	1	2	3	4	5
5. Decreased mood and self-esteem due to my nose	0	1	2	3	4	5
6. The shape of my nasal tip	0	1	2	3	4	5
7. The straightness of my nose	0	1	2	3	4	5
8. The shape of my nose from the side	0	1	2	3	4	5
9. How well my nose suits my face	0	1	2	3	4	5
10. Overall appearance of my nose	0	1	2	3	4	5
11. The overall symmetry of my nose	0	1	2	3	4	5
12. How good my nose looks in photos	0	1	2	3	4	5
13. The overall attractiveness of my nose	0	1	2	3	4	5

Fig. 2. Standardized Cosmesis and Health Nasal Outcomes Survey (SCHNOS).

consensus statement based on a panel of functional rhinoplasty experts regarding diagnosis and management of nasal valve collapse.[11] The consensus concluded that there is a paucity of high-quality evidence for nasal valve compromise. In the absence of rhinitis, there is no role for medical management, with the mainstay of treatment being surgical. In terms of therapeutic management, they concluded that a surgical procedure that is, targeted to support the lateral nasal wall/alar rim is a distinct entity from procedures that correct a deviated nasal septum or hypertrophied turbinate. In some cases, septoplasty with or without turbinate surgery can treat NVC without surgery to support the lateral nasal wall/alar rim. In some cases, turbinate surgery alone can treat NVC without surgery to support the lateral nasal wall/alar rim. In some patients, nasal strips can be used therapeutically with nasal valve collapse. The statement also concludes that PROMs are more important than objective measures.

In terms of dynamic valve collapse, or LWI, multiple techniques have been described but there is no widely adopted treatment approach. One study aiming to establish an algorithm for dynamic collapse depending on the location of collapse was published by Vaezeafshar and colleagues[40] in 2018. A total of 44 patients underwent open septorhinoplasty to repair dynamic valve collapse (group 1) and were compared with age and sex-matched controls undergoing cosmetic rhinoplasty (group 2). Collapse at the level of the external valve (zone 2) was treated with alar rim grafts, and collapse at the level of the internal valve (zone 1) was treated with lateral crural strut grafting. NOSE scores in both groups significantly improved after surgery ($P<.001$ and $P = .018$), although the improvement in group 2 was not clinically significant. Mean preoperative LWI grades were higher in group 1 for each zone ($P<.001$ and $P = .001$) but were similar between groups for each zone postoperatively. Postoperative LWI scores significantly decreased in group 1 to levels similar to that of group 2 patients. A positive linear correlation was noted between NOSE and LWI scores, with the strongest correlation between preoperative zone 1 LWI and NOSE scores ($R = 0.68$). Lateral crural strut grafts were used for zone 1 LWI and alar rim grafts were used for zone 2 LWI. Typical graft placement for treatment of zone 1 and zone 2 LWI is shown in **Fig. 3**.

Dorsal reduction procedures in the primary rhinoplasty setting can result in destabilization of the nasal midvault and subsequent compromise of the INV. An attractive option that has been described is the autospreader flap, which creates a flap based on the ULC rather than requiring graft harvest.[12] Saedi and colleagues[12] conducted a

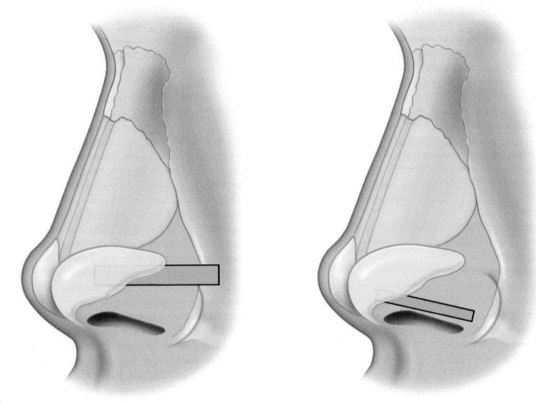

Fig. 3. Left panel: lateral crural strut graft. Right panel: Alar rim graft.

randomized controlled trial of 66 primary rhinoplasty candidates undergoing dorsal reduction. Patients in the control group underwent a similar dissection to the autospreader group; however, excess ULC that might serve as the spreader flap was simply excised and the free edge was sutured directly to the septum.[12] All patients and one of the authors measuring outcome data were blinded to the treatment method.[12] There was no difference between the two groups in both acoustic rhinomanometry measures, as well as patients' subjective responses to surgery as measured by VAS4. However, the study did not compare the autospreader technique to the spreader graft technique.

Nasal Septum

In 2015, the American Academy of Otolaryngology published a Clinical Consensus Statement on septoplasty with or without turbinate reduction.[27] Septoplasty is usually performed through a standard left hemitransfixion incision and the guidelines clearly mention that external approaches should be considered when anterior septal deformities are present.[27] In this paper, we classify anterior deviations as part of the nasal valve.

Therefore we recommend traditional endonasal septoplasty for non-L strut deformities.

A recent double-blind randomized controlled trial was performed on patients with nasal obstruction and severe septal deviation and found no significant effect of intranasal steroids on nasal obstruction as compared with placebo.[41] Surgery, however, was associated with significant sustained improvement in nasal obstruction.[41] The cost-effectiveness of surgery versus steroid use has also been demonstrated, when evaluated from a patient quality-of-life perspective (Teti and Most).

Caudal septal deviations present a particular problem, given the importance of maintaining tip support, and the primacy of the caudal septum to the nasal valve area. A recent survey showed that the most commonly used techniques to repair the caudal septum are the swinging door, extracorporeal septoplasty (ECS), cartilage scoring, and splinting using cartilage.[42] Modified ECS is the authors' technique of choice and is shown in **Fig. 4**.[43,44] Full ECS was extensively described by Gubisch.[45] In a large series, the revision rate was 9% but decreased by use of camouflage grafts to mask settling at rhinion, as it is difficult to reform the bony-cartilaginous attachment at

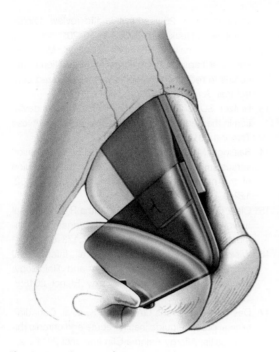

Fig. 4. Anterior septal reconstruction.

the keystone.[45] The technique was further modified including the use of polydioxanone plates, grafting techniques, limited dorsal septal removal, and methods to better secure the cartilage to reduce dorsal irregularities.[46] A recent meta-analysis compared conventional ECS in 16 studies (51.6%), and modified ECS in 15 studies (48.4%), showing a significantly decreased rate of dorsal irregularities but equivalent functional results.

Nasal Turbinates

Inferior turbinate hypertrophy is a frequent occurrence in patients with nasal obstruction and septal deviation and can be an independent cause of nasal obstruction.[27] Several randomized controlled trials have shown that inferior turbinoplasty is an effective adjunct to septoplasty.[27] However, conservative techniques are generally recommended due to the associated risks of inferior turbinoplasty(eg, atrophic rhinitis, bleeding, or adhesions).[27]

A recent systematic review of turbinectomy techniques revealed the absence of scientific data on the outcomes of turbinate outfracture.[47] Of all the turbinate reduction techniques evaluated in the literature, only submucosal resection and radiofrequency ablation provide long-lasting results, preservation of turbinate function, and low complication rates.[47]

In cases with isolated inferior turbinate hypertrophy, without septal deviation, and nasal

obstruction, it is recommended to trial medical therapy first, as described in the following section.[48,49]

Rhinitis, Rhinosinusitis, and Other Inflammatory Conditions

Comprehensive management of rhinitis, rhinosinusitis, and other inflammatory conditions is beyond the scope of this text. Briefly, the current international consensus statement on the management of allergic rhinitis, the most common type of rhinitis, recommends allergen avoidance, intranasal steroids, or oral antihistamines as treatments of allergic rhinitis.[16] Turbinate reduction is reserved for allergic rhinitis patients refractory to medical treatment.[16] Other types of rhinitis such as rhinitis medicamentosa, infectious rhinitis, food- and alcohol-induced rhinitis, and others, are all treated in a specific fashion.

The management of rhinosinusitis is usually medical at first, with topical steroids, antibiotics, and oral steroids being used depending on the type of rhinosinusitis that the patient is suffering from.[17,50]

Autoimmune, granulomatous, or vasculitic conditions affecting the nose are all treated differently, often times with systemic immunosuppressants.[16]

Other Conditions

Malignant neoplastic conditions causing nasal obstruction are best treated in a multidisciplinary fashion with various treatment such as radiation therapy, chemotherapy, or surgery, depending on the type of cancer.[51] Choanal atresia is usually treated with surgery.[52] Hypertrophied adenoids in adults are rare and should be initially managed medically with surgery reserved to refractory cases.[53]

SUMMARY

In conclusion, nasal airway obstruction is very common, affecting up to half of the population and results in significantly decreased quality of life. It may involve the nasal valve area, nasal septum, inferior turbinates, sinonasal mucosa, or nasopharynx. History and physical examination, including nasal endoscopy, help make a precise diagnosis. Treatment is tailored to the specific condition that is, causing nasal airway obstruction, with many patients suffering from multilevel obstruction. Use of PROMs is increasingly considered standard of care in patients undergoing rhinoplasty of all types, and the SCHNOS is currently the well-validated and widely adopted.

CLINICS CARE POINTS

- Nasal valve obstruction is treated with rim grafts in zone 2 and lateral crural strut grafts in zone 1
- Caudal septal deviations are usually treated with anterior septal reconstruction
- Posterior septal deviations are treated with septoplasty
- Turbinate hypetrophy is initially managed medically. Refractory hypertrophy is treated with submucous resection.

REFERENCES

1. Mohan S, Fuller JC, Ford SF, et al. Diagnostic and therapeutic management of nasal airway obstruction: advances in diagnosis and treatment. JAMA Facial Plast Surg 2018;20:409–18.
2. Valero A, Navarro AM, Del Cuvillo A, et al. Position paper on nasal obstruction: evaluation and treatment. J Investig Allergol Clin Immunol 2018;28:67–90.
3. Stewart M, Ferguson B, Fromer L. Epidemiology and burden of nasal congestion. Int J Gen Med 2010;3:37–45.
4. Kimmelman CP. The problem of nasal obstruction. Otolaryngol Clin North Am 1989;22:253–64.
5. Rhee JS, Weaver EM, Park SS, et al. Clinical consensus statement: diagnosis and management of nasal valve compromise. Otolaryngol Head Neck Surg 2010;143:48–59.
6. Grymer LF, Hilberg O, Elbrond O, et al. Acoustic rhinometry: evaluation of the nasal cavity with septal deviations, before and after septoplasty. Laryngoscope 1989;99:1180–7.
7. Guyuron B, Uzzo CD, Scull H. A practical classification of septonasal deviation and an effective guide to septal surgery. Plast Reconstr Surg 1999;104:2202–9 [discussion 2202–12].
8. Sedwick JD, Lopez AB, Gajewski BJ, et al. Caudal septoplasty for treatment of septal deviation: aesthetic and functional correction of the nasal base. Arch Facial Plast Surg 2005;7:158–62.
9. Rudy S, Moubayed SP. Most SP: lateral wall insufficiency after septal reconstruction. Facial Plast Surg 2017;33:451–2.
10. Tsao GJ, Fijalkowski N, Most SP. Validation of a grading system for lateral nasal wall insufficiency. Allergy Rhinol (Providence) 2013;4:e66–8.
11. Rhee JS, Arganbright JM, McMullin BT, et al. Evidence supporting functional rhinoplasty or nasal valve repair: a 25-year systematic review. Otolaryngol Head Neck Surg 2008;139:10–20.
12. Saedi B, Amali A, Gharavis V, et al. Most SP: spreader flaps do not change early functional outcomes in reduction rhinoplasty: a randomized control trial. Am J Rhinol Allergy 2014;28:70–4.
13. Reitzen SD, Chung W, Shah AR. Nasal septal deviation in the pediatric and adult populations. Ear Nose Throat J 2011;90:112–5.
14. Salihoglu M, Cekin E, Altundag A, et al. Examination versus subjective nasal obstruction in the evaluation of the nasal septal deviation. Rhinology 2014;52:122–6.
15. Clark DW, Del Signore AG, Raithatha R, et al. Nasal airway obstruction: prevalence and anatomic contributors. Ear Nose Throat J 2018;97:173–6.
16. Wise SK, Lin SY, Toskala E, et al. International consensus statement on allergy and Rhinology: allergic rhinitis. Int Forum Allergy Rhinol 2018;8:108–352.
17. Desrosiers M, Evans GA, Keith PK, et al. Canadian clinical practice guidelines for acute and chronic rhinosinusitis. Allergy Asthma Clin Immunol 2011;7:2.
18. Devi CP, Devi KM, Kumar P, et al. Diagnostic challenges in malignant tumors of nasal cavity and paranasal sinuses. J Oral Maxillofac Pathol 2019;23:378–82.
19. Eggesbo HB. Imaging of sinonasal tumours. Cancer Imaging 2012;12:136–52.
20. Calvo-Henriquez C, Chiesa-Estomba C, Lechien JR, et al. The recumbent position affects nasal resistance: a systematic review and meta-analysis. Laryngoscope 2021 [online ahead of print].
21. Roithmann R, Demeneghi P, Faggiano R, et al. Effects of posture change on nasal patency. Braz J Otorhinolaryngol 2005;71:478–84.
22. Camacho M, Zaghi S, Certal V, et al. Inferior turbinate classification system, grades 1 to 4: development and validation study. Laryngoscope 2015;125:296–302.
23. Most SP. Trends in functional rhinoplasty. Arch Facial Plast Surg 2008;10:410–3.
24. Fung E, Hong P, Moore C, et al. The effectiveness of modified cottle maneuver in predicting outcomes in functional rhinoplasty. Plast Surg Int 2014;2014:618313.
25. Das A, Spiegel JH. Evaluation of validity and specificity of the cottle maneuver in diagnosis of nasal valve collapse. Plast Reconstr Surg 2020;146:277–80.
26. Spataro E. Most SP: measuring nasal obstruction outcomes. Otolaryngol Clin North Am 2018;51:883–95.
27. Han JK, Stringer SP, Rosenfeld RM, et al. Clinical consensus statement: septoplasty with or without inferior turbinate reduction. Otolaryngol Head Neck Surg 2015;153:708–20.

28. Fairley JW, Durham LH, Ell SR. Correlation of subjective sensation of nasal patency with nasal inspiratory peak flow rate. Clin Otolaryngol Allied Sci 1993;18: 19–22.

29. Hirschberg A, Rezek O. Correlation between objective and subjective assessments of nasal patency. ORL J Otorhinolaryngol Relat Spec 1998;60:206–11.

30. Lam DJ, James KT, Weaver EM. Comparison of anatomic, physiological, and subjective measures of the nasal airway. Am J Rhinol 2006;20:463–70.

31. Sipila J, Suonpaa J, Silvoniemi P, et al. Correlations between subjective sensation of nasal patency and rhinomanometry in both unilateral and total nasal assessment. ORL J Otorhinolaryngol Relat Spec 1995;57:260–3.

32. Wang DY, Raza MT, Goh DY, et al. Acoustic rhinometry in nasal allergen challenge study: which dimensional measures are meaningful? Clin Exp Allergy 2004;34:1093–8.

33. Ishii LE, Tollefson TT, Basura GJ, et al. Clinical practice guideline: improving nasal Form and function after rhinoplasty executive summary. Otolaryngol Head Neck Surg 2017;156:205–19.

34. Stewart MG, Witsell DL, Smith TL, et al. Development and validation of the nasal obstruction symptom evaluation (NOSE) scale. Otolaryngol Head Neck Surg 2004;130:157–63.

35. Moubayed SP, Ioannidis JPA, Saltychev M. Most SP: the 10-item standardized Cosmesis and health nasal outcomes survey (SCHNOS) for functional and cosmetic rhinoplasty. JAMA Facial Plast Surg 2018;20:37–42.

36. Kandathil CK, Patel PN, Spataro EA. Most SP: examining preoperative expectations and postoperative satisfaction in rhinoplasty patients: a single-center study. Facial Plast Surg Aesthet Med 2020 [online ahead of print].

37. Okland TS, Patel P, Liu GS. Most SP: using nasal self-esteem to predict revision in cosmetic rhinoplasty. Aesthet Surg J 2021;41(6):652–6.

38. Spataro EA, Kandathil CK, Saltychev M, et al. Most SP: correlation of the standardized Cosmesis and health nasal outcomes survey with psychiatric screening tools. Aesthet Surg J 2020;40:1373–80.

39. Manahan MA, Fedok F, Davidson C, et al. Evidence-based performance measures for rhinoplasty: a multidisciplinary performance measure set. Plast Reconstr Surg 2021;147:222e–30e.

40. Vaezeafshar R, Moubayed SP. Most SP: repair of lateral wall insufficiency. JAMA Facial Plast Surg 2018;20:111–5.

41. Rudy SF, Kandathil C, Spataro EA, et al. Most SP: effect of nasal steroids on nasal obstruction in septal deviation: a double-blind randomized controlled trial. Facial Plast Surg Aesthet Med 2020;22:243–8.

42. Voizard B, Theriault M, Lazizi S, et al. North American survey and systematic review on caudal Septoplasty. J Otolaryngol Head Neck Surg 2020;49:38.

43. Most SP. Anterior septal reconstruction: outcomes after a modified extracorporeal septoplasty technique. Arch Facial Plast Surg 2006;8:202–7.

44. Surowitz J, Lee MK. Most SP: anterior septal reconstruction for treatment of severe caudal septal deviation: clinical severity and outcomes. Otolaryngol Head Neck Surg 2015;153:27–33.

45. Gubisch W. The extracorporeal septum plasty: a technique to correct difficult nasal deformities. Plast Reconstr Surg 1995;95:672–82.

46. Spataro EA, Saltychev M, Kandathil CK. Most SP: outcomes of extracorporeal septoplasty and its modifications in treatment of severe L-strut septal deviation: a systematic review and meta-analysis. JAMA Facial Plast Surg 2019;21:542–50.

47. Sinno S, Mehta K, Lee ZH, et al. Inferior turbinate hypertrophy in rhinoplasty: systematic review of surgical techniques. Plast Reconstr Surg 2016;138: 419e–29e.

48. Batra PS, Seiden AM, Smith TL. Surgical management of adult inferior turbinate hypertrophy: a systematic review of the evidence. Laryngoscope 2009;119:1819–27.

49. Ye T, Zhou B. Update on surgical management of adult inferior turbinate hypertrophy. Curr Opin Otolaryngol Head Neck Surg 2015;23:29–33.

50. Fokkens WJ, Lund VJ, Hopkins C, et al. European position paper on rhinosinusitis and nasal polyps 2020. Rhinology 2020;58:1–464.

51. Ferrari M, Orlandi E, Bossi P. Sinonasal cancers treatments: state of the art. Curr Opin Oncol 2021; 33:196–205.

52. Galluzzi F, Garavello W, Dalfino G, et al. Congenital bony nasal cavity stenosis: a review of current trends in diagnosis and treatment. Int J Pediatr Otorhinolaryngol 2021;144:110670.

53. Rout MR, Mohanty D, Vijaylaxmi Y, et al. Adenoid hypertrophy in adults: a case series. Indian J Otolaryngol Head Neck Surg 2013;65:269–74.

The Principles and Practice of Endonasal Rhinoplasty
Special Topics for Clinics in Plastic Surgery Journal

Ariel N. Rad, MD, PhD[a,b,*], Matthew A. Bridges, MD[c,d],
Mark B. Constantian, MD[e,f,g]

KEYWORDS

- Endonasal rhinoplasty • Closed rhinoplasty • Airway obstruction • Nasal tip graft • Spreader graft
- Dorsal hump reduction • Radix graft • Supratip deformity

KEY POINTS

- Endonasal rhinoplasty, or closed rhinoplasty, aims to minimize surgical dissection, structural disequilibrium, and scar burden, thus limiting unpredictable secondary deformity.
- Endonasal rhinoplasty, or closed rhinoplasty, aims to preserve intrinsic ligamentous support throughout the nasal skeleton, thus obviating the need for techniques that reconstruct them and make the nose unnaturally rigid.
- The entire surgical plan can be constructed preoperatively and all key intraoperative decisions can be made from the nasal surface with the skin sleeve intact.
- Four anatomic variants lead to all 3 patterns of secondary deformity: nasal disproportion or imbalance, supratip deformity, and airway compromise.
- Most primary nasal deformities can be corrected with only 4 techniques: radix/dorsal grafts, tip grafts, spreader grafts, and alar wall grafts.

INTRODUCTION
Equilibrium and Balance

Regardless of preference for open or closed technique, rhinoplasty surgeons endeavor to achieve ethnically appropriate nasal balance and proportions and an open airway. Toward these goals, the surgeon's analysis and planning should lead to predictable and reproducible results with minimal risk of secondary deformity and reoperation.

This mandates that the surgeon respect the dynamic equilibrium of forces within the nose and that s/he identifies and avoids pitfalls. Equilibrium is a crucial concept: preoperative nasal shape represents not a static structure but rather a dynamic sum of balanced, opposing forces within and between the nasal soft tissues and their underlying support. At the start of a rhinoplasty, the nose is equilibrated, that is, the sum of all forces equals

[a] Private Practice, Plastic Surgery (SHERBER+RAD), 1101 15th Street, Northwest, Suite #100, Washington, DC 20005-5002, USA; [b] Department of Plastic Surgery, The Johns Hopkins Hospital, Baltimore, MD, USA; [c] Private Practice, Facial Plastic Surgery (Commonwealth Facial Plastic Surgery), 1 Park West Circle, Suite #200, Midlothian, VA 23114, USA; [d] Department of Otolaryngology-Head & Neck Surgery, Virginia Commonwealth University School of Medicine; [e] Private Practice, Plastic Surgery, 19 Tyler Street, Suite #302, Nashua, NH 03060-2979, USA; [f] Department of Surgery, Division of Plastic and Reconstructive Surgery, University of Wisconsin School of Medicine and Public Health, Madison, WI, USA; [g] Department of Plastic Surgery, University of Virginia Medical School, Charlottesville, VA, USA
* Corresponding author. 1101 15th Street, Northwest, #100, Washington, DC 20005.
E-mail address: dr.rad@sherberandrad.com

Clin Plastic Surg 49 (2022) 33–47
https://doi.org/10.1016/j.cps.2021.07.004
0094-1298/22/© 2021 Elsevier Inc. All rights reserved.

zero. Surgical dissection and skeletal reduction disrupt this equilibrium which, like the ripple effect of a stone thrown into a pond, induces soft tissue and skeletal changes until the nose re-establishes a net zero balance of forces. Greater dissection, particularly with wide dissection and degloving, induces greater instability, like a large boulder thrown into a pond produces large "waves" which, in the nasal sense, disrupt equilibrium in a less controllable fashion with higher risk of secondary deformity. Soft tissue scar contracture adds further unpredictability overtime despite a good result early on. Therefore, the surgeon must control the postoperative equilibrium by limiting dissection (ie, scar), by permitting soft tissue contraction only where it is most predictable (eg, over the bony and cartilaginous dorsa) and by minimizing contraction where it is less predictable (eg, the lower nasal third). In doing so, the surgeon immediately gains greater control over the postoperative result and its long-term stability. In no other esthetic surgery than in rhinoplasty is the concept "less is more" more applicable.

Visibility

Much controversy in rhinoplasty theory is centered on visibility. Residents and novice surgeons resonate with the concept that one must "see," in the traditional sense of binocular vision, the skeletal structures on which s/he is operating. Open surgery is based on the premise that "if the nasal skeleton is right, then the nose will be right," which presumes that nasal skin is an inanimate tablecloth, devoid of intrinsic contractility, passively taking on the underlying skeletal contour. If the skin acted this way (which it does not), then one might expect the risk of deformity to be more or less equivalent regardless of open or closed technique. However, the incidence of secondary deformity requiring corrective surgery after open rhinoplasty is 3 to 5 times higher as compared with closed.[1] This disparity is explained by the fact that elasticity of the skin sleeve, in concert with soft tissue scar contractility, exerts tensioning forces on the nasal skeleton and accounts for up to 50% of the final result.[2] Eliminating this variable by open dissection significantly reduces a surgeon's ability to assess nasal shape intraoperatively often leading to deformities such as low dorsum, blunt/rounded and inadequately projected tip, elevated supratip, and retracted columella and/or alar rims, despite a seemingly good result "on table." While wide undermining of soft tissues in facelifting may be well tolerated because of the rigidity of the facial skeleton, the high rate of secondary revision after open rhinoplasty tells us that wide degloving is not tolerated in the nose because of its lack of rigidity. To counteract this, open techniques that make the lower nasal cartilages more rigid have been reported.[3] On balance, the susceptibility of the nose to disequilibrating forces and scar contracture mandates leaving the skin sleeve intact as much as possible. Furthermore, by doing so, the surgeon has "true visibility" of nasal shape, just as the patient will see it, in its most equilibrated state. Paradoxically, total degloving of the nasal skeleton reduces the surgeon's visibility of the true nasal contour despite "better" visibility of underlying structures. Limited endonasal exposure is both adequate and by design: the surgeon dissects structures only to the degree that is essential, and no more, to create the desired contours at the skin surface. As nasal contour is the product of both skeletal shape and its investing soft tissues, only with the skin sleeve intact over the nasal skeleton and the functional nasal layers undisrupted can the surgeon "read" its effects and adjust for them.

ANALYSIS
Rhinoplasty as a "Right Brain" Operation

Endonasal rhinoplasty is not the same as open rhinoplasty performed through a keyhole. The mindset is different and it is a "right-brain" endeavor, that is, one in which the surgeon must translate many complex esthetic concepts into a unified vision for the end result. How to arrive at the "right" unified vision is the exercise requiring diligent study and practice particularly in identifying preoperative deficiencies (such as low radix and inadequate tip projection), which is more difficult than identifying excesses (such as dorsal hump, wide nasal base, etc.). Right brain function can be cultivated by analytical exercises and by studying silhouettes of patient profiles (**Fig. 1**).[2] This allows us to see relative excesses and deficiencies more readily.

Ethnic Variation and Patient Preference

Rhinoplasty is a challenging operation not only due to the dynamic nature of surgical changes but also because esthetic ideals are highly personal and must be ethnically appropriate. Respecting patient preference and ethnic variations is crucial (**Fig. 3**), and to apply blindly a preconceived esthetic ideal to every nose would invariably lead to unhappy patients. Just as a rigid nose is unnatural, a rigid algorithm cannot be applied to such decision-making, as these decisions are highly variable and patient-dependent.

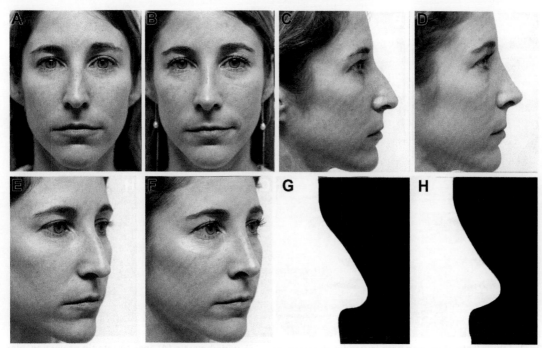

Fig. 1. Woman with low radix, dorsal hump (*C,E*), upper/middle vault asymmetry (*A*), and inadequate tip projection (*C*) treated with endonasal rhinoplasty with dorsal/radix grafts, spreader grafts, tip grafts. Note the correction of the dorsal aesthetic lines (*B,D*) and upward rotation of the tip with dorsal resection and tip grafting (*D,F*). Silhouette analysis of the lateral preoperative (*G*) and postoperative (*H*) views demonstrate the corrections. Intraoperative views are shown in **Fig. 2**. Postoperative images demonstrate 8-month results by author (ANR).

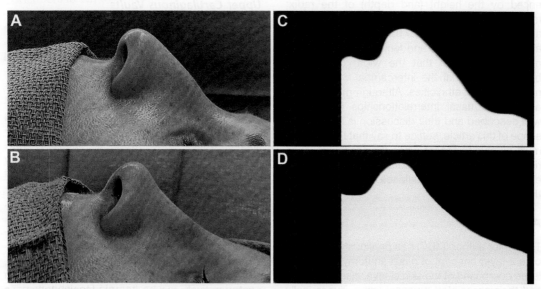

Fig. 2. "On-table" preoperative (*A*) and postoperative (*B*) nasal contours should be esthetically balanced, and contours and grafts should look and feel perfect. With the skin sleeve intact, esthetic assessment is more accurate than when a degloved skin envelope has been redraped over the nasal skeleton. Comparison of silhouettes (*C, D*) is instructive for training "right brain" analysis.[2] Eight-month postoperative views are shown in Fig. 2. Results by ANR.

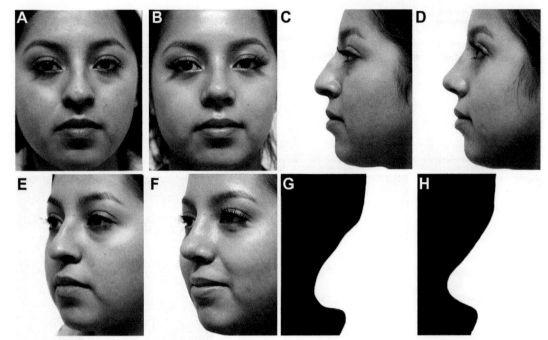

Fig. 3. Ethnic (Latina) woman with low radix, dorsal hump (*C,E*), wide/boxy tip (*A*), inadequate tip projection, alar cartilage malposition and alar rim retraction (*C,E*). Following endonasal rhinoplasty, dorsal reduction, dorsal/radix grafts, spreader grafts, and tip grafts (*B,D,F*). Nasofacial relationships are ethnically appropriate and proportionate. Silhouette analysis of the lateral preoperative (*E*) and postoperative (*F*) views demonstrate the corrections. Postoperative images demonstrate 9-month results by author (ANR).

Nasal Proportion

Nasal and nasofacial proportions entail optical illusions. For example, profile balance is highly influenced by the height (and depth) of the radix; middle vault width should balance with the upper and lower nasal thirds; alar base width should balance with other nasal and facial proportions. The neoclassical canon that the width of the alar base should equal the intercanthal width[4] does not apply to all ethnicities. Although many "ideal" angles and nasal interrelationships have been well described and their discussion is beyond the scope of this article, suffice to say that the surgeon must be able to assess when the nose "just looks right." It is the overall nasofacial proportion with ethnically appropriate balance for each patient that matters.

ANATOMY

The senior author (MBC) has previously published on a 2-layer concept of nasal anatomy. The outer layer, composed of the skin sleeve, alar cartilages, and their associated mucosal lining, dynamically slides over the inner layer composed of the bony and upper cartilaginous vaults, the nasal septum, and their associated linings. This critical anatomic relationship is disrupted as soon as the surgeon

degloves the alar cartilages through a transcolumellar incision.[2]

Upper Cartilaginous Vaults

The upper cartilaginous vault is composed of the upper lateral cartilages and their intimate apposition with the dorsal septal edge. The functional importance of this anatomic area is that it comprises the internal nasal valves whose patency depends on the height and width of the middle vault roof. Resection of the middle vault roof during hump reduction destabilizes the upper lateral cartilages whose outer walls tilt medially, thus creating a characteristic "inverted V" deformity and internal nasal valve obstruction. Middle vault collapse virtually always occurs when the cartilaginous roof has been resected more than 2 mm, whether or not osteotomy has been performed. Although obvious esthetic and functional deformity is more obvious with thin skin, a thick soft tissue envelope may mask the esthetic deformity, and a patient's complaint of breathing obstruction postoperatively maybe its only manifestation. To avoid middle vault collapse and internal valvular incompetence, the surgeon can stabilize the middle vault with spreader grafts and/or a dorsal graft, each providing the same degree of functional mean nasal airflow improvement as documented by a level II outcome study.[5]

Middle and Lower Cartilaginous Vaults

The upper lateral cartilages articulate with the cephalic margins of the lateral crura in the scroll region. This articulation is a "watershed" area between the internal and external nasal valves, and radical surgery in this area can have problematic esthetic and functional consequences. Radical alar cartilage resection can compromise middle vault support and may leave an external deformity typified by deepening and lengthening of the alar creases. External valvular competence can be compromised particularly in patients whose lateral crura are cephalically rotated[6] (see section 4.3). However, airway support provided by an intact cartilaginous roof is more critical to airway function than support provided by the lower lateral cartilages.

Tip and Supratip

Tip shape and projection are dictated by the middle and lateral crura. True tip projection has nothing to do with the distance from alar base to tip. Tip projection is defined relative to the septal angle and is deemed "adequate" when the tip lobule extends past the anterior septal angle.[6] Dr Jack Sheen realized that true tip projection comes from within the tip, that is, intrinsic, rather than from extrinsic forces.[7] While tip suturing techniques can work in certain circumstances such as with orthotopic lateral crura, in the presence of anatomic variants suturing can create peridomal concavity, alar rim retraction, distortion of the soft triangle, or displacement of the lateral crura into the airway causing airway obstruction. Furthermore, surgical degloving of the tip complex reduces its stability, thus forcing the surgeon to rely on more complex structural methods to reestablish equilibrium and projection. However, even with restabilization, long-term stability is unpredictable. Conversely, the power of endonasal tip grafting lies in its simplicity and in the preservation of structural dome support (by avoiding excessive dissection) on which the grafts are placed. Equilibrium is minimally disturbed, thus stability is maximally preserved.

Septum and Turbinates

The septum should be assessed for deviation, buckling, fracture, and calcification due to prior trauma. Turbinates, if obstructing, may need out fracturing or conservative reduction.

FOUR ANATOMIC VARIANTS

Minimizing invasiveness is the sine qua non of the endonasal approach. In a retrospective analysis of 50 consecutive primary and 150 secondary rhinoplasty patients, 4 anatomic characteristics, specifically (1) low radix, (2) narrow middle vault, (3) alar cartilage malposition, and (4) inadequate tip projection, were identified by the senior author (MBC) as the most important anatomic findings for which surgical correction is crucial.[6] At least one of these 4 anatomic traits was present in each of the 150 secondary patients in one series, and 78% of the secondary patients and 58% of the primary patients had 3 or all 4 traits.[5] The most common grouping in both primary and secondary patients is the triad of low radix, narrow middle vault, and inadequate tip projection (40% and 28%, respectively).

Low Radix/Low Dorsum

First described by Sheen,[7] the diagnosis of a low radix is made when the visual "starting point of the profile," that is, the inflection point at which the contour changes from concave to convex, is caudal to the level of the upper lash margin with the patient's eyes in primary gaze (note that this applies to most Caucasians, but radix height needs to be balanced against nasal base size; for example, it would be lower in many Asians.) A low radix was present in 32% of primary patients and 93% of secondary patients in one series[5] and it creates an imbalance in nasal proportions where the upper nose appears too small for its nasal base. A low radix can create the appearance of a pseudohump (**Fig. 4**). If solely the dorsum is lowered, the nasal base appears disproportionately too large. In this scenario, the surgeon has 2 treatment options: either tip reduction or dorsal/radix augmentation to balance the nasal base. Tip reduction would yield suboptimal results because the skin sleeve has limited contractility. Dorsal/radix augmentation is more predictable and therefore preferable. Elevating a low radix requires less aggressive dorsal reduction which favors stability of the middle vault, tip equilibrium of internal stresses, and optimal nasal balance (**Fig. 5**). Conversely, failure to recognize the low radix or low dorsum invariably leads to deformities from imbalance, disproportion, and disequilibrium.

Narrow Middle Vault

If the middle vault width is 75% or less than that of the upper or lower nasal thirds, then a narrow middle vault is diagnosed.[5] Originally described by

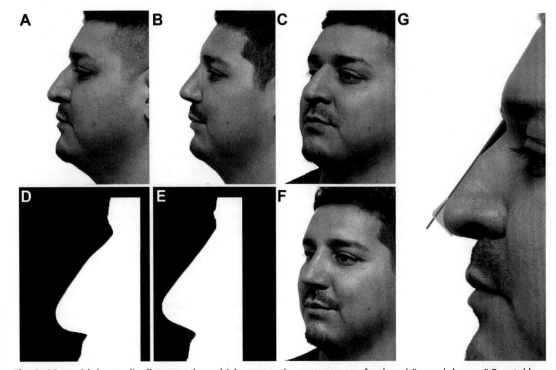

Fig. 4. Man with low radix disproportion which creates the appearance of a dorsal "pseudohump." Frontal bossing and a deep nasofrontal angle exacerbate the depth of the radix. Preoperatively (*A, C*), the patient also has inadequate tip projection and alar retraction. Following endonasal rhinoplasty, septoplasty, with layered septal cartilage grafts placed in the radix, conservative rasping of pseudohump (without significant reduction), dorsal and spreader grafts, tip grafts, nasal bone osteotomy and infracture (*B, F*). In (*G*), extension of a straight line (*red*) from supra tip to the radix demarcates the region of the radix to be grafted (*blue* filled area), and tip projection that is required (*green* filled area). Note that downward gaze lowers the lash line, which may confuse the diagnosis of low radix. Silhouette analysis of the lateral preoperative (*D*) and postoperative (*E*) lateral views demonstrates the corrections. Postoperative images demonstrate 12-month results by author (ANR).

Sheen in conjunction with short nasal bones,[6] a narrow middle vault places the patient at increased risk for internal valvular obstruction, which can exist preoperatively or may be produced by dorsal resection in the absence of spreader grafts. Surgical resection of the bilateral roofs of the upper lateral cartilages and their articulation with the anterior septal edge (as in dorsal hump reduction) leads to instability of the lateral cut edges of the upper laterals which then tilt inward, pinching the internal nasal valves, and producing a characteristic inverted "V deformity." Airflow obstruction is severe: rhinomanometric studies indicate that valvular obstruction is 4 times more common than pure septal obstruction in primary rhinoplasty patients and 12 times more common in secondary patients; reconstruction of incompetent, internal valves by dorsal or spreader graft doubles nasal airflow.[8] While "spreader flaps" have been described, that is, redundant upper lateral cartilage edges downturned into the internal valve interval and suture fixated to the septal edge, no airway measurements have yet been performed that demonstrate their functional efficacy or superiority to spreader grafts.[9]

Alar Cartilage Malposition

Alar cartilage (or lateral crural) malposition refers to cephalically rotated lateral crura whose long axes run toward the medial canthi instead of toward the lateral canthi[6] (the orthotopic configuration) (**Fig. 6**). The esthetic appearance of a tip lobule with this anatomy is a round or boxy shape and characteristic "parentheses" deformity on frontal view. Functionally, malpositioned lateral crura provide suboptimal alar support and so is a leading cause of external valvular incompetence.[5,6] First recognized by Sheen,[7] alar cartilage malposition is common and present in up to 50% of primary patients and 80% of secondary patients and has important esthetic and functional consequences if not identified and surgically corrected. Worsening of the deformity follows a predictable "ripple effect" especially when an intracartilaginous incision is made at its

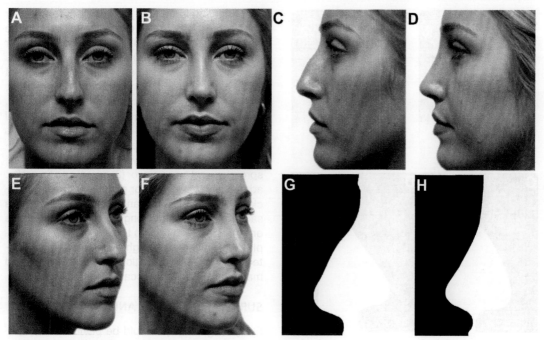

Fig. 5. Woman with subtle low radix disproportion, moderate dorsal hump, mild alar cartilage malposition, and inadequate tip projection (*A, C, E*) treated with endonasal hump reduction, radix/dorsal grafts, spreader grafts, alar wall grafts, and tip grafts, nasal bone osteotomy and infracture (*B, D, F*). Silhouette analysis of the lateral preoperative (*G*) and postoperative (*H*) views demonstrates the corrections. Postoperative images demonstrate 12-month results by author (ANR).

usual location but ends up transecting the lateral crura along its short axis, rather than reducing its cephalic margin along its long axis, possibly unbeknownst to the surgeon if s/he has not

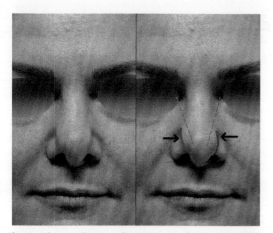

Fig. 6. Alar cartilage malposition results in "parentheses" deformity (*red lines*) and external nasal valve insufficiency/collapse (*black arrows*) due to cephalically rotated lateral crura along an axis from tip to medial canthi (*blue dotted lines*). The traditional intercartilaginous incision can result in inadvertent transection of lateral crura. External nasal valves require reinforcement with alar wall grafts.

identified this deformity preoperatively. Treatment of lateral crura malposition requires either (1) resection and relocation, or (2) autogenous cartilage grafting to support the external valves.

Inadequate Tip Projection

Inadequate tip projection is present in 31% of the primary patients and 80% of the secondary patients[5] and is crucial to achieve a straight profile line. An inadequately projecting tip may exist equally with a low dorsum (**Fig. 7**) or high dorsum (**Fig. 8**), and regardless of dorsal height, a straight profile line is not possible without adequate tip projection.

Tips with inadequate "intrinsic" cartilage strength cannot project beyond the septal angle and will appear to "fall off" of the angle with a rounded or deformed supratip. And, when investing soft tissues are stripped from the middle crura, intrinsic support decreases further. Open dissection strips the middle crura of intrinsic ligamentous and cartilaginous support structures, and thus destabilizes the tip. The surgeon must therefore rely on extrinsic methods to reconstruct these structures.[3,10,11] However, these have not been shown to produce a long-term stable outcome. Alar cartilages, and their investing soft tissues, carry a

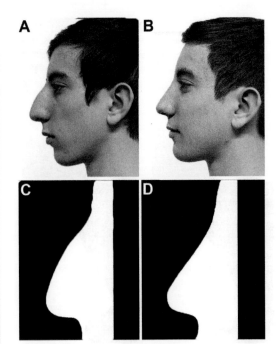

Fig. 7. Man with high dorsum, poor tip projection, and nasofacial disproportion (*A*) treated with endonasal approach, dorsal reduction, dorsal, radix and tip grafts, and chin augmentation with silicone implant (*B*). Note that dorsal reduction without tip grafting would have resulted in supratip deformity and suboptimal nasal disproportion. Silhouette analysis of the lateral preoperative (*C*) and postoperative (*D*) views demonstrates the corrections. Postoperative images demonstrate 12-month results by author (ANR).

larger responsibility for caudal nasal support than may be obvious. This becomes evident with futile attempts to reduce the dorsum/septal angle to compensate for inadequate tip projection and, predictably, the tip lobule falls with it, potentially worsening the deformity unless the middle crura are lengthened and their ligamentous attachments to themselves and to surrounding structures are preserved.

Summary

Tissue excesses are much more readily noticed than tissue deficiencies and so identification of these anatomic variants preoperatively can be difficult unless one's attention is directed specifically to look for them. These 4 anatomic deficits do not always require treatment. For example, the low radix must always be assessed relative to nasal base size: if the base is small, dorsal resection may improve optimal balance. However, the deficits do provide cautionary signs and failure to recognize them can lead to 3 patterns of

secondary deformity: (1) nasal disproportion or imbalance, (2) supratip deformity (or soft tissue collapse pattern), and (3) airway compromise (or skeletal collapse pattern). Radix and dorsal grafts correct the imbalance pattern. Tip grafts correct inadequate projection and supratip deformity, which comprise the soft tissue collapse pattern. Spreader and alar wall grafts support the internal and external valves, respectively, the components of the skeletal collapse pattern. Nearly every rhinoplasty follows 1 of only 2 strategies: (1) radix, spreader, and tip grafts, or (2) dorsal and tip grafts, adding alar wall grafts for external valvular insufficiency. Because radix and dorsal grafts are the same graft in different lengths, the surgeon needs only master 4 graft types to solve almost all rhinoplasty problems. Although not easy, these 2 strategies make the operation comprehensible and manageable even for occasional nasal surgeons.

SURGICAL PLANNING AND EXECUTION

Every surgical step should be planned for a specific reason. Incisions and dissection strategies should follow from each step and the rationale for its use is irrefutable. Recognizing the 4 anatomic variants, all visible on the surface, allows the surgeon to make a diagnosis and set a surgical plan. Therefore, the entire surgical strategy can be set preoperatively and the need for dorsal, radix, alar wall, or tip grafts should be planned. The only decisions made intraoperatively are not qualitative but only quantitative, depending on graft availability and quality.

Sequence of Steps

Analysis

- Identify the 4 critical anatomic variants/traps (low radix/low dorsum, inadequate tip projection, narrow middle vault, and alar cartilage malposition)
- Evaluate not only the septum and turbinates but also the preoperative competence of the internal and external nasal valves, as well as the potential intraoperative valvular incompetence created by dorsal or alar cartilage reduction

Surgery

- Step 1: Resect deformities; create spreader graft tunnels
- Step 2: Septoplasty; turbinate modification as indicated
- Step 3: Grafts as indicated: dorsum, radix, spreader, tip, alar walls as indicated
- Step 4: Osteotomy and infracture as indicated

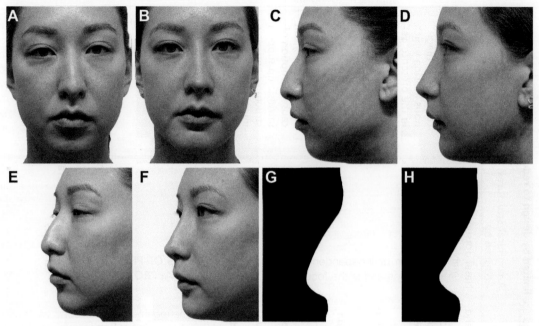

Fig. 8. Woman with low radix, dorsal pseudohump, poor tip projection, and disproportion of nose and mentum (*A*, *C*, *E*). Following endonasal approach with layered radix and tip grafts, conservative dorsal rasping, cephalic trim of alar cartilages, as well as sliding genioplasty (*B*, *D*, *F*). Note that dorsal reduction without tip grafting would have resulted in worsened nasal and nasofacial disproportion and supratip deformity. Silhouette analysis of the lateral preoperative (*G*) and postoperative (*H*) views demonstrate the corrections. Postoperative images demonstrate 10-month results by author (ANR).

Incisions

An exhaustive description of incisions is beyond the scope of this article; a summary is provided in **Table 1**.

Step 1: Resect Deformities and Create Spreader Graft Tunnels

The workhorse incision is intercartilaginous through which blunt scissor dissection gives the surgeon access to the dorsum, radix, septal angle, upper lateral cartilages, and cephalic margin of the lower lateral cartilages (**Fig. 9**). Care should be taken not to skeletonize widely the bony dorsum as this can predispose to lateral displacement of a planned dorsal graft. A Foman rasp is used to roughen the surface of the radix for better graft adherence or to deepen a high radix. Dorsal reduction is performed with rasping of the bony vault. To deepen a high radix, 4 to 6 mm straight osteotomes may be used and then rasping to smooth cut edges. Sharp resection of the cartilaginous dorsum is done with a #11 blade (the tip broken off to prevent skin injury). Once the dorsal line is set, bilateral spreader graft tunnels are created in the submucoperichondrial plane along the cut anterior septal edge using a Cottle elevator. Cephalic margins of the lateral crura are trimmed retrograde (as needed). If alar cartilage malposition was diagnosed preoperatively, the cephalically malpositioned portions of the lateral crura are resected and replaced within the alar walls at the external nasal valves. Nasal shortening via membranous and/or caudal septal resection, as well as medial footplate modification, can be made through a transfixion incision.

Step 2: Septoplasty

The Killian incision gives access for septoplasty and should be done only after dorsal and/or caudal septal resection is satisfactory. Septoplasty should be planned with a minimum 12- to 15-mm-wide contiguous L-strut with undissected mucoperichondrium attached. Bilateral mucoperichondrial flaps are elevated over the resection specimen taking particular care not to dissect lining and potentially enter the spreader graft tunnels. Accidental stripping of soft tissue between tunnels and septal flaps can cause spreader graft displacement making suture fixation necessary (and difficult). Septal cartilage is harvested in 2 strips with angled Knight septal scissors, taken across the articulation with the perpendicular plate of the ethmoid to provide the longest possible graft. Ideally, the septal fragment is harvested

Table 1
Intranasal incisions used in endonasal rhinoplasty provide direct access to target structures and are limited by design to reduce dissection and morbidity

Incision	Relative Importance/ Usefulness	Anatomical Guides	Purpose	Anatomical Structures Accessed by	Cautions
Intercartilaginous incision	****	1. Starts at the lateral aspect of the caudal ULC 2. Extends within the interval between the caudal ULC and the cephalic margin of the ULC 3. Ends at the septal angle	1. Dorsal reduction and augmentation 2. Reduction of the cephalic margin of the lateral crura of lower lateral cartilages 3. Reduction of the caudal margin of the upper lateral cartilage 4. Radix augmentation 5. Spreader graft placement	Nasal dorsum cephalic margin of the lateral crura of the LLC caudal edges of the ULC septal angle	1. Excessively cephalic incision placement can result in inadvertent intracartilaginous incision which, in the presence of alar cartilage malposition can transect the lateral crura thus worsening external valvular support (see "Four Anatomic Variants, Section 4.3")
Infracartilaginous incision	***	1. Starts approximately 2 mm cephalad from the alar margin and at the soft triangle inflection 2. Extends parallel to the alar margin 3. Ends 4–20 mm lateral (length depending on whether only tip grafting is needed or dome delivery/ECR technique is done, respectively)	1. Tip augmentation and/or modification 2. Alar rim grafts 3. External nasal valve grafts 4. Dome delivery and/or ECR technique[15],*	1. Nasal domes 2. Alar rim 3. External nasal valve	1. *Dome delivery can cause disruption of intrinsic tip support structures and may impair efforts to augment the tip
Transfixion incision	**	1. Starts at septal angle 2. Extends parallel to the caudal septal margin 3. Ends at level of posterior septal angle	1. Reduction of membranous or caudal septum 2. ECR technique[15],* 3. Tongue-in-groove medial crural advancement technique**	1. Membranous and cartilaginous septum 2. Septal angle 3. Columella/Medial crura of lower lateral cartilages	

Killian incision	***	1. Starts approximately 12–15 mm cephalad from, and posterior to, the caudal septal margin 2. Extends parallel to the caudal septal margin, through unilateral mucoperichondrium and septal cartilage 3. Ends at maxilla	1. Septoplasty 2. Harvest of perpendicular plate of the ethmoid	1. Access to mid-portion of cartilaginous septum, Ethmoid bone, Vomer	1. A septal cartilaginous "L-strut" must be contiguously intact and be at least 12 mm wide. 2. The mucoperichondrium overlying the L-strut must be preserved, both for stability and spreader graft tunnels
Nasal floor incision	**	1. 5 mm stab incision over pyriform aperture	1. Lateral "low to high" nasal bone osteotomy 2. Maxillary augmentation	1. Pyriform aperture/nasal bone 2. Anterior maxilla	1. In nasal bone osteotomy, use curved guarded osteotomes 2. In maxillary augmentation, take care not to over dissect the pocket for maxillary graft

Abbreviations: ECR, endonasal complete release[15]; LLC, lower lateral cartilages; ULC, upper lateral cartilages.

* = rarely useful
** = sometimes useful
*** = very useful
**** = essential

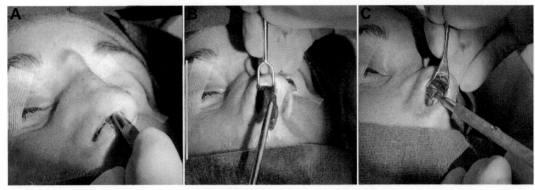

Fig. 9. Limited skeletonization of the dorsum and radix through unilateral endonasal intercartilaginous incision (*A*, tip of Freer elevator at radix), cartilaginous dorsal hump resection specimen (*B*), and bilateral spreader graft tunnels (*C*, Freer elevator inserted at septal angle and extends to mid-vault). Images by author (ANR).

with the ethmoid bone attached. Grasping the specimen at the ethmoid/cartilage articulation with a Killian septal forceps allows harvest in one long piece yielding approximately 25 to 30 mm. The posterior septal cartilage strip is done by gentle separation from the Vomerine groove using a narrow straight osteotome or periosteal elevator. Mucoperichondrial flaps are closed with mattress 4-0 Chromic. However, before complete closure, the surgeon should take inventory of the quality and quantity of graft material and determine the amount that is needed for grafting; possible excess cartilage may be banked within the septal flaps as a "back up" in case secondary rhinoplasty becomes necessary. Communicating, bilateral mucosal tears can lead to septal perforations postoperatively. However, initial practice on "straight forward" primary septorhinoplasty facilitates dexterity. Indeed, learning and becoming facile with the finesse of endonasal septoplasty reaps tremendous rewards in avoiding the vagaries of open septoplasty: disruption of critical intrinsic support structures in the middle vault and its articulations with the alar cartilages increases the chance of secondary deformity. In contrast, approaching the septum via a separate incision endonasally preserves intrinsic stability thus reducing risk.

Partial inferior turbinectomy, defined as a trim of the anterior edge sufficient to obtain 3 mm clearance to the septum or nasal floor, is valuable adjunctive airway treatment if indicated. Rhinomanometric data by the senior author (MBC) suggest that aggressive turbinate treatment is unnecessary in most patients if septal and valvular causes have been adequately relieved.[8] Turbinate outfracture may suffice in patients whose voluminous turbinates contain significant cystic bone and in whom adequate airway size can be achieved by crushing with the septal forceps and without

resection. When resection is necessary, biopsy forceps allow smaller, more incremental changes than angled scissors. The raw surfaces left will contract and epithelize, further reducing the size of the remaining turbinate. Conservatism is best as over-resection is not correctible.

Step 3: Grafts

Graft material yielded from septoplasty should be inventoried, assessed for quality, and then prioritized according to need: the best pieces are reserved for radix or dorsal grafts; other grafts can be fashioned from the remaining pieces. The surgeon should endeavor for "hand in glove" fit of all grafts to avoid the need for suture fixation. Following graft placement, contours should look and feel perfect.

Spreader grafts
With dorsal reduction or preoperatively diagnosed narrow middle vault, spreader grafts are essential. Acting as spacers, spreader grafts prevent the collapse of the upper lateral cartilages onto the septum and consequent internal valve obstruction. Spreader grafts may be symmetric, whereas with septal deviation or middle vault asymmetry, one graft may need greater width and/or curvature to counterbalance the anatomic deviation. Spreader grafts are inserted into tight tunnels along the undissected dorsal septal strut. When properly performed, grafts are secured in the pockets usually with a single transfixing suture at the caudal end adjacent to the septal angle to close the tunnels.

Radix/dorsal grafts
Soft tissue swelling noted intraoperatively can mask a low radix identified preoperatively. Therefore, the surgeon is generally well served to stay with his/her preoperative plan for dorsal and radix

augmentation. A dorsal graft, with adequate length, edges beveled and its substance lightly crushed, as with a Sheen-Constantian morselizer (Marina Medical), should be fashioned to extend from radix to, and past, the bony-cartilaginous junction of the middle vault. The graft should not be palpable after placement and should taper seamlessly to the distal dorsum. Edges that are too thick can create supratip deformity. For greater proximal dorsal elevation, grafts may be layered and fixated to one another with an absorbable suture.

Tip grafts

Customarily the final grafts to be placed, tip grafts increase tip lobule projection, effectively increasing middle crural length. Careful scissor dissection through a single infracartilaginous incision directly over the domes gives access and must be done conservatively as over dissection can cause grafts to shift. The pliability (ie, solid, bruised, or crushed) and number of grafts selected are dictated by how much projection is needed, and by the thickness of the skin. Thicker skin requires more solid grafts to apply greater tension; a "buttress" graft, composed of solid cartilage or ethmoid can be placed to support overlying bruised or crushed cartilage grafts. Conversely, thin skin requires soft grafts. Multiple grafts placed sequentially through a very short, unilateral infracartilaginous incision evenly distribute tension under the skin and avoid issues with irregularities.

There are multiple advantages to using tip grafts via an endonasal approach placed into a precise pocket over the domes. As they do not require exposure of the tip via delivery techniques, the patient's intrinsic tip support remains undisturbed. The effect is seen immediately on the table and is persistent postoperatively if the tip skin is adequately supported against postoperative change (**Fig. 10**). Also, in addition to providing instant intrinsic tip projection to achieve a straight dorsum, they improve definition by tensioning the skin. Even in cases where the tip is relatively broad and/or bifid, tip grafts are frequently sufficient to create a tip that looks narrower. Finally, if problems arise after healing, revision becomes a much simpler endeavor than if the lower lateral cartilages had been extensively modified primarily.

Alar wall grafts

Alar grafts are crucial to address alar cartilage malposition (variant or risk factor #3) for which lateral alar concavity and external valve incompetence are esthetically and functionally common preoperative findings. Alar grafts can easily be placed through a small incision made perpendicular to the rim. The lining is dissected to create a pocket that spans the area of collapse. With respect to graft material, septal cartilage or remnant lateral crural cartilage resected from its cephalic malposition is most often used. In the absence of these sources, conchal bowl ear cartilage is ideal due to the convex contour which nicely conforms to this area, and lightly bruised rib cartilage works very well.

Osteotomy and Infracture

Osteotomy achieves 2 goals: reducing bony vault width (**Fig. 11**) and closing the open nasal roof. Because the bony vault may remain unopened after conservative dorsal resections, it is the former of these 2 objectives that is probably more important. Nasal bone osteotomy destabilizes the nasal framework, causing nasal lengthening. Therefore, before performing any osteotomy, the surgeon should be sure that one is necessary. If the lower nasal third is already appropriately wider than the bony vault, narrowing the upper nose further may be counterproductive by making the nasal base appear larger. If there is a high septal deviation, bilateral osteotomies may create a newly asymmetric nose because one nasal bone will move medially farther than the other. In the elderly patient (in whom comminution of the nasal bones may occur), the patient who wears heavy eyeglasses, or the patient with nasal bones extending less than one-third the distance to the septal angle (in whom middle vault width depends partially on bony vault width), the surgeon may wish to omit osteotomy.

DISCUSSION

The grand aim of all science is to cover the greatest possible number of empirical facts by logical deductions from the smallest possible number of hypotheses or axioms.
—Albert Einstein, quoted in Nash 1963, p. 173

The beauty of endonasal surgery is its simplicity. Resident and novice surgeons are often overwhelmed by the many varied open techniques required for mastery. Taking a "beginners mind," one must ask why such a difference in simplicity versus complexity? The answer is rooted in the disequilibrium concept: open and closed proponents share the common view that a surgically-induced scar burden and its associated contracture have deleterious effects on nasal stability. Although the former counteracts this by adding structural rigidity and stiffness to

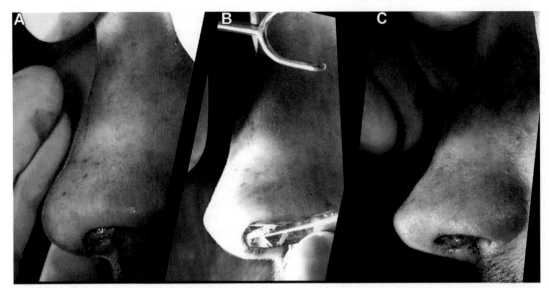

Fig. 10. With the skin sleeve undissected, the surgeon is able to accurately assess tip shape before tip grafting (*A*). Limited dissection with a sharp iris scissor over nasal domes through a unilateral infracartilaginous incision mimics the desired tip shape (*B*). The final contour after endonasal placement of cartilage grafts should show excellent tip projection which predictably will remain because intrinsic tip support has been preserved (*C*). Images by author (ANR).

the nose,[12] it is at the expense of unnatural stiffness, prolonged tip edema, bulk, greater need for grafting material, greater complexity of techniques in the form of columellar struts, septal extension grafts, lateral crural strut grafts,[3,10–12] a higher risk of secondary deformity, and a visible scar. The proliferation in the peer-reviewed literature of open structural rhinoplasty techniques speaks to the vagaries and complexity of open rhinoplasty. Thus begging the question: alternatively, and more simply, is it better to reduce surgical dissection thus reducing scar burden and the risk of associated deformities? Furthermore, applying Occam's razor as a guide (ie, the principle that, of 2 explanations that account for all the facts, the simpler one is more likely to be correct),

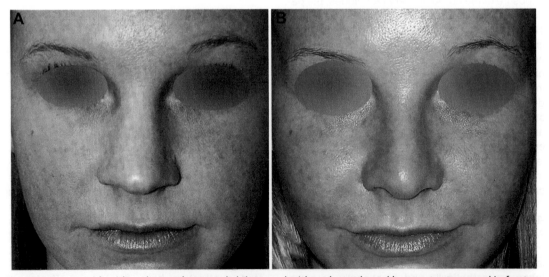

Fig. 11. Woman with widened upper bony vault (*A*) treated with endonasal nasal bone osteotomy and in fracture (and buccal fat pad resection) (*B*). Note, supratip has also been modified with cephalic trim, and the alar base modified with rim excisions. Postoperative image demonstrates 24-month postoperative results by author (ANR).

this leads us to the latter conclusion, that reducing scar burden, the sine qua non of the endonasal approach, is best. Therefore, it is the view of the authors that endonasal rhinoplasty achieves the ideal trifecta of simplicity, minimal scar burden, and "true" visibility.

Learning rhinoplasty can be a confusing endeavor for the novice rhinoplasty surgeon.[13] However, Sheen's principles of "observation, realization, and change,"[14] which allow us to question what we do, why we do it, and how we can improve our understanding and therefore our techniques, cannot be overemphasized.

CLINICS CARE POINTS

- Limiting surgical dissection only to that which is absolutely necessary, rather than complete degloving of the nasal skeleton, is essential to limit the risk of secondary deformity.

- Leaving the skin sleeve intact over the nasal skeleton allows the surgeon to recognize and react to surface skin-level changes; conversely, stripping the skin sleeve from the skeleton removes this important feedback.

- Endonasal rhinoplasty simplifies an otherwise complex operation as only 4 techniques are needed to address most primary rhinoplasties: radix grafts, dorsal grafts, spreader grafts, and tip grafts (alar wall grafts are occasionally needed).

- Reconstruction of both internal and external valvular incompetence triples or quadruples airflow in most patients without concomitant septoplasty or turbinectomy.

- The entire surgical plan can be constructed preoperatively and all key planning and intraoperative decisions can be made from the nasal surface.

DISCLOSURE

Dr M.B. Constantian receives royalties from Taylor and Francis and from Thieme for his textbooks, and from Marina Medical Company for designing surgical instruments. He also receives royalties from Quality Medical Publishing for his instructional surgical videos. All amounts are nominal.

REFERENCES

1. Constantian MB. Differing characteristics in 100 consecutive secondary rhinoplasty patients following closed versus open surgical approaches. Plast Reconstr Surg 2002;109:2097.
2. Constantian MB. Rhinoplasty: craft and magic. St. Louis: Quality Medical; 2009. p. 9.
3. Toriumi DM, Asher SA. Lateral crural repositioning for treatment of cephalic malposition. Facial Plast Surg Clin N Am 2015;23(1):55–71.
4. Bashour M. History and current concepts in the analysis of facial attractiveness. Plast Reconstr Surg 2006;118:741.
5. Constantian MB. Functional effects of alar cartilage malposition. Ann Plast Surg 1993;30:487.
6. Constantian MB. Four common anatomic variants that predispose to unfavorable rhinoplasty results: a study based on 150 consecutive secondary rhinoplasties. Plast Reconstr Surg 2000;105:316.
7. Sheen JH, Sheen AP. Aesthetic rhinoplasty. 2nd edition. St. Louis: Mosby; 1987. p. 988–1011.
8. Constantian MB, Clardy RB. The relative importance of septal and nasal valvular surgery in correcting airway obstruction in primary and secondary rhinoplasty. Plast Reconst Surg 1996;98:38.
9. Saedi B, Amaly A, Gharavis V, et al. Spreader flaps do not change early functional outcomes in reduction rhinoplasty: a randomized control trial. Am J Rhinol Allergy 2014;28:70–4.
10. Rohrich RJ, Durand PD, Dayan E. Changing role of septal extension versus columellar grafts in modern rhinoplasty. Plast Reconstr Surg 2020;145(5):927e–31e.
11. Gunter JP, Friedman RP. Lateral crural strut graft: technique and clinical applications in rhinoplasty. Plast Reconstr Surg 1997;99(4):943–52.
12. Byrd HS, Andochick S, Copit S, et al. Septal extension grafts: a method of controlling tip projection shape. Plast Reconstr Surg 1997;100:999–1010.
13. Constantian MB, Martin JP. Why can't more good surgeons Learn rhinoplasty? Aesthet Surg J 2015;35(4):486.
14. Constantian MB. Personal interview of Dr. Jack Sheen.
15. Gassner HG, Mueller-Vogt U, Strutz J, et al. Nasal tip recontouring in primary rhinoplasty: the endonasal complete release approach. JAMA Facial Plastic Surgery 2013;15(1):11–6.

The External Rhinoplasty Approach

Ali Totonchi, MD[a,b,*], Bahman Guyuron, MD[c,d]

KEYWORDS

• Primary rhinoplasty • Open approach • External rhinoplasty

KEY POINTS

• A thorough patient analysis and examination is the cornerstone of a successful rhinoplasty.
• Dynamics of rhinoplasty: understanding the primary and secondary effects of each surgical maneuver will help to achieve a more consistent outcome.
• Open approach will give the surgeon good understanding of the deformity and, therefore, facilitates the reconstruction.

BACKGROUND

The nose is a complex three-dimensional structure with critical structural and functional roles; its relationship to surrounding structures is, in part, responsible for a harmonious, pleasing visage as a whole. There are many variables and dimensions that can be adjusted to alter the esthetic appearance, structural components, and functional role of the nose and many tools and maneuvers available to the rhinoplasty surgeon to adjust these numerous variables. Although every rhinoplasty operation should be individualized, a systematic order and algorithm may be helpful in operative planning as well as establishing a logical progression of steps and maintaining stability. While each adjustment may have a primary anticipated effect, it will invariably have a secondary impact.

Patient Assessment

The process of rhinoplasty begins with patient evaluation. Arguably, the foundation of a successful rhinoplasty is established at the initial patient visit including a thorough, accurate evaluation of the nose; its relation to the rest of the patient's face; identification of appropriate and realistic goals given the patient's anatomy; clear

communication; and mutual understanding and agreement of surgical goals between the patient and the surgeon. A vital part of any successful rhinoplasty is the detection of the functional abnormalities. This begins with keen observation of mouth breathing which often is unbeknown to the patients and ends with circumspect examination of the internal and external nasal valves, septal deviation, and enlargement of the turbinates. Meticulous preoperative photo-documentation is crucial, and life-size-based planning or computer-generated images of potential postoperative goals may be helpful in facilitating patient-surgeon discussion and establishing matching and achievable operative goals.

History

Important components of a complete history include medical, surgical, family, and social history as well as thorough review of all prescription and nonprescription medications. Of particular interest is whether there has been any previous nasal trauma or surgery. A history of diabetes, connective tissue disease, anticoagulation, or a bleeding or clotting disorder should be noted. Smoking significantly impedes healing and can lead to scarring, skin necrosis, and a poor outcome. A

[a] Case Western Reserve University, MetroHealth Hospital, 2500 Metrohealth Drive, Cleveland, OH 44109, USA; [b] Craniofacial Deformity Clinic; [c] Zeeba Clinic, 29017 Cedar Rd, Lyndhurst, Ohio, 44124, USA; [d] Case Western Reserve University, Cleveland, OH, USA
* Corresponding author. Case Western Reserve University, MetroHealth Hospital, 2500 Metrohealth Drive, Cleveland, OH 44109, USA.
E-mail address: TOTONCHIMD@GMAIL.COM

Clin Plastic Surg 49 (2022) 49–59
https://doi.org/10.1016/j.cps.2021.07.010
0094-1298/22/© 2021 Elsevier Inc. All rights reserved.

psychiatric history may help the surgeon understand a patient's motivation for cosmetic surgery. If a patient's motives are self-driven rather than driven by pressure from peers or a significant other, the patient is more likely to be satisfied with the ultimate surgical outcome. In addition to motivation, it is important to elicit a clear picture of the patient's desires and expectations from rhinoplasty. This should be considered in the surgeon's nasal analysis and proposal of surgical goals and limitations with thorough counseling and establishment of reasonable goals. History of sinus infections, sinus headaches, or migraine headaches should be documented in depth.

PHYSICAL EXAMINATION

Physical examination should include a thorough facial analysis characterizing the nasal structures themselves and their relationship to the face as a whole. A careful intranasal examination should also be performed, including inspection of the septum, turbinates, nasal valves, and an assessment of nasal breathing. Finger palpation is an essential component of the examination.

Only in idealized drawings is the face completely symmetric, and strict symmetry of the nose and the face should not be anticipated. The nose should occupy the middle third of the face horizontally and the middle fifth of the face vertically. The nose itself may be divided into thirds vertically. Generally, the upper third comprises the nasal bones, the middle third comprises the upper lateral cartilages, and the lower third comprises the tip and the lower lateral cartilages. Deviations from the ideal figure should be accurately localized, and surgical correction of these variations should address the appropriate structures.

An important feature is the smooth, unbroken, and symmetric brow-tip esthetic line, which is described as a "gentle sweeping line from the medial brow to the lateral nasal wall to the tip defining point;" the ideal shape of this esthetic line in a female nose is that of an hourglass, narrowing in the middle and flaring at the top and bottom.[1]

Numerous proportions and relationships have been described to characterize the ideal nose. In the frontal view, the ideal nasal length is two-third that of the midface, measured from the glabella to the alar base, and equal to the vertical length of the chin, measured from the stomion to the menton.[2] The width of the alar base should approximate the intercanthal distance and may be up to, but not more than, 2 mm wider,[1] so long is the intercanthal distance is normal. The radix should be at the level of the supratarsal crease.

In the lateral view, the nasofrontal angle should be approximately 115° to 130°,[3] and the radix should be 4- to 6-mm deep. In females, the dorsum should extend as a straight line until reaching the supratip break, which esthetically separates the dorsum from the tip unit. Ideally, the nasolabial angle should be 93° to 98° for men and 95° to 100° for women, although this angle varies somewhat based on the height of the patient. In general, shorter individuals may have a more obtuse angle while taller individuals may have a more acute angle. In the lateral view, the alar base should be 2 mm above the line between the lower and middle third of the nose.[3] The lateral tip projection can be measured from the alar-cheek junction to the tip defining point.[2]

The alar-columellar relationship should be carefully evaluated from the lateral view. When viewed from this aspect, the upper border of the nostril is formed by the alar rim, and the lower border is formed by the columellar rim. Gunter described a method of analyzing this relationship. A line is drawn which approximates the long axis of the nostril: the ala should be 1 - 2 mm above this line, and the columella 1 to 2 mm below this line. If the columellar rim is less than 1 to 2 mm from this line, the columella is considered to be retracted; conversely, if the distance is greater than 1 to 2 mm, the columella is considered to be "hanging." If the ala is less than 1 to 2 mm from this axis, it is considered to be a hanging ala; if it is greater than 1 - 2 mm from this axis, it is considered a retracted ala.[4,5]

The alar-columellar relationship and alar rim deformities should also include analysis from the alar base view. The ideal base view is an equilateral triangle with each ala forming the sides of the triangle and the alar base width forming the remaining side. A concave ala is present when the lateral border of the ala is medial to the line of the equilateral triangle, whereas when it extends lateral to the line of the triangle, it should be considered convex.[6]

The ideal nostril is oval shaped, wider than the columella, and should be almost parallel to the vertical axis of the columella in the Caucasian nose. The length of the columella should be twice the height of the infratip lobule. The alae should insert at a soft angle to the cheek with a slight curve medially. Disharmonies of the alar base can be in either the vertical or horizontal plane, and careful analysis is critical, as surgical correction of these deformities differ depending on the nature of the deformity.[3]

The relationship of the nose to surrounding facial structures affects the perception of nasal features. A sloping forehead may give the illusion of overprojection of the nasal tip, whereas a flattened forehead may give the illusion of an underprojected nasal tip. Similarly, an underprojected chin may make the nose appear relatively overprojected and vice versa.

The esthetics of the nasal tip may be defined by several relationships, many of which are quite subtle. The angle at which the lateral and medial crura of the lower lateral cartilages meet should be about 30° on either side. The ideal nasal tip should be well defined. Subtle variations in anatomy may make it appear boxy or bulbous. Wide lateral crura may blunt dome definition resulting in a boxy tip. A greater than 30° angle between the lateral and medial crura or divergent domes can result in a bulbous-appearing tip.[1]

Physical examination should include palpation of the bony and cartilaginous components of the nasal dorsum to understand the relationships between them. The tip recoil test is performed by placing gentle pressure on the tip to assess the strength of the lower lateral cartilages. An intranasal examination should be performed to identify deviations of the nasal septum, turbinate hypertrophy, and any internal causes of nasal obstruction. The Cottle or modified Cottle maneuver is performed to assess nasal valve collapse.

Although the most thoroughly studied and well-described ideal nasal esthetics pertain to the Caucasian nose, much individual variety exists, and these ideals cannot be indiscriminately applied to all noses, particularly in different ethnicities such as the African, Asian, Middle Eastern, or Hispanic noses.[7–10]

Rhinoplasty Dynamics

The nose is a three-dimensional centerpiece on the face with critical structural and functional roles. There are many variables and dimensions that can be adjusted to alter the esthetic appearance, structural components, and functional role of the nose. There are many tools and maneuvers available to the rhinoplasty surgeon to adjust these numerous variables. While each adjustment may have a primary anticipated effect, such as increasing tip projection or reducing a dorsal hump, it will invariably have consequences, desirable or undesirable, to another variable nasal dimension.[11]

Adjusting the height at the radix or the caudal aspect of the dorsum will have different effects on several facial dimensions. Lowering the radix will frequently result in the appearance of increased intercanthal distance and increased nasal length. Augmenting the dorsum at the radix will appear to reduce the intercanthal distance and shorten the nose. In contrast, reducing the height of the dorsum more caudally can have the opposite effect giving the nose a shorter appearance and the illusion of greater cephalic rotation of the tip. Similarly, reduction of the caudal dorsum will cause the intercanthal distance to appear wider, while augmenting the dorsum will cause the intercanthal distance to appear narrower. Reducing the caudal dorsum may also reduce the tip projection as the caudal septum has an important role in supporting tip projection. Osteotomies can result in a narrower appearing nose and intercanthal distance.[11]

Numerous procedures may be used to adjust tip projection and width; however, not every procedure is appropriate for every patient. For example, an overprojected tip can be reduced with a cephalic trim of the lower lateral cartilages only if the cephalic portions of the lower lateral cartilages are actually the highest projecting part of the caudal tip. If this is not the case, securing the footplate of the medial crura to the caudal septum can decrease or increase tip projection depending on the location on the septum to which they are secured. Reducing tip projection may result in the appearance of a relatively widened alar base and bowed columella. Several maneuvers are frequently used to both increase tip projection and the angle of cephalic tip rotation. Placement of a columellar strut, anchoring the medial crura to the caudal septum, approximating the medial crura foot plates, and advancing the nasal spine can all result in the appearance of increased cephalic rotation and projection. Advancing the nasal spine may also shorten the upper lip. Care must be taken to choose the appropriate procedure for the anatomic constraints presented by each patient.[11]

The astute nasal surgeon will be aware of these effects in planning for rhinoplasty to anticipate the most appropriate and effective maneuvers for a specific patient's anatomy, to make adjustments when needed during surgery, and to assess the results of their adjustments postoperatively.

Operative Approach

External approach (open) rhinoplasty

Although every rhinoplasty operation should be individualized to each patient's particular anatomic indications, a systematic order and algorithm may be helpful in operative planning as well as establishing a logical progression of steps and maintaining stability. Local anesthesia using lidocaine with epinephrine should be carefully but judiciously infiltrated into all the areas of the nose to be dissected, but not adding so much volume that the features and subtle nuances of anatomy are masked. We prefer the administration of 1 in

200,000 epinephrine solution in lidocaine to minimize the systemic effects of the epinephrine followed after 5 minutes by 1 in 100,000 epinephrine solution to maximize the local vasoconstriction. Between the injections, we also place oxymetazoline-soaked packings inside the nostrils and around the septum to boost the effects of epinephrine (**Fig. 1**).

Numerous variations of the columellar incision exist. The authors use a midcolumellar stair-step incision while other surgeons might prefer an inverted-V or 5-cornered incision which is connected with bilateral marginal incisions placed at the caudal border of the lower lateral cartilages. Care is taken not to violate the soft-tissue triangles. Dissection of the skin-soft-tissue envelope is performed in the subperichondrial avascular plane directly over the cartilage of the lower lateral cartilages, then the upper lateral cartilages; keeping the dissection in this plane will allow the surgeon to avoid the neurovascular structures near the nasal tip.[8] The dissection is then continued cephalically to the caudal aspect of the nasal bones at which point a periosteal elevator is used to elevate the periosteum of the nasal bones in the nasion region (see **Fig. 1**).

As previously noted, each operation should be individualized to address each patient's anatomy. As required, the radix is addressed first, either by reducing it with a guarded burr if it is overprojected or by placing radix grafts if it is underprojected.

Then, the bony and cartilaginous dorsum is addressed. Preoperative evaluation of the dorsum should have identified whether there is an excess or deficiency of the dorsum. The skin is thinnest at the rhinion or bony-cartilaginous junction and becomes thicker cephalically toward the radix and caudally toward the nasal tip. Therefore, a slight prominence should exist at the upper portion of the upper lateral cartilage to compensate for the thinner skin to create a straight profile. Any cartilage or bony hump in excess of this should be removed.[12]

The upper lateral cartilages are released from the septum, preserving the underlying mucoperichondrium, thereby minimizing chances of postoperative internal valve narrowing. Any significant prominence of the cartilaginous and bony dorsum is addressed together using sharp dissection and an osteotome or a rasp. For a larger dorsal hump, a Rubin osteotome may be used to reduce the bony hump en bloc.[13,14] The bony dorsum can be further reduced or smoothed with rasping.[13] Precise cartilage reduction can be achieved by removing consecutive thin slices with a 15 blade until reaching the desired profile. After dorsal hump reduction, the patient may be left with an

"open roof deformity" where the lateral nasal bones and upper lateral cartilages are no longer touching the septum. This deformity is corrected later in the procedure with osteotomies and spreader grafts. When the dorsum is deficient, grafts can be placed to create a pleasing esthetic.

If there is significant septal deviation, the septum is addressed at this time either from the dorsal/open approach or intranasally through a hemitransfixion or Killian incision. Also at this time, if cartilage grafting is anticipated, septal cartilage can be harvested; as the old adage wisely professes, "Where the septum goes so goes the nose ...". Several indications exist for septoplasty in septorhinoplasty: obstructed nasal breathing associated with septal deviation, dorsal deviation associated with deviation of the anterior septum, and for harvest of graft material for other aspects of the rhinoplasty.

When septoplasty is performed from the dorsal approach, the anterior septal angle is identified: The lower lateral cartilages are retracted laterally and downward, and the septum is identified caudal to its attachment to the upper lateral cartilage. The perichondrial envelope is dissected from the septal cartilage in the subperichondrial plane, and if not already performed or as dissection proceeds, the upper lateral cartilages are released from the septum to provide adequate visualization of the more posterior septum. Preservation of the mucoperichondrium provides support and ultimately reduces internal valve collapse.

Once the septal cartilage and bone is exposed, it is assessed to determine which portion of the septal cartilage must be resected or weakened to relieve the deviation. One should also consider how much cartilage grafting material should be harvested. An important principle guiding septoplasty or septorhinoplasty is to maintain the structurally supportive "L-strut" comprising dorsal and caudal septum. We recommend leaving at least a 1.5, preferably 2 - 2.5, cm dorsal strut to maximize the degree of support. If significant deviation exists in the L-strut, this may be corrected and stabilized with unilateral or bilateral spreader grafts[4] or septal rotations suture (An effectively placed horizontal mattress suture [eg, 4-0 PDS (Ethicon, Bridgewater, New Jersey)] may correct mild deviations of the L-strut.). Gruber and colleagues demonstrated that a 10-mm wide and 0.5-mm thick piece of cartilage with a curvature may be adequately straightened with a horizontal mattress suture placed with an 8-mm longitudinal spacing with the knot on the convex side.[15]

If there is a spur or deviation involving the bony septum either superiorly in the perpendicular plate

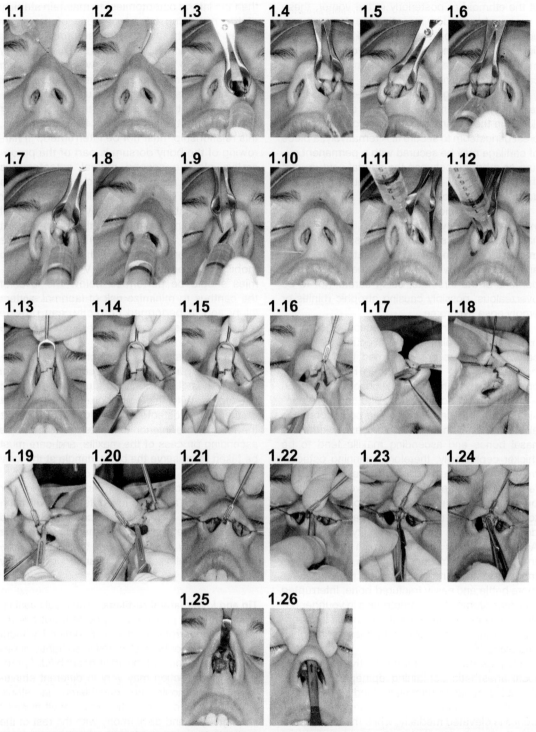

Fig. 1. Steps of open rhinoplasty approach. Systematic nose injection, starting from each side of nasion (1, 2), then subcutaneous and submucosal part of the nasal bone (3, 4, 5, and 6), dorsal septum (7, 8, and 9), alar base (10), and caudal septum (11 and 12). Steps of open nasal incision, stair step incision design and cut (13–15), nostril and side incisions (16–20). Dissection of skin and subcutaneous pocket starting in columellar area and hemostasis (21–23), subperichondrial dissection of lower lateral cartilages (24–25), subperiosteal dissection of the dorsum and rasping (25–26).

of the ethmoid or posteriorly in the vomer, these may be addressed by resecting the deviated portions. Caution should be exercised during resection of the perpendicular plate, avoiding rocking motions, as CSF leak may occur as a rare complication of septorhinoplasty.

If the inferior edge of the caudal L-strut has been released from the maxillary crest, it can be repositioned in the midline and sutured to the maxillary crest periosteum to secure it. Alternatively, a piece of cartilage may be secured with a permanent suture as a bridge between the caudal septum and the nasal spine if there is not enough length for adequate projection.[16]

If the septorhinoplasty is being performed to improve nasal airway obstruction, inferior turbinate hypertrophy should be addressed with submucosal resection, inferior turbinate outfracture, and/or conservative resection of the hypertrophic portions of the turbinate, being careful not to be overzealous, possibly causing atrophic rhinitis or empty nose syndrome.

Once satisfactory dorsal projection is achieved, osteotomies are planned and executed as necessary. Osteotomies are performed to narrow the bony dorsum, to close an open roof deformity created by dorsal hump reduction, or to straighten a crooked bony dorsum. Recalling anatomic considerations, the ideal width of the bony dorsum is about two-third that of the alar base width. The nasal bones and ascending maxilla tend to be thicker cephalically; therefore, planning osteotomies higher may help to minimize the narrowing effect on the internal nasal valve and nasal breathing. However, if the osteotomy is carried too high or if the medial and lateral osteotomies do not meet, a rocker deformity may result. Another anatomic consideration in osteotomy is the patient age: Younger patients tend to have more flexible bone while older patients have more brittle and easily fractured bone. Interrupted "postage stamp style" osteotomies in younger patients may be less effective if they result in greenstick fracture, and their nasal bones spring back into place.[12]

It is important to perform effective injection of local anesthetic containing epinephrine before the osteotomies to minimize bleeding and postoperative swelling. The periosteum of the nasal bones is elevated medially, while the lateral periosteum is left attached to the bone to provide stability to the segment of bone after lateral osteotomy during the healing period. If significant hump reduction has been performed, a formal medial osteotomy may be unnecessary.

In general, medial osteotomies should be performed first, followed by vertical osteotomies, then the lateral osteotomies, to maintain stability of the remaining lateral portions of the nasal bones for each succeeding osteotomy. Medial osteotomies are usually performed intranasally by seating the osteotome between the septum and the upper lateral cartilage at the caudal edge of the nasal bone. As the upper lateral cartilages obtain their structural support from their connection to the underside of the nasal bones, this relationship must not be interrupted.[3] If narrowing of the bony dorsum is part of the preoperative plan, a second medial osteotomy is performed to remove the excess bone as a wedge. Medial osteotomy is followed with vertical (anteroposterior) osteotomy at the level of the medial canthal ligament (the deepest part of frontonasal suture laterally) to connect the lateral osteotomy with medial osteotomy and mobilize the bony segment.[2] Vertical osteotomies should be performed below the level of the canthus to minimize risk of lacrimal system injury and, if performed correctly, can provide more precise control of nasal bone positioning.[17]

The lateral osteotomy is performed in a continuous fashion in a caudal to cephalic direction through nostril incisions and using a guarded osteotome. With this approach, the inferior limit of the lateral osteotomy should be just above the level of the inferior turbinate insertion in the ascending process of the maxilla, and care must be taken to preserve the bony triangle at the level of the piriform aperture at the caudal aspect of the maxillary bone. Staying above the inferior turbinate, as in a high-to-low osteotomy, will minimize risk of nasal airway compromise and address a wide bony base at the same time; the alternative way is to infracture the inferior turbinate to minimize the chance of airway compromise.

Tip and lower lateral cartilages The ideal nasal tip should be well projected, supported, not overrotated or underrotated, and well defined without being bulbous or have skin that is so tightly pulled over the cartilage that the tip appears bifid. Appropriate tip projection may vary in different ethnicities. This should be considered in ethnic rhinoplasty as overprojection may result in racial incongruity[7,9] and disharmony with the rest of the patient's face.

Various cartilaginous trimming, grafting, and suture techniques may achieve nasal tip definition and correct mild tip deviations. Conservative trimming of the lateral crus may be performed to even out asymmetries. It is imperative to leave a minimum 6 mm of strip of the lateral crus to preserve enough strength to prevent buckling.[15]

The domes should be about 4.5 mm in width, and the width of overall tip should be around 8 to 11 mm, with the average being 9 mm. The thicker the soft tissues of the tip are, the narrower the tip should be. A lateral crural mattress suture may be used to strengthen the lateral crus or to straighten convexities of the ala, either after over-resection or in the setting of weak cartilage. For the lower lateral cartilage, typically about 6-mm wide and 0.5-mm thick, a mattress suture may be placed with 6-mm spacing between the two loops of the stitch. Multiple stitches may be placed along the length of the lower lateral cartilage for added strength.[15] The same concept may be used to provide a subtle increase in strength for the columella. A columellar-septal suture strengthens the columella when only a mild weakness is present that does not require grafting.[15]

Dome stitches may be used to not only create more definition of the nasal tip but also to correct mild deviations or asymmetries by bringing together divergent intermediate crura.[16] If there is any chance of knots protruding into the skin, absorbable monofilament PDS is preferred. If sutures are placed deep in a location with no risk of extrusion or visibility, nylon is also a viable option.[15] A hemitransdomal stitch is placed through the vestibular skin and traverses the most cephalic end of the dome and attempts to evert the lateral crus. A transdomal suture is a horizontal mattress suture that brings together the medial and lateral crura of one of the lower lateral cartilages.[18] When placing this stitch, care must be taken to avoid causing the lateral crus to invert as it may result in concavity of the ala. Also, if the lateral bite of the stitch is not placed laterally enough, it may result in counterrotation and decrease in projection. A transdomal stitch placed appropriately laterally should increase tip rotation, projection, and definition.[13] An interdomal stitch approximates the medial crura together and is set back from the tip several millimeters.[15]

In profile, the domes should rise about 6 mm beyond the dorsum. This projection should be increased to 8 mm or even more on noses with thick skin. As previously described, in the ideal profile view of the nose, the ala sits 1 - 2 mm above the long axis of the nostril, and the columella 1 - 2 mm below it. It is vital to identify the correct anatomic problem: When a hanging ala is present, this should be correctly distinguished from retracted columella so that the appropriate problem is addressed.[5] If a mild alar retraction exists (<2 mm from the long axis of the nostril), an alar rim graft will not only correct this deformity but also will correct the concavity commonly associated with the retraction. On noses with wide bases and mild alar retraction, a small wedge of alar skin may be resected, and the remaining ala repositioned inferiorly. If greater than 2 mm of retraction exists, a V-Y advancement, a composite graft, or an intercartilaginous graft may be required between the upper and lower lateral cartilages on that side.[11] These maneuvers can lower the ala 4 - 8 mm. A hanging ala may be corrected by excising a small wedge of vestibular skin intranasally or by resecting a strip of cartilage at the caudal edge of the lateral crus of the lower lateral cartilage. A hanging columella can be corrected by resecting a thin strip of the caudal cartilaginous septum or by securing the medial crura to the caudal septum in a tongue-in-groove configuration.[19] Columellar retraction can be addressed by columellar strut or septal extension grafting.[5]

The base view of the nose should approximate an equilateral triangle. If there is convex ala protruding from the triangle, debulking of soft tissue, trimming lateral crura, or placing dome spanning sutures may correct this. Concave ala may be corrected by alar rim or strut grafting with cartilaginous grafts on top of or deep into the lateral crus, respectively, depending on the severity of the concavity[6].

Grafts Autologous graft material is preferable to alloplastic implants because the latter is significantly more prone to infection and extrusion. Common choices of graft material include septal cartilage, conchal cartilage, rib cartilage, and temporalis fascia. Cadaveric irradiated cartilage and alloplastic materials such as Medpore (Stryker, Portage, Michigan), silicone, and Gortex (Delaware, USA) are used by some surgeons. For most primary rhinoplasties, septal cartilage is preferred and has several advantages: It is readily accessible and, in the same operative field, abundant (in patients who have not undergone septoplasty) and strong, which is ideal for supportive grafts. Auricular conchal cartilage can be harvested without additional preparation if its use is anticipated and the ear is prepped into the operative field. Some surgeons prefer a preauricular incision, whereas others prefer a postauricular incision for graft harvest. A significant amount of cartilage may be harvested without compromising the structural or esthetic appearance of the ear as long as a few millimeters of rim is left in place along the conchal wall. Conchal cartilage is curved and significantly weaker than septal cartilage thus making it less suited for supportive strut grafts and better for alar reconstruction. Potential donor site morbidity includes auricular hematoma or perichondritis, although their risk can be minimized by the use of antibiotics and a bolster dressing.

Rib cartilage may be necessary for significant nasal reconstructive procedures. The rib provides an abundant source of graft material, but it carries the minor disadvantage of requiring a second harvest site and potentially causing a pneumothorax. The most common source of costal cartilage for grafting in females is the 6th and 7th rib cartilages because the incision can be hidden in the inframammary crease. Costal cartilage carries the risk of warping once it is in place. The effect of warping can be minimized by keeping the cartilage in saline for 30 to 60 minutes after harvest, determining in which direction twist will occur, and anticipating warp when carving the cartilage. A warping prevention suture described by us could be used to minimize the potential for a revision surgery. After deciphering the direction of the warping following placing the cartilage in saline solution, a 4 to 0 or 5 to 0 PDS suture is passed back and forth on the convex side of the cartilage from one end to the other end and tied tight enough to straighten the warped cartilage. This suture negates the need for the use of K-wire. Perichondrium, native fascia, or temporal-parietal fascia harvested from the patient can be laid over cartilage grafts to camouflage irregularities. Multiple layers of fascia can be laid on top of each other with each layer of fascia resulting in 0.5 mm of augmentation[20] although additional layers of fascia may prolong postoperative swelling. For bulk, any of the aforementioned cartilages can be diced and wrapped in fascia. These fascia-wrapped cartilage grafts can add volume in areas such as the dorsum but have little utility as supportive grafts.[20] We prefer placement of diced cartilage using a 1-cc insulin syringe in an ideally prepared pocket without fascia. Alloplastic material such as Medpore, a high-density polyethylene, is theoretically biocompatible, and intentionally placed pores allow fibrovascular ingrowth which serves to prevent graft migration. However, the risks of extrusion and infection and the fact that it is often difficult to remove because of the fibrovascular ingrowth make it less ideal than autologous graft materials.[21]

Spreader Grafts

Spreader grafts may be indicated when there is mid-vault nasal obstruction to widen the internal nasal valve, to augment an overly narrow dorsum, to support a deviated L-strut, to fill a defect from dorsal hump reduction, or when there is an inverted-V deformity. We believe that anytime a large-enough hump is removed to create an open roof, the use of spreader grafts becomes mandatory, otherwise an inverted-V deformity will ensue months or years later. The ideal material for a spreader graft is septal cartilage. Costal cartilage, layered or folded conchal cartilage, or the medial edge of the upper lateral cartilages (spreader flap) may also be used. Typically the cartilage is cut into strips approximately 5 mm high and 30 mm long, spanning the cartilaginous dorsum. If there is a curve in the graft cartilage, it can be scored and oriented so that the two pieces counteract the other curve. The graft is secured with at least two mattress sutures. The mattress sutures each traverse 5 layers securing both pieces to the septum medially and the upper lateral cartilages laterally.[16]

Supportive Grafts

The columellar strut graft is the most commonly used graft. The ideal material for a columellar strut is septal cartilage. It can be placed to help support the tip and overcome ptosis and over-rotation of the tip. The medial crura of the lower lateral cartilage can be secured to the graft to prevent hanging columella.[2]

For dorsal augmentation and increased tip projection with adequate support, onlay grafting may be performed. Adequate healthy skin must be present at the tip, as this graft may stretch the skin increasing the risk of skin necrosis. The ideal graft material is either septal cartilage or a straight segment of rib.[2]

A lateral crural strut graft can be placed to correct a prior concavity of the base view of the ala or to counteract the effect of dome sutures that may lead to concavity. A pocket is dissected on the deep surface of the lateral crus of the lower lateral cartilages beneath the vestibular skin intranasally. The graft cartilage is placed in the pocket and secured to the lateral crura using mattress sutures.

Alar rim grafts, fashioned from septal or costal cartilage, may be used to support the nasal valve or cosmetic purpose, and it is ideally placed in a pocket at the lowest part of the alar rim. Cephalic placement on the lower lateral cartilage will stent open the internal nasal valve while caudal placement on the lower lateral cartilage will stent open the external nasal valve.[21] Once the appropriate placement is done, the graft is secured with a suture that will be used to repair the rim incision.

The ideal alar rim smoothly transitions from the tip defining point to the nasofacial insertion, the contour and strength of which are determined by the lateral crus of the lower lateral cartilage. The lower lateral cartilage is in a position close to the rim more medially, but laterally, it is in a more cephalic position as it moves away from the alar margin: This lack of rigid support can lead to scarring, retraction, and/or unpredictable asymmetry. The alar rim graft, placed along the alar margin, is a powerful graft capable of directly altering the contour and strength of the alar margin. Indications include correction of alar flare, cephalic malposition and inadequate alar support, and correction of dynamic margin collapse.[17] On patients with cephalically oriented lower lateral cartilages, the lateral crura are dissected and transposed caudally.

Several types of tip grafts can be used to create a more-defined-appearing tip and/or to achieve slight increase in projection of the nasal tip. A shield or onlay graft is cut or prepared using the tip punch device designed by our group and placed as an onlay graft on top of the lower lateral cartilages or as a shield graft.[22] A tip graft is created from a horizontal piece of cartilage that crosses both domes with beveled edges laterally. The tip graft can be used to correct minor tip asymmetries. An infralobular graft can be attached to the septal cartilage to increase columellar show in noses with a retracted columella. After placement of a columellar strut, an onlay to the nasal tip is supported by the columellar strut and overlies both domes. A subdomal graft can be used to correct a pinched dome appearance or set the distance between the domes. The subdomal graft is placed after dissecting a tunnel under the domes and secured with 6 to 0 Vicryl suture. Septum is the ideal location for donor site, and the dimension of the graft is $1 \times 1 \times 8$ mm.[23]

ALAR BASE ADJUSTMENTS

Alar adjustments should be reserved for the last step after all the tip refinement and supportive grafts have been completed. An overprojected nasal tip or hypoplastic maxilla may give the illusion of narrowed alar width. Similarly, an underprojected tip or protruding maxilla may give the illusion of widened alar width. These issues must be ruled out before considering adjusting the alar base positions.[3] Ala that are displaced cephalically can be repositioned by resecting an ellipse of skin around the alar base and repositioning the ala medially; this will bring it to a more medial and caudal position. Wedge excisions according to the appropriate abnormality can remove a part of nasal sill, ala, or both. V to Y advancement and inverted-T excision for wide and thick alae are other maneuvers that can be useful in certain patients.[10]

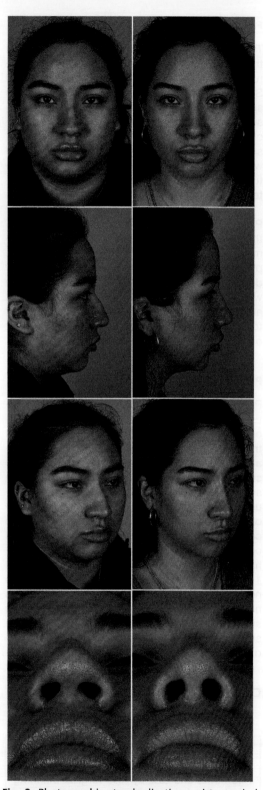

Fig. 2. Photographic standardization assists surgical planning and allows accurate preoperative and postoperative comparison, thereby facilitating the surgeon's self-assessment and critique allowing continual refinement of surgical technique.

FINAL STEPS

Typically, if septoplasty has been performed and there is a mucosal incision, it is closed with interrupted 5 to 0 chromic sutures, and intranasal Silastic or Doyle (Medtronics, Dublin, Ireland) splints are placed. Some surgeons prefer quilting sutures to reapproximate the opposing mucoperichondrial flaps in the absence of the removed septal cartilage. The columellar incision is closed with interrupted 6 to 0 fast-absorbing catgut sutures. Marginal incisions are closed with interrupted 6 to 0 fast-absorbing catgut sutures.

The dorsum is taped with Steri-Strips (3M, Saint Paul, Minnesota). If osteotomies were performed, the dorsum is splinted with a Denver Splint (Summit Medical , Saint Paul, Minnesota) or a thermoplastic splint. If a rib graft has been used for dorsal grafts, it may have been secured in place with K-wires: These are pulled through the splint and secured in place until they are removed at 2 to 3 weeks postoperatively. Sample of a patient operated by these steps is shown in **Fig. 2**.

POSTOPERATIVE CARE

Postoperative care varies among surgeons. Patients are counseled about the potential for postoperative bleeding, which can be self-limited and treated with oxymetazoline spray. In the immediate postoperative period (24 - 48 hours), patients should keep their head elevated to minimize swelling. Patients should avoid exercise or strenuous activity for 2 - 4 weeks postoperatively. Postoperative antibiotic prophylaxis may be considered if intranasal splints have been placed or an ear bolster is used after conchal cartilage harvest. Sutures and splints are removed at 1 week postoperatively. Although it is not always necessary or indicated, postoperative steroids have been observed to be effective in decreasing swelling.[24] Perioperative steroids have been shown to decrease periorbital edema in the immediate postoperative period.[25]

CLINICS CARE POINTS

- Preoperative identification of the nasal deformities and case-by-case surgical planning is the key for success.
- Open rhinoplasty provides better visualization of the deformities and, therefore, improves the consistency.

- Rhinoplasty is the surgery of millimeters, and so every move should be executed perfectly to achieve good results.

DISCLOSURE

The authors declare no conflict of interest.

REFERENCES

1. Woodard CR, Park SS. Nasal and facial analysis. Clin Plast Surg 2010;37(2):181–9.
2. Hobar PC, Adams WP, Mitchell CA. Lengthening the short nose. Clin Plast Surg 2010;37(2):327–33.
3. Ponsky D, Guyuron B. Alar base disharmonies. Clin Plast Surg 2010;37(2):245–51.
4. Gunter JP, Rohrich RJ, Friedman RM. Classification and correction of alar-columellar discrepancies in rhinoplasty. Plast Reconstr Surg 1996; 97(3):643–8.
5. Hackney FL. Diagnosis and correction of alar rim deformities in rhinoplasty. Clin Plast Surg 2010;37(2): 223–9.
6. Guyuron B. Alar rim deformities. Plast Reconstr Surg 2001;107(3):856–63.
7. Rohrich RJ, Bolden K. Ethnic rhinoplasty. Clin Plast Surg 2010;37(2):353–70.
8. Porter JP, Olson KL. Analysis of the African American female nose. Plast Reconstr Surg 2003; 111(2):620–6.
9. Toriumi DM, Pero CD. Asian rhinoplasty. Clin Plast Surg 2010;37(2):335–52.
10. Milgrim LM, Lawson W, Cohen AF. Anthropometric analysis of the female Latino nose. Revised aesthetic concepts and their surgical implications. Arch Otolaryngol Head Neck Surg 1996;122(10): 1079–86.
11. Guyuron B. Dynamics of rhinoplasty. In: Guyuron B, editor. Rhinoplasty: Expert consult premium edition. 1st edition. Philadelphia: Saunders; 2012. p. 61–102.
12. Dobratz EJ, Hilger PA. Osteotomies. Clin Plast Surg 2010;37(2):301–11.
13. Toriumi DM. Structural approach to primary rhinoplasty. Aesthet Surg J 2002;22(1):72–84.
14. Simons RL, Greene RM. Rhinoplasty pearls: value of the endonasal approach and vertical dome division. Clin Plast Surg 2010;37(2):265–83.
15. Gruber RP, Chang E, Buchanan. Suture techniques in rhinoplasty. Clin Plast Surg 2010;37(2):231–43.
16. Stepnick D, Guyuron B. Surgical treatment of the crooked nose. Clin Plast Surg 2010;37(2):313–25.
17. Boahene KDO, Hilger PA. Alar rim grafting in rhinoplasty: indications, technique, and outcomes. Arch Facial Plast Surg 2009;11(5):285–9.

18. Guyuron B, Behmand RA. Nasal tip sutures part II: the interplays. Plast Reconstr Surg 2003;112(4): 1130–45.

19. Kridel RW, Scott BA, Foda HM. The tongue-in-groove technique in septorhinoplasty. A 10-year experience. Arch Facial Plast Surg 1999;(4):246–56.

20. Daniel RK. Rhinoplasty: dorsal grafts and the designer dorsum. Clin Plast Surg 2010;37(2): 293–300.

21. Weber SM, Baker SR. Alar cartilage grafts. Clin Plast Surg 2010;37(2):253–64.

22. Guyuron B, Jackowe D. Modified tip grafts and tip punch devices. Plast Reconstr Surg 2007;120(7): 2004–10.

23. Guyuron B, Poggi JT, Michelow BJ. The subdomal graft. Plast Reconstr Surg 2004;113(3):1037–40.

24. Gurlek A, Fariz A, Aydogan H, et al. Effects of different corticosteroids on edema and ecchymosis in open rhinoplasty. Aesthet Plast Surg 2006;30(2): 150–4.

25. Kara CO, Gokalan I. Effects of single-dose steroid usage on edema, ecchymosis, and intraoperative bleeding in rhinoplasty. Plast Reconstr Surg 1999; 104(7):2213–8.

Nasal Tip Support and Management of the Tip Tripod Complex

Sebastian Sciegienka, MD[a],*, Andrea Hanick, MD[b], Emily Spataro, MD[c]

KEYWORDS

- Rhinoplasty • Tripod • Columellar strut graft • Septal extension graft • Tongue-in-groove

KEY POINTS

- The major and minor support mechanisms of the nasal tip must be restored during rhinoplasty surgery for acceptable cosmetic and functional outcomes.
- Analysis of the nasal tip and how rhinoplasty techniques change projection and rotation are critical factors in nasal tip surgery.
- The columellar strut graft, septal extension graft, and tongue-in-groove suture technique are methods to augment the nasal tip, and each has advantages and disadvantages in nasal tip surgery.

INTRODUCTION

Obtaining an aesthetically pleasing yet structurally sound nasal tip is one of the most challenging aspects of primary and revision rhinoplasty. As the major tip support mechanisms of the nose and management of the nasal tip and tripod complex centers around the lower lateral cartilages, proper understanding of surgical anatomy and techniques involving the lower lateral cartilages is essential for optimal cosmetic and functional results. Several methods of tip support and augmentation have been previously described, the best of which rely on predictability and optimal control of nasal tip position for achieving desired outcomes.[1] Three of the most popular techniques used by rhinoplasty surgeons include the columellar strut graft, the septal extension graft, and the tongue-in-groove suture, and are the focus of the following discussion.

BASICS OF NASAL TIP SUPPORT

A strong knowledge of major and minor tip support mechanisms is required to understand factors that may disrupt tip support as well as surgical techniques affecting the tripod complex (**Fig. 1**).[2] Specifically, the nasal tripod complex is a concept related to the lower third of the nose. The 3 legs of the tripod are composed of the conjoined medial crura forming one leg and the right and left lateral crus forming the second and third legs (**Fig. 2**). The nasal tip sits at the apex of the tripod. The complex rests on the anterior nasal spine and is supported by lateral soft tissue attachments to the sesamoid cartilages, upper lateral cartilages, and nasal pyramid, as well as by midline attachments to the caudal septum.[3] Successful tip augmentation should center around maintaining the integrity and appearance of the nasal tripod complex. More recently, rhinoplasty surgeons

Conflict of Interests/Disclosures: The authors have no conflicts of interest and did not receive any specific grant from funding agencies in the public, commercial, or not-for-profit sectors.

[a] Department of Otolaryngology – Head and Neck Surgery, Washington University School of Medicine, 600 South Euclid Avenue, P.O. Box 8115, St Louis, MO 63110, USA; [b] 1000 W. Nifong Building 3, Suite 100 Columbia, MO 65203, USA; [c] 1044 N. Mason Road, Medical Building 4, Suite L10, Creve Coeur, MO 63141, USA
* Corresponding author. 660 South Euclid Avenue, Campus Box 8115, St. Louis, MO 63110
E-mail address: ssciegienka@wustl.edu

Clin Plastic Surg 49 (2022) 61–70
https://doi.org/10.1016/j.cps.2021.07.005
0094-1298/22/© 2021 Elsevier Inc. All rights reserved.

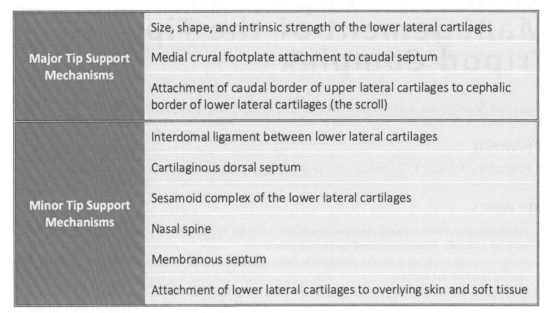

Major Tip Support Mechanisms	Size, shape, and intrinsic strength of the lower lateral cartilages
	Medial crural footplate attachment to caudal septum
	Attachment of caudal border of upper lateral cartilages to cephalic border of lower lateral cartilages (the scroll)
Minor Tip Support Mechanisms	Interdomal ligament between lower lateral cartilages
	Cartilaginous dorsal septum
	Sesamoid complex of the lower lateral cartilages
	Nasal spine
	Membranous septum
	Attachment of lower lateral cartilages to overlying skin and soft tissue

Fig. 1. Major and minor tip support mechanisms.

have included the septum in the definition of the traditional "nasal tripod" and include its use and augmentation as critical components of successful nasal tip surgery.[4]

The factors that lead to nasal tip deficiency can be congenital or secondary to open rhinoplasty or trauma to the nose. Any innate or created deficiency in nasal tip support mechanisms leads to relative weakness in the nasal tip and very likely unwanted cosmetic changes. For example, short or weak medial crura lead to loss of supratip definition, whereas unstable or cephalically malpositioned lateral crura can lead to nasal obstruction with inspiration due to external valve collapse.[5] Open rhinoplasty techniques routinely violate the major tip support mechanisms, namely the medial crural footplate attachment to the caudal septum and the scroll area. Therefore, restoring these mechanisms is always of utmost importance during nasal tip surgery.

Because of the destructive nature of certain open rhinoplasty techniques, some surgeons advocate for the preservation of tip ligament support as an alternative.[6] Traditionally the interdomal and intercrural ligaments are divided in open septorhinoplasty; this allows access to the anterior and caudal septum, but it disrupts the natural relationship and symmetry of the lower lateral cartilages and can lead to unfavorable postoperative results.[6] The interdomal ligament is a relatively discreet structure that connects the 2 middle crura at the cephalic junction of the infralobular segment, whereas the intercrural ligament connects long segments of the lower lateral cartilages

to one other and to the septum.[6] Preservation of these ligaments involves subcutaneous dissection from the transcolumellar incision to the intermediate crura then transitioning to a subperichondrial dissection.[6] The caudal septum is then palpated and accessed superiorly, keeping the ligaments intact. Septal work and placement of grafts can then be performed through the passageway between the septum and posterior aspect of the medial crura.[6] At the end of the operation, the tip can be addressed using suture techniques described later in this text.

But before performing a surgery to correct nasal tip support and its effect on tip position in accordance with the tripod complex, one must be comfortable with a detailed analysis of the nasal tip.

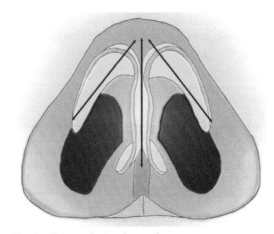

Fig. 2. The nasal tripod complex.

ANALYSIS OF THE NASAL TIP

As with any surgery, a thorough physical examination and the formulation of a differential diagnosis for a nasal deformity is key to success in rhinoplasty. The practice of diagnosing nasal tip deformities beneath intact skin is one of the more challenging aspects of rhinoplasty and often takes years of experience to become consistently accurate.[7] The basics of nasal tip analysis should serve as a foundation for these endeavors.

The "Ideal" Tip

Although there are some factors that always contribute to a more aesthetically pleasing tip, constant societal and cultural shifts in what is considered most "beautiful" make the definition of an ideal tip elusive. In addition, what may be accepted as ideal may not be consistent with patient wishes, making clear communication of surgical goals essential. In general, across sex and ethnicity, the nose and nasal tip should be as symmetric as possible. Even small asymmetries can draw marked, unwanted attention to the nose.

General

The assessment of the nasal tip should first focus on whether the tip is altered due to deficiencies of the nasal tripod itself or due to caudal septal issues such as causal septal deviation, fractures in the septum, or lack of septal support. These septal defects can cause deprojection or underrotation of the tip, fooling the surgeon into thinking that the lower lateral cartilages are to blame. To identify lower lateral cartilage deformity, one should examine for a bulbous tip, asymmetries localized to the lateral crura, and distortion of the soft tissue triangle. Tip deformity secondary to septal defect will present with asymmetry of the tip on both sides and can be accompanied with alar asymmetries. In practice, many patients will present with defects in both, particularly in the case of trauma to the nose.[7]

Next, the nasal base should be examined. From this angle a triangle between the tip and ala bilaterally is formed. The most anterior third of the triangle should be composed of the infratip lobule, and the posterior two-thirds should comprise the columella and nostrils. Some consider the posterior third to be reserved for the separate nasal sill.[8] This angle is also ideal for determining whether the tip deviates from midline and, if so, to what extent.[7]

Projection

Projection is the term used to describe how far anterior the tip of the nose is from the rest of the face and nasal dorsum as seen in oblique and lateral view. There are several methods for assessing tip projection. The Goode method asserts that if the nasofacial angle is between 36 and 40°, the length measured to the tip defining point will be 0.55 to 0.60 of the length of the dorsum.[9] The Crumley method expanded on Goode's analysis to describe the ideal nasal tip position using a 3:4:5 triangle, where one side of the triangle is formed from the nasofrontal angle through the alar crease, the second side is a perpendicular line to the first side that goes through the tip defining point, and the last side connects these 2 lines along the dorsum.[10] The Simons method states that the length measured from the subnasale to the tip defining point should be equal to that of the length from the subnasale to the vermillion border of the upper lip.[11] No one method is superior to others, and an experienced clinician will use multiple in order to estimate ideal projection for a given patient. Other useful standards are that the nasofrontal angle should be between 115 and 130°, the nasofacial angle should be between 30 and 40°, and there should be about 2 to 4 mm of columellar show.[12]

Rotation

Rotation is the term used to describe the position of the columella of the nasal tip in relation to the upper lip and the position of the infratip lobule segment relative to the columella as viewed laterally. Classically the nasolabial angle, the angle between the columella of the nose and the upper lip, is used to describe rotation. One must be cautious when using the nasolabial angle to estimate tip rotation because it can be severely skewed in cases of a hanging or retracted columella, in traumatic noses, or in those with upper lip retraction or protrusion.[7] In these cases other methods should be used. A second method uses the nostril axis line, a line drawn along the long axis of the nostril, in relation to the facial plane or a line perpendicular to the Frankfurt horizontal line. Similarly, the line drawn from the anterior columella to the subnasale can be used in relation to the facial plane or a line perpendicular to the Frankfurt horizontal line.[13]

Several different standards exist in the literature for ideal tip rotation, speaking to the subjective nature of what is considered "ideal." However, aesthetically pleasing nasolabial angles should be 90 to 100° in men and 95 to 115° in women.[13,14] Overrotation and underrotation imply angles that are over the upper end of these ranges or under the lower end of these ranges, respectively. Ethnicity, age, height, facial features, and societal norms all play a major role in determining what level of tip rotation is "ideal." As any aspect of rhinoplasty, a discussion about the patient's goals and expectation must occur before surgery.

METHODS OF RESTORING OR AUGMENTING TIP SUPPORT

Since the first modern rhinoplasty was performed and documented in 1887, various surgical methods have been developed to restore or augment the nasal tip and tripod complex. An in-depth discussion of every method is beyond the scope of this summary; however, some important techniques bear mentioning.

Many suture techniques involving the medial crura have been described for strengthening and changing the shape of the nasal tip. The transdomal or interdomal suture is a horizontal mattress suture that is used to narrow the dome and nasal tip. The intradomal suture provides tip strength, symmetry, and refinement, and it can also result in about 1 mm of increased tip projection.[15] The septocolumellar suture technique involves suturing the 2 medial crura to the caudal septum with the aim of reconstituting and sustaining nasal tip support and augmenting tip rotation and projection. This suture is often performed after endonasal rhinoplasty approaches, as the attachment of the medial crura to the caudal septum is frequently violated[16]. Lateral crural strut grafts are rigid cartilage grafts that secured the underside of the lateral crura and can span the length from the dome to the alar side wall or piriform aperture. As they strengthen the lateral crura, a major tip support mechanism, they can also increase tip support, in addition to correcting a boxy tip, external valve collapse, alar retraction, and lateral crura deformities.[17] Lastly, tip grafts of varying sizes and thickness can be used to increase the projection and change rotation; however, they typically do little to increase the strength of the nasal tip. Each of these techniques is important to keep in the rhinoplasty surgeon's armamentarium, but the remainder of this discussion focuses on columellar strut grafts, septal extension grafts, and the tongue-in-groove technique.

COLUMELLAR STRUT GRAFTS

With the popularization of external rhinoplasty techniques in the twentieth century, columellar strut grafts became common and are considered by some to be the primary treatment of a weak nasal tip.[18] The columellar strut graft is a small, rectangular piece of rigid cartilage or bone that is placed in the soft tissue pocket between the medial crura and is typically secured in place with sutures (**Fig. 3**). The graft can be placed

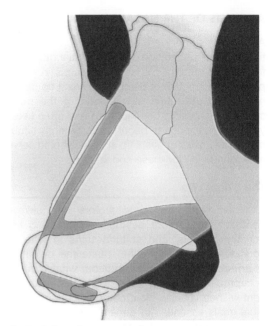

Fig. 3. Columellar strut graft.

with both endonasal and open approaches. During an endonasal approach, retrograde dissection is performed until a small pocket is created between the medial crura. The graft is placed and secured to the medial crura using suture. An open approach gives the surgeon more flexibility and control in placement of the graft. For patients with good projection and strong but asymmetric lower lateral cartilages, a short floating strut graft will reinforce and realign the lower lateral cartilages but will not increase tip projection. Conversely, patients with weak but symmetric lower lateral cartilages and poor tip projection may benefit from a long floating strut, which both adds strength to the nasal tripod and provides projection to the nasal tip.[19] Because of the columellar strut graft's close relationship to the midline leg of the nasal tripod, it is easy to see how this graft can affect tip position. Furthermore, recently Bucher and colleagues showed that significant tip projection and rotation is an attainable goal using a columellar strut graft alone if that is the surgical goal.[20]

A second vital principle to understanding columellar strut grafts is to be aware of how they change the shape of the columella itself. The columella is important not only as midline structural support but also important aesthetically. The columella needs to be balanced with the alar rim and neither be retracted nor have too much show.[12] When placing columellar strut grafts, one must avoid causing a retracted columella, a discontinuous contour, or excessive width. Retraction typically occurs when the graft has been improperly shaped or placed within the midline pocket. Discontinuous contours are seen when the graft is placed at an improper angle to the nasal spine or if the graft is too short. A wide columella is encountered when the graft itself is too thick but can be corrected using full-thickness horizontal mattress sutures through the columella to narrow it. Lastly, "clicking" against the anterior nasal spine has been reported and in the most extreme instances is audible to others.[4]

SEPTAL EXTENSION GRAFTS

The septal extension graft was described by Byrd and colleagues in 1997 as a more reliable way of controlling tip projections, rotation, and shape.[21] It is similar to columellar strut grafts in that it adds support to the medial crura; however, this method is more useful in patients with weak cartilages, a plunging tip, caudal septal deficiency, overrotated or shortened noses, or retracted alae. By securing structural support to the already stable nasal septum, strengthening and shaping the tip becomes more predictable and the height and length of the septal cartilage can be corrected.[21]

At its core, a septal extension graft is a piece of rigid cartilage that is sutured to the native septum. Classically the graft is sutured to the native anterior caudal septum to allow control of tip position (**Fig. 4**). The graft should be larger than necessary when suturing it into place. Then the surgeon can methodically trim the graft to reach the desired

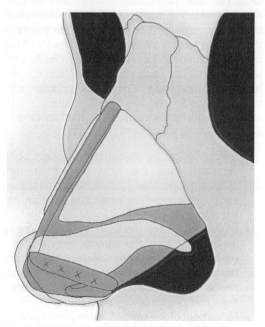

Fig. 4. Septal extension graft.

outcome. Ptotic tips can be corrected by including a longer inferior portion of the graft to support and rotate the tip up. Short, overrotated noses can benefit from longer superior grafts to derotate the nose and increase the length of the nose. When the anterior septum is relatively weak, other methods to strengthen the graft are necessary such as stabilizing on extended spreader grafts or using excess cartilage for additional support.[21–23]

Many variations on the septal extension graft exist. Although they differ in the shape and fixation points along the cartilaginous septum, they all should extend past the anterior septal angle and into the interdomal space to be effective. The extended spreader graft is a variation of the septal extension graft used in the setting of midvault collapse or nasal valve stenosis to increase both the internal nasal valve angle and tip projection and rotation simultaneously. The grafts should be placed so a portion extends past the anterior dorsum; the tip complex can then be sutured to the graft itself to achieve desired rotation and projection (**Fig. 5**).[21] Septal batten grafts can also be used to add rotation and projection to the nasal tip, but they do not require nearly the amount of cartilage as extended spreader grafts. They are placed just distal to the upper lateral cartilage and must be securely sutured to a strong septum. In addition, a unilateral septal batten graft can be helpful if asymmetries in the anterior septum are causing tip deviation.[4]

TONGUE-IN-GROOVE SUTURE TECHNIQUE

The tongue-in-groove technique gained popularity in 1999, when Kridel illustrated the technique. He demonstrated positive functional and cosmetic results using the technique in his patients over a 10-year period.[24] The technique involves repositioning both medial crura in relation to the caudal septum by suturing the 2 together in specific ways. The *tongue* refers to the caudal boarder to the septum and the *groove* refers to the space created between the medial crura (**Fig. 6**). It can be performed through a hemitransfixion, full transfixion, or external rhinoplasty approach. Since it was first described, it has been implemented to reduce columellar show, narrow a widened columella, correct tip ptosis, enhance tip support, and change both projection and rotation.[25,26]

To properly perform the tongue-in-groove technique, one must first assess the nose and address any deficiencies that would hinder its success. The medial crura's integrity, symmetry, and width should be noted along with the status of the caudal

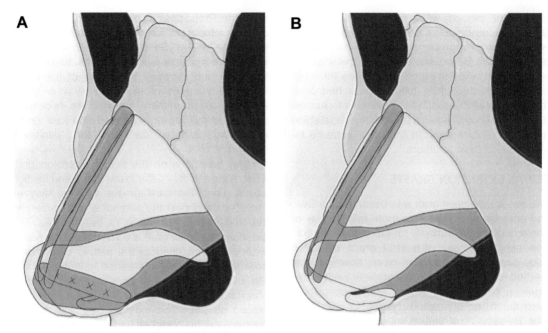

Fig. 5. Extended spreader grafts with (*A*) and without (*B*) septal extension graft.

septum. As such, the method is best for patients whose caudal septum is midline or brought to the midline and for the patients with sufficient caudal septal length.[27,28] If the septum is not midline or of sufficient length, measures should be taken to correct this before proceeding, including anterior septal replacement grafts or the addition of a septal extension graft.[18]

Next, the suture is placed. One can place a suture in several locations depending on the goals of surgery. Regarding the symmetry of the lower lateral cartilages, suture entry can be on either the lateral or the medial surface of the medial crus, but all sutures must be placed while keeping

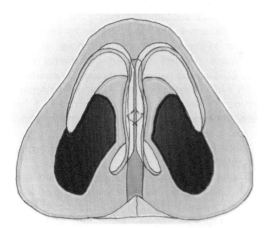

Fig. 6. Tongue-in-groove suture technique.

the external contours of the cartilages in mind.[18] It is critical to keep the suture entry and exit points at the same relative positions in the crura bilaterally, both in relation to the caudal edge of the medial crura and the tip defining points. By keeping the distances equal bilaterally, the external columella and the infratip lobule will be symmetric. In addition, varying the point of fixation on the medial crura can alter projection, rotation, and tip stiffness.[18] Next, one must consider the suture position on the septum. The position of the suture in the septum has no effect on the symmetry of the columella or infratip lobule, but it can alter tip projection, rotation, and columellar show. The following is a summary of how the 4 variables (stiffness, projection, rotation, and columellar show) interplay with differences in medial crura and septal suture fixation position.[18]

- Movement of the medial crura fixation point vertically, from the base toward the tip, causes an increase in stiffness and rotation and a decrease in projection. Columellar show is unaffected.[18]
- Movement of the medial crura fixation point horizontally, from the anterior aspect of the medial crura toward the posterior aspect of the medial crura, causes an increase in columellar show and decrease in rotation. Stiffness and projection are unaffected.[18]
- Movement of the septal fixation point horizontally, from the anterior septum toward the

posterior septum, causes an increase in rotation and decrease in columellar show. Projection and stiffness are unaffected.[18]

• Movement of the septal fixation point vertically, from the anterior nasal spine toward the tip, causes an increase in projection and rotation. Stiffness and columellar show are unaffected (**Fig. 7**A,B).[18]

Over the last 2 decades the popularity of the tongue-in-groove technique has grown both in practice and in the literature as evidenced by the many publications characterizing its use and quantifying its results. Tongue-in-groove suture technique has been demonstrated to significantly increase tip rotation and significantly reduce alar-columellar disproportion.[29] Notably, some investigators have demonstrated interval decrease in the initially achieved tip rotation over time, citing decreases in tip rotation of approximately 7°.[13,30] These changes may be affected by techniques including suture selection.[26] Although the utility of the tongue-in-groove suture technique for controlling tip rotation and projection has been well established, its longevity and other nuances bear further evaluation.

COMPARISON OF TECHNIQUES

As new techniques to strengthen and shape the nasal tip have been developed over the years, several comparisons between these methods have been made to describe which are best in various situations. However, one should note that rhinoplasty typically uses a combination of techniques to provide the best cosmetic and functional results. One should not be limited to using a single technique.

Despite its relatively long history, the popularity of columellar strut grafts has decreased, in part due to the popularization of the septal extension graft. Both enable the surgeon to increase projection and rotation of a nose, but opponents of the columellar strut argue that it cannot provide nearly the positional control that is obtained with use of a septal extension graft. In fact, some believe that the single most important limitation to a columellar strut over a septal extension graft is the lack of control of nasal tip rotation[4]. In addition, wound contraction forces are thought to be better mitigated by septal extension grafts due to its attachment to the septum, which is adherent to the nasofacial skeleton. Weeks to months after rhinoplasty surgery using a columellar strut, patients may complain of "clicking" when the patient smiles or wiggles the nose. This clicking manifests from the rubbing of the free-floating graft against the anterior nasal spine and does not occur with secured septal extension grafts.[1]

Despite some of these drawbacks, the columellar strut graft does have advantages over a septal extension graft. First, it is often not necessary to disrupt as many attachments to the medial crura or dissect as much nasal tissue in order to

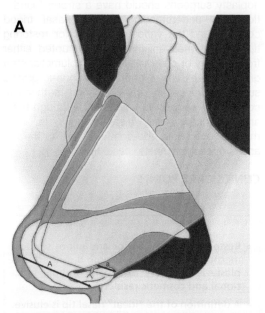
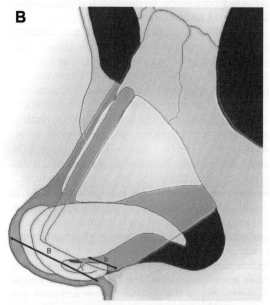

Fig. 7. (*A*)Tongue-in-groove suture with septal component toward nasal spine (a) resulting in decreased projection and rotation (A). (*B*) Tongue-in-groove suture with septal component toward nasal tip (b) resulting in increased projection and rotation (B).

place a columellar strut effectively compared with a septal extension graft[1]; this may be beneficial when the goal is to provide only minor changes to rotation or projection of the nose. It is also accepted that a columellar strut graft will provide some level of tip support without overstiffening the nasal tip.[4] Conversely, the septal extension graft can create a firm nasal tip that can feel unnatural. The septal extension graft can also lead to columellar or nostril asymmetry if it is placed on either side of the septum or a pinched nasal tip resulting from too robust of a graft.[27] In general, septal extension grafts should not be used on noses with heavy lower lateral cartilages and normal or excessive tip projection.[4]

Recent literature has attempted to quantify differences in the 2 grafts, particularly when considering tip position. Shaw-Martinez and colleagues looked at 106 patients who underwent either columellar strut (floating only) or caudal septal extension graft to increase tip projection and analyzed photographs based on tip projection, nasal length, the Goode ratio, and tip rotation in a blinded fashion. They found that the columellar strut group had about 5% derotation compared to about 1% in the caudal septal extension graft group at least 12 months from the surgical date. Interestingly, tip projection, nasal length, and the Goode ratio decreased similarly in both groups.[1] Akkus and colleagues compared the long-term stability of projection and rotation of the 2 grafts in 36 patients and found that both methods increased nasal projection significantly, but the septal extension graft provided more stable tip position and less derotation after 16 to 24 months.[31]

The tongue-in-groove technique has become more popular since it was first described. The growing number of proponents argue that it allows for superior control of the nasal tip when making both large and small adjustments.[25] Compared with the aforementioned tip strengthening methods, it also generally does not rely on healing and tissue contracture for the final surgical result. As each stitch can be assessed easily and immediately, the surgeon has the advantage of instant feedback and does not rely on "guess-work." Furthermore, the technique is largely reversible. If a stitch does not have the desired effect, it is simple to remove and try again. As with other methods, it can also be performed in open and closed rhinoplasty and is easily combined with other rhinoplasty techniques. However, the tongue-in-groove does have some drawbacks. The technique can cause overstiffening of the tip and overretraction of the columella.[18]

Similar to the columellar strut and septal extension graft, there is a growing base of literature comparing the tongue-in-groove technique with other rhinoplasty methods. Dobratz and colleagues studied how the tongue-in-groove, columellar struts, and septal extension grafts affected the strength of the tip both in cadavers and clinically. In cadavers, the tongue-in-groove and septal extension graft provided greater strength than columellar strut grafts; however, there were no statistical difference between techniques regarding tip position in 40 live patients after at least 1 year.[32] Karaiskakis and colleagues compared the results of the tongue-in-groove technique and the columellar strut technique in a retrospective cohort of 33 patients. The tongue-in-groove technique led to more rotation but less skin sensitivity on the nasal tip when compared with the columellar strut graft technique. Both techniques lead to high chance of patient-reported, subjective tip rigidity. Aesthetic results were similar in both groups when evaluated by the patients themselves and by an independent and blinded group of 3 plastics surgeons.[33] Demir also compared the tongue-in-groove and columellar strut graft results in 28 patients and found that both significantly increased nasal projection and nasal tip rotation to a similar extent at least 6 months after surgery.[34]

SUMMARY

Control of the nasal tip to achieve excellent structural and cosmetic outcomes is one of the most challenging aspects of rhinoplasty surgeries. Rhinoplasty surgeons should have a strong foundation and understanding of the nasal tripod complex and the various methods for restoring tip support mechanisms when disrupted either from surgery or other means. The columellar strut graft, septal extension graft, and tongue-in-groove suture technique are well-described methods to control and support the nasal tip. Although there are advantages and disadvantages to each method, one should be comfortable with the nuances of each to master nasal tip surgery.

CLINICS CARE POINTS

- Restoration of the major and minor support mechanisms of nasal tripod during rhinoplasty is necessary to obtain optimal functional and cosmetic results.

- A definition of the "ideal" nasal tip is elusive. There are several factors that dictate tip aesthetics including projection and rotation, but patients' desires and expectations should be heavily weighted in preoperative consultation.

- Columellar strut grafts are small, floating pieces are rigid cartilage that are placed between the medial crura in open or closed rhinoplasty. They are most beneficial when the nasal tip needs only minor adjustments in rotation and projection.
- Septal extension grafts are pieces of rigid cartilage sutured to the native septum. They allow for significant change to rotation and projection and give the tip more structural support. Compared with columellar strut grafts, septal extension grafts allow the surgeon to alter the tip with increased control.
- The tongue-in-groove suture technique involves repositioning of the medial crura in relation to the caudal septum with suture to achieve both large and small changes in projection and rotation. It allows for superior control of the nasal tip and can easily be used with other rhinoplasty techniques.

REFERENCES

1. Sawh-Martinez R, Perkins K, Madari S, et al. Control of nasal tip position: quantitative assessment of columellar strut versus caudal septal extension graft. Plast Reconstr Surg 2019;144(5):772e–80e.
2. Tardy ME. Surgical anatomy of the nose. Chicago: Lippincott Williams & Wilkins; 1990.
3. Westreich RW, Lawson W. The tripod theory of nasal tip support revisited: the cantilevered spring model. Arch Facial Plast Surg 2008;10(3):170–9.
4. Rohrich RJ, Durand PD, Dayan E. Changing role of septal extension versus columellar grafts in modern rhinoplasty. Plast Reconstr Surg 2020;145(5):927e–31e.
5. Cerkes N. Nasal tip deficiency. Clin Plast Surg 2016; 43(1):135–50.
6. Marcus JR, Thomas AB, Levites HA. Tip ligament preservation and suspension: why and how? Facial Plast Surg Clin North Am 2021;29(1):47–58.
7. Balaji N. Assessment of the nasal tip. Textbook of nasal tip rhinoplasty. 1st edition. Cham: Springer International Publishing; 2020. p. 41–65.
8. Kridel RW, Castellano RD. A simplified approach to alar base reduction: a review of 124 patients over 20 years. Arch Facial Plast Surg 2005;7(2):81–93.
9. Goode R. A method of tip projection measurement. In: Powell HB, editor. Proportions of the esthetic face. New York: Thieme-Stratton Inc; 1984. p. 15–39.
10. Crumley RL, Lanser M. Quantitative analysis of nasal tip projection. Laryngoscope 1988;98(2):202–8.
11. Simons RL. Nasal tip projection, ptosis, and supratip thickening. Ear Nose Throat J 1982;61:452–5.
12. Gunter J, Rohrich R, Friedman R, et al. Importance of the alar-columellar relationship. Dallas

13. Antunes MB, Quatela VC. Effects of the tongue-in-groove maneuver on nasal tip rotation. Aesthet Surg J 2018;38(10):1065–73.
14. Tasman AJ, Lohuis PJ. Control of tip rotation. Facial Plast Surg 2012;28(2):243–50.
15. Gruber RP, Chang E, Buchanan E. Suture techniques in rhinoplasty. Clin Plast Surg 2010;37(2): 231–43.
16. Tezel E, Ersoy B. Tip-oriented closed rhinoplasty built on septocolumellar suture and a new caudal septal graft technique. Ann Plast Surg 2016;77(3): 264–71.
17. Cochran CS, Sieber DA. Extended alar contour grafts: an evolution of the lateral crural strut graft technique in rhinoplasty. Plast Reconstr Surg 2017; 140(4):559e–67e.
18. Spataro EA, Most SP. Tongue-in-groove technique for rhinoplasty: technical refinements and considerations. Facial Plast Surg 2018;34(5):529–38.
19. Rohrich RJ, Hoxworth RE, Kurkjian TJ. The role of the columellar strut in rhinoplasty: indications and rationale. Plast Reconstr Surg 2012;129(1):118e–25e.
20. Bucher S, Kunz S, Deggeller M, et al. Open rhinoplasty using a columellar strut: effects of the graft on nasal tip projection and rotation. Eur Arch Otorhinolaryngol 2020;277(5):1371–7.
21. Byrd HS, Andochick S, Copit S, et al. Septal extension grafts: a method of controlling tip projection shape. Plast Reconstr Surg 1997;100(4):999–1010.
22. Toriumi DM, Checcone MA. New concepts in nasal tip contouring. Facial Plast Surg Clin North Am 2009;17(1):55–90, vi.
23. Toriumi DM. Caudal septal extension graft for correction of the retracted columella. Oper Tech Otolayngol Head Neck Surg 1995;6(4):311–8.
24. Kridel RW, Scott BA, Foda HM. The tongue-in-groove technique in septorhinoplasty. A 10-year experience. Arch Facial Plast Surg 1999;1(4): 246–56 [discussion 257–8].
25. Datema FR, Lohuis PJ. Tongue-in-groove setback of the medial crura to control nasal tip deprojection in open rhinoplasty. Aesthet Plast Surg 2015;39(1): 53–62.
26. Kridel RWH, Delaney SW. Commentary on: effects of the tongue-in-groove maneuver on nasal tip rotation. Aesthet Surg J 2018;38(10):1074–7.
27. Aksakal C. Comparing the effects of tongue-in-groove and septocolumellar suture with short and floating columellar strut of open rhinoplasty on nasal tip rotation and projection. J Oral Maxillofac Surg 2021;79(2):474.e1–11.
28. Williams EF. Alar-columellar disharmony using the tongue-in-groove maneuver in primary endonasal rhinoplasty. Arch Facial Plast Surg 2012;14(4): 283–8.

rhinoplasty: nasal surgery by the masters. St. Louis: Quality Medical Publishing Inc; 2002. p. 105–16.

29. Shah A, Pfaff M, Kinsman G, et al. Alar-columellar and lateral nostril changes following tongue-in-groove rhinoplasty. Aesthet Plast Surg 2015;39(2): 191–8.

30. Delarestaghi MM, Jahandideh H, Sanaei A, et al. "Modified tongue-in-groove": a new tip-plasty technique and comparison of its effect on correction of the nasolabial angle with the columellar strut technique. Br J Oral Maxillofac Surg 2020;58(5):602–7.

31. Akkus AM, Eryilmaz E, Guneren E. Comparison of the effects of columellar strut and septal extension grafts for tip support in rhinoplasty. Aesthet Plast Surg 2013;37(4):666–73.

32. Dobratz EJ, Tran V, Hilger PA. Comparison of techniques used to support the nasal tip and their long-term effects on tip position. Arch Facial Plast Surg 2010;12(3):172–9.

33. Karaiskakis P, Bromba M, Dietz A, et al. Reconstruction of nasal tip support in primary, open approach septorhinoplasty: a retrospective analysis between the tongue-in-groove technique and the columellar strut. Eur Arch Otorhinolaryngol 2016;273(9): 2555–60.

34. Demir UL. Comparison of tongue-in-groove and columellar strut on rotation and projection in droopy nasal tip: contribution of a cap graft. J Craniofac Surg 2018;29(3):558–61.

Tip Reduction and Refinement Maneuvers

Matthew Novak, MD, Justin Bellamy, MD, Rod Rohrich, MD*

KEYWORDS

- Rhinoplasty • Tip reduction • Deprojection • Tip refinement • Tip grafts • Tip suturing
- Nasal anatomy

KEY POINTS

- Tip reduction and refinement require a thorough understanding of the dynamic nasal anatomy and implementation of the tripod concept to explain the relationship between tip projection, rotation, and nasal length.
- To achieve favorable and consistent results, factors contributing to tip overprojection must be diagnosed accurately and addressed appropriately through an incremental approach.
- After achieving the appropriate reduction, the desired projection and rotation of the tip must be set and the structural support restored.

INTRODUCTION

The achievement of a well-defined and appropriately projected nasal tip is paramount to success in rhinoplasty. In contrast to antiquated destructive techniques, the popular modern approaches to managing the nasal tip have seen increased efforts to conserve the native anatomy by sparing cartilage and emphasizing structural support in conjunction with suture technique tip refinement.[1–8] In significantly overprojected or deformed tips, however, cartilage transection may be required. An algorithmic and graduated approach should be applied to identify patients who would benefit from this technique. Furthermore, in patients who require more aggressive techniques to deproject the tip, restoration of structural integrity increasingly becomes a priority.

To achieve consistent and reproducible results, a thorough understanding of the anatomic factors contributing to the overprojected and deformed nasal tip is imperative. Subtle variations in soft tissue characteristics, cartilaginous framework, and tip support have a profound impact on the final, long-term result.[9] Each factor must be assessed individually and addressed incrementally.

Successful tip reduction and refinement relies on a detailed nasal analysis preoperatively and intraoperatively, followed by precise operative execution. This article reviews the pertinent anatomy, analysis, approach, and surgical technique for nasal tip deprojection and refinement.

HISTORY

Surgical techniques aimed at deprojecting the nose inevitably affect the anatomic structure of the nasal tip. Addressing the projection of the nose without considering the contour of the tip yields undesired and inconsistent results. As such, a variety of surgical techniques have been described to address nasal projection while simultaneously controlling the tip.

In 1931, Joseph[10] first described deprojecting the nose by shortening the medial and lateral crura. Safian[11] subsequently suggested domal excision, which prompted the description of multiple modifications of scoring and weakening the nasal dome.[12–14] Finally, techniques ranging from full-thickness columellar and alar base excision to cartilage division and set back have been described.[15,16] Although favorable results can be

Dallas Plastic Surgery Institute, Dallas, TX, USA
* Corresponding author. Dallas Plastic Surgery Institute, 9101 North Central Expressway, Suite 600, Dallas, TX.
E-mail address: rod.rohrich@dpsi.org

Clin Plastic Surg 49 (2022) 71–79
https://doi.org/10.1016/j.cps.2021.08.004

achieved with manipulation of the lower lateral cartilages (LLCs), disruption of the fibrocartilaginous structure of the tip is not without risks. In particular, a weakened or anatomically altered tip is subject to migration and contour deformity.

This concept of tip support is well illustrated by the tripod concept as described by Jack Anderson in 1969.[17] As a conceptual tool to understand tip dynamics, the original tripod concept describes the cartilaginous structure of the nasal tip as that of a tripod. The paired lateral crura of the LLC serve as the lateral legs and the conjoined medial crura serve as a central leg. The apex of the resulting tripod forms the tip unit. This entire construct is reinforced by ligamentous attachments and the caudal septum, sometimes referred to as the fourth leg, or "tetrapod concept."[18] Additional support to the tip also is provided by the cephalic upper lateral cartilage (ULC) at the scroll region and fibrofatty tissue at the base of the columella.

As a means to preserve the structure of the nasal tip tripod and maintain tip topography, rhinoplasty surgeons have evolved from the predominantly destructive tip reshaping techniques of the mid to late twentieth century to less destructive modifications of the existing tip cartilages with suture techniques.[19–22] This paradigm shift changed the focus to reversible suture techniques as a means to preserve structural integrity and limit use of visible grafts.[1,2,5–7,23–26]

Not surprisingly, there is no single maneuver that allows for successful sculpting, projection, and rotation of the nasal tip. A combination of maneuvers is required for optimal tip control, each with advantages and disadvantages. For example, lateral crural steal and transection techniques have the advantage of increased flexibility at the cost of decreased intrinsic structural support.[27,28] The septal extension graft (SEG) was introduced by Byrd and colleagues and adds both support and shaping flexibility by adding a central post upon which to stabilize and tension the LLCs.[29] Recent descriptions of tip shaping technique have combined and expanded on these principles because control of tip projection, rotation, and shape remain key components in modern rhinoplasty.

ANATOMY

Precise and reproducible results in the management of the nasal tip begin with a detailed understanding of the underlying and interrelated anatomy that contribute to tip projection, rotation, and shape. The bony, cartilaginous, and soft tissue tripod that contributes to projection of the tip can be divided in to major and minor tip support structures. Major structures include fibrous connections of the lateral crura to the ULC and medial crura to the caudal septum and maxillary spine, abutment of the lateral crura at the pyriform rim, and the interdomal suspensory ligament. Minor structures include fibrous attachments of the alar cartilage to the dorsum, skin, and the membranous septum.[2,30,31] Although these factors provide the structural support for projection and rotation of the tip, aberrations can result in underprojection or overprojection and rotation.

Furthermore, perceived overprojection of the tip must be defined preoperatively as true overprojection versus pseudo-overprojection, because the difference influences surgical management. To rule out pseudo-overprojection, nasal and nonnasal factors must be excluded as causes of perceived overprojection.[8] The nasal factors contributing to the appearance of overprojection are composed of the anatomic characteristics of the nose above the tip.

Nasal factors contributing to pseudo-projection:

1. Deep nasofrontal angle
2. Low radix
3. Deficient dorsum/saddle nose deformity

The nonnasal factors that give the illusion of overprojection are related to the anatomic facial characteristics above and below the nose.

Nonnasal factors contributing to pseudo-projection:

1. Sloping forehead
2. Anterior maxilla
3. Short upper lip
4. Micrognathia/deficient chin

These nasal and nonnasal factors require careful attention to rule out pseudo-overprojection as the cause of perceived overprojection.

Regarding the shape of the nasal tip, the paired LLCs are composed of medial, middle, and lateral crura. It is the relationship between these 3 crura and the overlying skin that ultimately determines nasal tip appearance. Anatomically, the paired LLCs have an interdomal angle of divergence of 30°, domal arc width of 4 mm or less, and distance between the tip-defining points of 5 mm to 6 mm.[32,33] The ideal orientation of the lateral crura is straight and everted, with the caudal edge projecting anterior to the cephalic edge. Widening of the domal arc or angle of divergence contributes to a boxy appearance. Redundant lateral crura contribute to a bulbous tip with domal fullness, whereas malformation in orientation can result in a variety of tip deformities including alar notching, a pinched tip, or other asymmetries.

Another anatomic characteristic to note early in the nasal analysis is skin thickness. Specifically, skin thickness should be assessed on the nasal tip as it is the main limitation in what can be accomplished in tip projection and definition.[34] For example, rigid tip grafts on a patient with thin skin may be palpable or visible postoperatively. Conversely, a weak tip graft on a patient with thick skin may not define the tip as desired and add unwanted volume.

Beyond identifying the factors contributing to projection, rotation, and shape of the tip, the structures contributing to the anatomy surrounding the tip also must be considered. The supratip break is formed by the relationship between the cephalic edge of the LLC and the caudal edge of the ULC in the scroll region. In the ideal nasal tip, the caudal edge of the LLCs sits higher in relation the cephalic edge. This correlates to a posteriorly oriented cephalic margin of the dome, which results in tip-defining points with the correct positioning and projection.

Finally, the infratip lobule is defined superiorly by the tip-defining points, the soft tissue triangles laterally, and the columellar-lobular junction inferiorly.[32] A point placed at the infratip and connected to points at the supratip and paired tip-defining points creates a diamond formed by opposing equilateral triangles. This relationship is a hallmark of the ideal nasal tip. Redundancy of the middle crura can contribute to infratip lobular excess, whereas redundancy in the medial crura may contribute to excess columellar show and disturbances in the alar-columellar relationship.

ANALYSIS AND DIAGNOSIS

Complete nasal analysis includes evaluation of the nose in the frontal, lateral, and basal views.[35] From the frontal view and focusing on the nasal tip, the dorsal aesthetic lines should be assessed. Originating on the supraorbital rims, the dorsal aesthetic lines traverse medially and converge at the medial canthal ligaments and diverge at the keystone area, finally ending at the nasal tip. The ideal width matches the tip-defining point width or interphiltral distance. Next, light reflection and shadowing should be used to analyze the nasal tip for normal contour.[2] Bulbous, boxy, or pinched tips should be identified and differentiated.[33] Four key points should be assessed[9]:

1. Supratip break for fullness or asymmetry
2. Infratip lobule for excess projection or fullness
3. Left tip domal transition zone for excess fullness or concavity
4. Right tip domal transition zone for excess fullness or concavity

Additionally, on the frontal view the alar base width and symmetry should be noted because adjustments in alar base width may affect tip projection.

On lateral view, the nasal length, dorsum, tip projection and rotation, and supratip characteristics should be defined clearly. The ideal nasal length is equal to two-thirds the midfacial height.[9,36] The dorsum should be smooth and straight in men and smooth with a slight supratip break in women. The supratip break should be 2 mm to 3 mm above the tip-defining points and is determined by the balance between the dorsum and tip projection.[37] Next on lateral view, tip projection is assessed. Several methods have been described to diagnose true overprojection, each using ratios to compare the tip projection to fixed surrounding landmarks.[38–43] A commonly used method, as described by Byrd and Hobar, suggests that projection is two-thirds of the ideal nasal length or 50% to 60% of the tip lies anterior to the upper lip.[9,43] The degree of tip rotation varies and is determined by a nasolabial angle of 90° to 95° in men and 95° to 110° in women.

On basal view, the columella-to-lobule and nostril-to-tip ratios should approximate 2:1, creating an equilateral triangle from the paired alar bases to the nasal tip.[1,37] Alar flaring also is diagnosed from the basal view. Correction of alar flare with excision of the alar bases can result in loss of 1 mm to 2 mm of tip projection. This should be accounted for when setting the tip projection intraoperatively.[44,45]

SURGICAL TECHNIQUE

Operative techniques to address overprojection of the nasal tip simultaneously and invariably affect the rotation and shape of the tip. For this reason, an incremental approach to deprojection of the nasal tip is crucial to maximize predictability and avoid unnecessary maneuvers. The fundamental surgical steps that broadly describe the approach to nasal tip deprojection and refinement include intraoperative analysis to determine the cause(s) of overprojection, incremental correction of overprojection, rebuilding of the tip, and refinement if the tip.

Intraoperative Analysis

In patients diagnosed with true overprojection of the nasal tip, the nasal envelope is opened with a transcolumellar and bilateral infracartilaginous incisions. This allows for full exposure of the underlying nasal tip anatomy and analysis of each element contributing to tip projection and shape. The lateral crura are assessed for degree of convexity, length and width, position, and symmetry. The medial crura are assessed for symmetry, deviation, length, and strength. The presence of excessive dorsal and/or caudal septum is identified. The interdomal width, angle of divergence, and symmetry then are characterized.[44,46] These characteristics are critical for tip projection and definition.

Incremental Correction of Overprojection

As discussed previously, tip projection and rotation are interconnected and are products of multiple factors: length and strength of the LLCs, ligamentous and fibrous support, and tip support from the anterior septal angle. After wide exposure and intraoperative analysis, the first of the incremental steps in deprojecting the tip is release of the fibrous attachments of the medial crura to the septum and maxillary spine. This destabilizes the central arm of the tripod and thus decreases projection. The attachments of the scroll region can then be released in isolation or performed in conjunction with a cephalic trim. Subsequently, resection of excessive dorsal and caudal septum is performed. It is pivotal to perform this step prior to any graft harvest of the septum. Performing these steps in a reversed order risks inadvertent over-resection and destabilization of the septum.

If significant deprojection is required, the medial crura cartilage can be divided and overlapped (with or without resection) following placement of the SEG during the tip rebuilding phase of the operation.

Rebuilding the Tip

Cartilage grafts are used routinely to set the desired projection and re-establish support. Cartilage harvest is performed in open rhinoplasty after nasal cartilage exposure, anterior septal angle dissection, dorsal reduction, and completion of any adjunct interventions. In patients with unusable septal cartilage or those who have had a prior septoplasty, fresh frozen rib cartilage is preferred.[47]

The use of cartilage grafts to create or restore support to the tip paralleled the evolution of the tripod concept. By deconstructing and rebuilding the nose, structure is maintained, which improves predictability. Columellar strut and the SEGs serve to bolster the medial crura of the LLC to rotate and project the tip. Although the columellar strut is effective in unifying the nasal tip and maintaining position, it has not been shown to be as effective at maintaining projection.[48–50] Therefore, a columellar strut graft is used primarily in patients who have weak, asymmetric, or short LLC but otherwise have sufficient tip projection and rotation. Importantly, when using a columellar strut alone the surgeon must account for mild loss of projection during healing.

Conversely, an SEG can control tip projection, rotation, and shape effectively by securing the nasal tip to the septum. When using a SEG, the surgeon can expect the tip to remain where it is placed without need for compensatory overprojection. The stable central unit provided by a SEG allows tensioning of the lateral crura, which enables flattening, eversion, and optimization of LLC shape.

The SEG enables the surgeon to deconstruct the nose, resect dorsal and caudal septum, divide and manipulate the LLCs, and tension the new construct on a stable platform at the desired projection and rotation. The positioning of the SEG on the septum determines tip projection and rotation as follows:

- The batten-type SEG is placed unilaterally at the anterior septal angle, contralateral to any identified tip deviation.
  - Approximately 1 cm to 1.5 cm of septal-SEG overlap
  - The SEG should extend above the septum and beyond the expected final tip position.
- Angulation of the SEG is at 45° to 100° relative to the dorsum (**Fig. 1**A).
  - Angulation greater than or equal to 90° rotates and shortens the nose.
  - Angulation of 45° derotates and lengthens the nose.
- Four sutures are placed at the base of the SEG: 2 placed centrally to secure and 2 placed laterally to prevent rotation[51] (**Fig. 1**B).

After the SEG has been secured, modifications to the LLC (transection and overlap or use of the native LLC) are made, as indicated. If transection and neo-LLC creation is desired (as is the case with significant LLC redundancy at the desired projection), the native LLC are widely undermined to achieve mobility and exposure for division. Either the medial crura then are divided at their weakest point (which usually is the junction of the medial and middle crura), overlapped 3 mm to 6 mm, and repaired with 5-0 Vicryl suture before forming the tip complex, or alternatively, the new tip complex is secured to the SEG first and division is performed at the area of bowing and repaired.

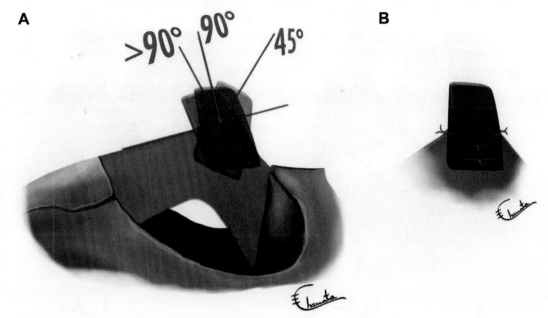

Fig. 1. (*A*) Angulation of the SEG relative to the dorsum sets tip rotation; 90° and greater yields increased rotation, whereas 45° derotates the nose. (*B*) The SEG is secured with 4 key sutures with adequate septal overlap to prevent movement. All figures previously have been published by Dr. Rohrich and he retains the copyright. Permission is granted to publish all included figures in this article, however, Dr. Rohrich requests the retention of his copyright to all of the figures. (*Courtesy of* Rod Rohrich, MD, Dallas, TX.)

Dividing medially rather than laterally avoids lateral alar notching while also the overlap provides the benefit of a thicker, strengthened medial support. The native LLC versus neo-LLC configuration is demonstrated in **Fig. 2**.

The native LLC or neo-LLC construct ultimately is tensioned to the SEG and set in the desired position before the skin is redraped to assess projection. Adjustments are made as required to accomplish ideal tip projection and rotation. Subsequent tip suturing techniques provide greatly improved shape, while the fixed-floating SEG maintains the tip position.

Refining the Tip

With the projection and rotation of the tip set and support re-established, additional transdomal and interdomal tip sutures are placed to achieve the ideal straight, everted, and diamond-shaped nasal tip (**Fig. 3**). Tip grafting seldom is performed in cases of deprojection. In general, visible tip grafts should be used only after maximizing all suturing and invisible grafting techniques. This situation is most likely to arise in men, secondary rhinoplasty, and ethnic patients with thick nasal skin.

The final step in achieving an optimally shaped and positioned nasal tip is management of the soft tissue. This component of the procedure involves closure of dead space created by changes in the osseocartilaginous framework. Medial crura footplate suturing and mattress sutures through the membranous septum and SEG are uniformly employed. Additionally, if significant redundancy of the septal mucosa is identified, a conservative wedge excision is performed. Finally, any skin redundancy at the columella, alar bases, and nostril sills then is excised.[44,52] In cases of considerable deprojection, excision at 1 or more of these areas is likely.

Putting it all together: 5 steps of rebuilding the tip

1. Secure the fixed-floating SEG along the caudal border of the septum.
   - SEG length sets projection (redrape to assess).
   - SEG angulation sets rotation and length (45°–100°).
   - LLC is brought to length manually at desired projection against the secured SEG to determine if transection is required.
2. The LLC or neo-LLC constructs is brought to length, stabilized with medial crura sutures, and secured to the SEG in a stepwise fashion.
   - The domal segments of each are secured to the SEG at desired projection.

A

B

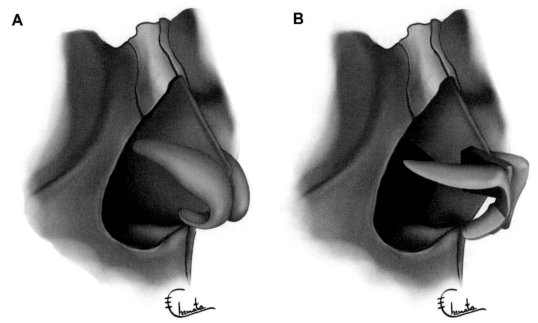

Fig. 2. (*A*) Native LLC configuration. (*B*) Neo-LLC configuration with flat, straight, everted lateral crura and medial crural transection/overlap. All figures previously have been published by Dr. Rohrich and he retains the copyright. Permission is granted to publish all included figures in this article, however, Dr. Rohrich requests the retention of his copyright to all of the figures. (*Courtesy of* Rod Rohrich, MD, Dallas, TX.)

- Excess or redundant SEG is trimmed flush to the new tip construct.
- Any discrepancies should be addressed before proceeding by either adjustment of the SEG or adjustments to the repaired LLC-construct.
3. Complete additional transdomal and interdomal tip suturing to achieve ideal tip aesthetics.
   - Superolateral obliquely oriented transdomal and horizontally oriented interdomal sutures both traverse the SEG and add additional support while shaping the tip (see **Fig. 3**).
   - Goal is a diamond shape with the caudal aspect more projected than the cephalic aspect.
4. Adjunct grafting is applied, as indicated.
   - Infratip butterfly grafts commonly are used to reduce soft triangle dead space.
   - Tip grafts may be added as needed for additional projection or tip softening.
   - Columellar strut grafts occasionally are added if required for volume (eg, retracted columella) or if dead space has been created from a downward angled SEG (eg, lengthening the nose with an SEG at 45°).
5. Advanced final tip shaping sutures are applied and soft tissue managed.
   - Alar equalization stitch: used to medialize the lateral crura at the supratip break

- Indicated if the lateral crura continue to bow laterally or peridomal fullness remains
- A 3-point horizontal mattress suture is passed through the midcolumella, each lateral crura medial margin (at the point of anticipated supratip break), and again through the starting point on the columella,

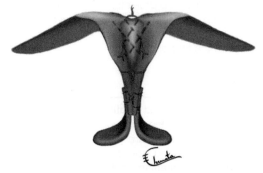

Fig. 3. Ideal diamond tip configuration with transdoman and interdomal sutures. Additionally, transection/overlap of the medial crura is shown after repair. All figures previously have been published by Dr. Rohrich and he retains the copyright. Permission is granted to publish all included figures in this article, however, Dr. Rohrich requests the retention of his copyright to all of the figures. (*Courtesy of* Rod Rohrich, MD, Dallas, TX.)

where it is tensioned and secured as to gently medialize the lateral crura.

- Supratip securing suture: used to further eliminate dead space and emphasize contour at the supratip break
  - Indicated only in thick-skinned or secondary rhinoplasty patients
  - A 3-point horizontal mattress cable suture, placed through the midcolumella, grasps the remnants of Pitanguy ligament on the underside of the nasal skin at the supratip break region, and again back through the columella, where it is gently tensioned and tied.
- Closure and excision of any redundant tissue of the mucosa, columella, alar bases, or nostril sills

SUMMARY

Reduction and refinement of the nasal tip require a thorough understanding of the dynamic anatomy, detailed preoperative and intraoperative nasal analysis, and an incremental operative approach. The tripod concept laid the foundation for managing projection and rotation of the nasal tip whereas parallel advances in the use of cartilage grafts have enabled surgeons to deconstruct and rebuild the nose without sacrificing structural support. Combining these maneuvers with tip suturing techniques and management of the soft tissue results in the straight, everted, and diamond-shaped ideal nasal tip. Adherence to this algorithmic approach is a basis for consistently excellent results.

CLINICS CARE POINTS

- The tripod concept is a helpful model for understanding the dynamic relationship between tip projection, rotation, and nasal length.
- Major structures of tip support include fibrous connection of the lateral crura to the ULC and medial crura to the caudal septum and maxillary spine, abutment of the lateral crura at the pyriform rim, and the interdomal suspensory ligament.
- Minor structures of tip support include fibrous attachments of the alar cartilage to the dorsum and skin and the membranous septum.
- Tip pseudo-overprojection must be ruled out preoperatively by assessing nasal and non-nasal contributing factors.

- When planning tip deprojection, it is essential to consider the contributing factors as the operative plan is developed. Each factor then must be addressed incrementally.
- The degree of tip deprojection that can be achieved is limited in a thick-skinned patient.
- The use of an SEG allows the tip to be deconstructed and rebuilt without sacrificing structural support.
- Final tip refinement after setting projection and rotation enables the achievement of the straight, everted, and diamond-shaped ideal nasal tip.

FINANCIAL DISCLOSURES

No funding was received for this article. Dr R. Rohrich receives instrument royalties from Eriem Surgical, Inc., and book royalties from Thieme Medical Publishing; he is a clinical and research study expert for Allergan, Inc.; Galderma; and MTF Biologics and the owner of Medical Seminars of Texas, LLC. Drs M. Novak and J. Bellamy have no financial disclosures.

REFERENCES

1. Sieber DA, Rohrich RJ. Finesse in nasal tip refinement. Plast Reconstr Surg 2017;140(2):10.
2. Toriumi DM. New concepts in nasal tip contouring. Arch Facial Plast Surg 2006;8(3):136–85.
3. Adamson PA, Funk E. Nasal tip dynamics. Facial Plast Surg Clin North Am 2009;17(1):29–40, vi.
4. Gruber RP, Weintraub J, Pomerantz J. Suture techniques for the nasal tip. Aesthet Surg J 2008;28(1): 92–100.
5. Cochran CS, Afrooz PN. A Simplified approach to nasal tip shaping: the five-suture technique. Plast Reconstr Surg 2020;145(4):938–42.
6. Behmand RA, Ghavami A, Guyuron B. Nasal tip sutures Part I: the evolution. Plast Reconstr Surg 2003; 112(4):1125–9.
7. Guyuron B, Behmand RA. Nasal tip sutures part II: the interplays. Plast Reconstr Surg 2003;112(4): 1130–45.
8. Lee MR, Geissler P, Cochran S, et al. Decreasing nasal tip projection in rhinoplasty. Plast Reconstr Surg 2014;134(1):41e–9e.
9. Rohrich RJ, Adams WP, Ahmad J, et al, editors. Dallas rhinoplasty: nasal surgery by the masters. 3rd edition. St. Louis, (MO): Quality Medical Publishing, Inc. ; CRC Press; 2014.
10. Nasenplastik und sonstige Gesichtsplastik, nebst einem Anhang über Mammaplastik und einige weitere Operationen aus dem Gebiete der ausseren

Körperplastik. By Prof. Dr. J. Joseph (Berlin). Imperial 8vo. Pp. 843 + xxxi, with 1718 illustrations, many in colour. 1931. Leipzig: Johann Barth and Curt Kabitzsch. RM. 242. Br J Surg 2005;19(74):341–2.

11. Safian J. Corrective rhinoplasty surgery. New York: P. Hoeber; 1935.

12. Smith TW. Reliable methods of tip reduction. Arch Otolaryngol 1978;104(10):564–9.

13. Kridel RWH, Konior RJ. Dome Truncation for management of the overprojected nasal tip. Ann Plast Surg 1990;24(5):385–96.

14. Brennan HG. Dome-splitting technique in rhinoplasty with overlay of lateral crura. Arch Otolaryngol 1983;109(9):586–92.

15. Davidson TM. Aesthetic plastic surgery, vols I & II. By T. D. Rees, 1,068 pp, illus, W.B. Saunders Co., Philadelphia, PA, 1980. Vol. I $75.00 (455 pp), Vol. II $85.00 (613 pp). Head Neck Surg. 1983;5(4): 372-373.

16. Foda HMT. Alar Setback technique: a controlled method of nasal tip deprojection. Arch Otolaryngol Neck Surg 2001;127(11):1341.

17. Larrabee WF. The tripod concept. Arch Otolaryngol - Head Neck Surg 1989;115(10):1168–9.

18. Regaladobriz A. Cephalo-crural suture: a new way to deal with supratip fullness. Aesthet Surg J 2005; 25(5):481–8.

19. McCollough EG, English JL. A new twist in nasal tip surgery: an alternative to the Goldman tip for the wide or bulbous lobule. Arch Otolaryngol - Head Neck Surg 1985;111(8):524–9.

20. Tardy M, Patt B, Walter M. Transdomal suture refinement of the nasal tip: long-term outcomes. Facial Plast Surg 1993;9(04):275–84.

21. Daniel RK. Rhinoplasty: creating an aesthetic tip. A preliminary report. Plast Reconstr Surg 1987;80(6): 775–83.

22. Daniel RK. Rhinoplasty: a simplified, three-stitch, open tip suture technique. Part I: primary rhinoplasty. Plast Reconstr Surg 1999;103(5):1491–502.

23. Tebbetts JB. Rethinking the logic and techniques of primary tip rhinoplasty. A perspective of the evolution of surgery of the nasal tip. Clin Plast Surg 1996;23(2):245–53.

24. Tebbetts JB. Shaping and positioning the nasal tip without structural disruption: a new, Systematic approach. Plast Reconstr Surg 1994;94(1):61–77.

25. Cochran CS, Sieber DA. Extended alar contour grafts: an evolution of the lateral crural strut graft technique in rhinoplasty. Plast Reconstr Surg 2017; 140(4):559e–67e.

26. Dosanjh AS, Hsu C, Gruber RP. The hemitransdomal suture for narrowing the nasal tip. Ann Plast Surg 2010;64(6):708–12.

27. Kridel RWH, Konior RJ. Controlled nasal tip rotation via the lateral crural overlay technique. Arch Otolaryngol - Head Neck Surg 1991;117(4):411–5.

28. Kridel RWH, Konior RJ, Shumrick KA, et al. Advances in nasal tip surgery: the lateral crural steal. Arch Otolaryngol - Head Neck Surg 1989;115(10):1206–12.

29. Byrd HS, Andochick S, Copit S, et al. Septal extension grafts: a method of controlling tip projection shape. Plast Reconstr Surg 1997;100(Supplement 1):999–1010.

30. Adams WP, Rohrich RJ, Hollier LH, et al. Anatomic basis and clinical implications for nasal tip support in open versus closed rhinoplasty. Plast Reconstr Surg 1999;103(1):255–61.

31. Soliemanzadeh P, Kridel RWH. Algorithm of surgical deprojection techniques and introduction of medial crural overlay. Arch Facial Plast Surg 2005;7:7374–80.

32. Rohrich RJ, Liu JH. Defining the infratip lobule in rhinoplasty: anatomy, pathogenesis of abnormalities, and correction using an algorithmic approach. Plast Reconstr Surg 2012;130(5):1148–58.

33. Rohrich RJ, Adams WP. The boxy nasal tip: classification and management based on alar cartilage suturing techniques. Plast Reconstr Surg 2001;107(7): 1849–63.

34. Cho GS, Kim JH, Yeo N-K, et al. Nasal skin thickness measured using computed tomography and its effect on tip surgery outcomes. Otolaryngol–Head Neck Surg 2011;144(4):522–7.

35. Brito ÍM, Avashia Y, Rohrich RJ. Evidence-based nasal analysis for rhinoplasty: the 10-7-5 method. Plast Reconstr Surg Glob Open 2020;8(2):e2632.

36. Gunter JP, Rohrich RJ. Lengthening the aesthetically short nose. Plast Reconstr Surg 1989;83(5):793–800.

37. Ghavami A, Janis JE, Acikel C, et al. Tip shaping in primary rhinoplasty: an algorithmic approach. Plast Reconstr Surg 2008;122(4):1229–41.

38. Simons R. Nasal tip projection, ptosis and supratip thicken- ing. Ear Nose Throat J 1982;61:452–5.

39. Baum S. Introduction. Ear Nose Throat J 1982;61: 426–8.

40. Powell N, Humphreys B. Proportions of the aesthetic face. New York: Thieme-Stratton; 1984.

41. Bailey B. Quantitative analysis of nasal tip projection. Laryngoscope 1993;103(12):1447–8.

42. Crumley RL, Lanser M. Quantitative analysis of nasal tip projection. The Laryngoscope 1988;98(2):202–8.

43. Byrd HS, Hobar PC. Rhinoplasty: a practical guide for surgical planning. Plast Reconstr Surg 1993; 91(4):642–54.

44. Rohrich RJ, Savetsky IL, Suszynski TM, et al. Systematic surgical approach to alar base surgery in rhinoplasty. Plast Reconstr Surg 2020;146(6): 1259–67.

45. Rohrich RJ, Malafa MM, Ahmad J, et al. Managing alar flare in rhinoplasty. Plast Reconstr Surg 2017; 140(5):910–9.

46. Rohrich RJ, Griffin JR. Correction of intrinsic nasal tip asymmetries in primary rhinoplasty. Plast Reconstr Surg 2003;112(6):1699–712.

47. Mohan R, Shanmuga Krishnan RR, Rohrich RJ. Role of fresh frozen cartilage in revision rhinoplasty. Plast Reconstr Surg 2019;144(3):614–22.

48. Sawh-Martinez R, Perkins K, Madari S, et al. Control of nasal tip position: quantitative Assessment of columellar strut versus caudal septal extension graft. Plast Reconstr Surg 2019;144(5):772e–80e.

49. Rohrich RJ, Durand PD, Dayan E. Changing role of septal extension versus columellar grafts in modern rhinoplasty. Plast Reconstr Surg 2020;145(5):927e–31e.

50. Ha RY, Byrd HS. Septal extension grafts revisited:: 6-year experience in controlling nasal tip projection and shape. Plast Reconstr Surg 2003;112(7): 1929–35.

51. Rohrich RJ, Savetsky IL, Avashia YJ. The role of the septal extension graft. Plast Reconstr Surg - Glob Open 2020;8(5):e2710.

52. Rohrich RJ, Afrooz PN. Revisiting the alar-columellar relationship: classification and correction. Plast Reconstr Surg 2019;144(2):340–6.

Dorsal Hump Reduction and Midvault Reconstruction

Bryan J. Pyfer, MD, MBA*, Andrew N. Atia, MD, Jeffrey R. Marcus, MD

KEYWORDS

- Rhinoplasty • Dorsal reduction • Hump reduction • Component reduction • Midvault reconstruction
- Spreader grafts • Spreader flaps

KEY POINTS

- Thorough preoperative examination is critical for determining the surgical plan; although the approach should be catered to each patient, well-established aesthetic ideals can serve as a starting point.
- A stepwise approach to deconstruct, reduce, and then reconstruct the nose should be used.
- Adequate reconstruction of the midvault is paramount to achieving optimal long-term functional and aesthetic results.
- The use of spreader grafts or spreader flaps, as determined by specific indications, helps maintain internal nasal valve patency and a pleasing dorsal profile.

INTRODUCTION

Rhinoplasty patients present with a wide variety of preoperative concerns, one of the most common of which is the nasal dorsum.[1] The dorsum is generally considered to be the area of the nose composed of the nasal bones superiorly, the anterior portion of the cartilaginous septum, and the upper lateral cartilages. Manipulation of the dorsum during rhinoplasty has tremendous impact on nasal function and cosmesis. The upper lateral cartilages are a critical component of the internal nasal valve as well as serve as a structural bridge between the rigid nasal bones superiorly and the more mobile lower lateral cartilages, tip, and alae inferiorly; rarely can one manipulate one part of the dorsum without causing changes in one or several other parts of the nose. These secondary changes must be anticipated and addressed at the time of the index operation to prevent negative long-term sequelae. This article describes the most relevant principles of management of the nasal dorsum, particularly as it pertains to conventional (nonpreservation) hump reduction and midvault reconstruction.

HISTORICAL CONTEXT AND BACKGROUND

Although it remains a matter of some debate, the father of modern cosmetic rhinoplasty is widely considered to be Jacques Joseph from Berlin, Germany, who first described his external reduction rhinoplasty technique in 1898.[2] As a means primarily to reduce a dorsal hump, his reduction rhinoplasty technique was originally described as a full-length en bloc resection of the apex of the nose, including the cartilage and its underlying mucosa, as well as the nasal bones superiorly (**Fig. 1**).

Reduction rhinoplasty in this manner was difficult to control and had high potential for both acute and long-term sequelae, both functionally and cosmetically. Particularly, these nasal reductions can result in asymmetry, open roof deformity, inverted V deformity, or an excessively wide or narrow midvault with subsequent internal valve

Division of Plastic, Maxillofacial, and Oral Surgery, Duke University Hospital, 40 Medicine Circle, DUMC 3974, Durham, NC 27710, USA
* Corresponding author.
E-mail address: Bryan.pyfer@duke.edu

Clin Plastic Surg 49 (2022) 81–95
https://doi.org/10.1016/j.cps.2021.07.011
0094-1298/22/© 2021 Elsevier Inc. All rights reserved.

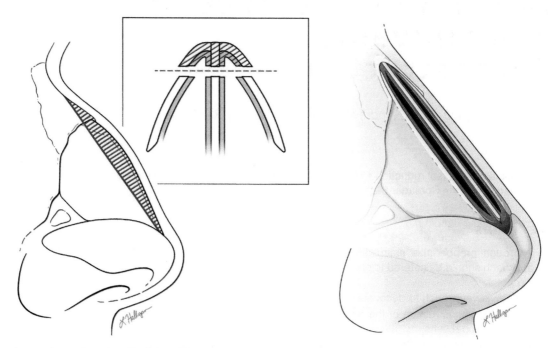

Fig. 1. The earliest described dorsal hump reductions were performed via en bloc resection of the apex of the nasal dorsum, including cartilage and bone with underlying mucosa. (Illustrated by Lauren Halligan, CMI; copyright Duke University; with permission under a CC BY-ND 4.0 license.)

narrowing and functional obstruction, among other issues.[3] At the time of Joseph, understanding of the nasal support construct concluded that the nasal bones, the midline cartilaginous septum, and the upper lateral cartilages were, in fact, fused. This no doubt was the reason that he described reduction of a single segment of dorsum. It was not until the 1950s that the theory began to be reconsidered, and even over the next several decades rhinoplasty experts continued to debate on the topic.[4–6]

By the 1980s, the nose was understood to be a construct of delicately interconnected but separate parts, namely nasal skin and soft tissue, paired upper and lower lateral cartilages, cartilaginous nasal septum, and paired nasal bones, all held closely together with dense fibrous attachments. Reduction rhinoplasty technique evolved from en bloc resection performed with endonasal (closed) technique to component reduction, with separation and reduction of only those individual parts responsible for causing the deformity.[7] Conceptually, the sequence was a stepwise deconstruction of the nasal components, with subsequent modification and reconstitution of those supportive elements. To accomplish this more structural approach, momentum shifted to open technique as the predominant exposure.[8] Until recently, where there is now a resurgence of interest in preservation techniques

often done endonasally, the open technique provided a means to facilitate deconstruction and reconstruction.

Component reduction has proven to be adaptable and precise; it can be carefully catered to individual variances in anatomy and in desired aesthetic result. Although some people may still refer to any dorsal reduction as the "Joseph Hump Reduction," most modern surgical techniques to address the dorsal hump are, in fact, different from those that Joseph originally described.

PREOPERATIVE EVALUATION

Effective hump reduction requires thorough preoperative patient evaluation. Although discussion of the full preoperative analysis of the nose before rhinoplasty is beyond the scope of this article, it is important to highlight some key considerations when evaluating the dorsum in particular. Addressing the nasal dorsum must consider each patient individually, especially with regard to the patient's gender, ethnicity, and functional or aesthetic concerns. Yet, there is an abundance of well-published and widely accepted aesthetic "ideals" as determined by centuries of facial metric analyses; these can serve as a starting point when evaluating the nasal dorsum.

Frontal Profile

From a frontal view of the face, the aesthetically ideal dorsum is straight; a straight line drawn from nasion to nasal tip should be vertical and should symmetrically bisect both sides of the nose. The outline of the nose should follow well-defined dorsal aesthetic lines. These diverging concave lines originate from the superomedial bony orbit and continue down the glabella to the keystone region, where they begin to gently diverge as they continue inferiorly to the middle crura of the lower lateral cartilages (**Fig. 2**). In addition, the width of the bony vault should be approximately 80% of the alar width, or 80% of the intercanthal distance[9] (see **Fig. 2**).

Lateral Profile

From a lateral view, one should evaluate the position of the radix, the nasofrontal angle, and the shape of the dorsum. The ideal vertical position of the radix for Caucasian and European noses is between the supratarsal fold and the margin of the upper eyelid,[10] although this is commonly as low as the mid-pupil in Asian or African American patients.[11,12] The radix should sit approximately 11 mm anterior to the corneal plane and 15 mm anterior to the medial canthus.[9] A deeper or lower radix would give the appearance of a short nose

and can exacerbate dorsal convexity. A shallow or high radix gives the appearance of a long nose.

The nasofrontal angle lies at the intersection of one line drawn tangential to the glabella through the nasion and another line drawn tangential to the nasal dorsum. The ideal angle for this ranges from 115° to 130°.[13] Last, the shape of the dorsum in men should follow a straight line from the radix to the nasal tip, and in woman should follow just 2 mm posterior to that line to account for a supratip break and resulting slight dorsal concavity (**Fig. 3**). Dorsal reduction is designed to accommodate the desire for supratip break by carefully planning the position of the tip-defining points (most projecting point of the tip at the genu) relative to the anterior septal angle. Therefore the 2 maneuvers that most strongly influence the supratip region and that must be balanced concurrently are dorsal reduction and support of the tip.

Dorsal humps come in many shapes and sizes, with some more cephalad and osseous in nature, some more caudal and cartilaginous in nature, and some with profound asymmetries (**Fig. 4**). In addition to visual inspection, preoperative palpation provides a set of expectations for the operating room and helps guide a surgeon's operative plan relative to the reconstruction stage following deconstruction and reduction. For instance, short nasal bones, weak or depressed upper lateral cartilages, and a tall thin dorsal

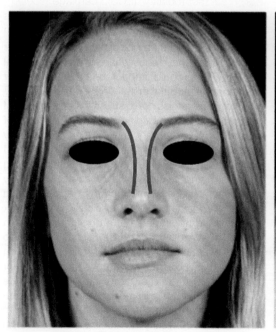
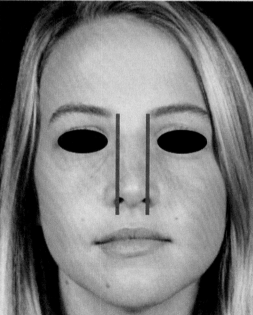

Fig. 2. The ideal nasal dorsum follows gently diverging dorsal aesthetic lines (*left*). The ideal width of the bony dorsum is 80% of the alar width, or 80% of the intercanthal distance (*right*).

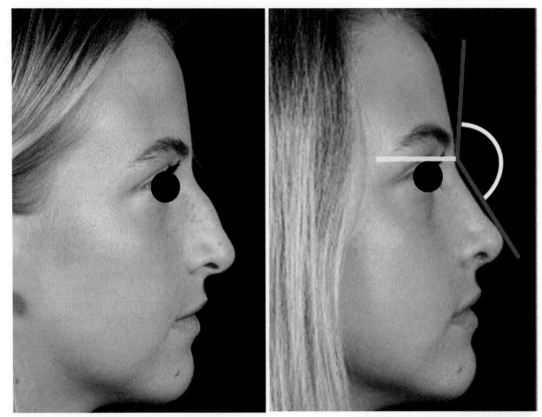

Fig. 3. Preoperative lateral facial profile with prominent dorsal hump (*left*). Postoperative lateral facial profile after open component reduction of the nasal dorsum (*right*). The ideal position of the radix lies between the supratarsal fold and the upper eyelid margin (*yellow line*). The optimal nasofrontal angle (*red lines*) is between 115 and 130°. The ideal female dorsum lies 2 mm behind a line drawn from the radix to the nasal tip, allowing for a gentle supratrip break and slight dorsal concavity.

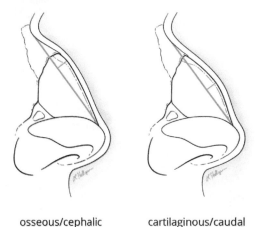

osseous/cephalic   cartilaginous/caudal

Fig. 4. Doral humps are usually a combination of cartilaginous and osseous components, but often one predominates. On the left is a hump more cephalad and osseous in nature, and on the right is more caudal and predominantly cartilaginous. (Illustrated by Lauren Halligan, CMI; copyright Duke University; with permission under a CC BY-ND 4.0 license.)

hump are all indications for placement of spreader grafts, which may require harvest from the nasal septum. This could impact one's approach or sequence of surgical maneuvers during the case.

It would be remiss not to stress the importance of a complete and thorough evaluation of all parts of the nose before surgery, even if the patient's only complaint is a dorsal hump. Insufficiencies of some parts of the nose may fool one into thinking a dorsal hump exists when it does not, or it may deceivingly cause a mild hump to appear much bigger than it actually is. Classically, a low radix can give the appearance of a dorsal hump, when the radix, in fact, needs to be raised. Those who currently advocate nonsurgical rhinoplasty with the use of fat or fillers take advantage of low or borderline low radix to camouflage the existence of a dorsal hump by filling cephalad to it.[14,15] Similarly someone with a ptotic nasal tip may appear to have dorsal convexity and complain of a dorsal hump, when in fact, they only need tip support. One must identify and address factors causing a "pseudo-hump" before committing to reduce the dorsum so that the dorsum is not over-reduced[16] (**Figs. 5** and **6**, **Table 1**).

GOALS AND CONSIDERATIONS

The goals of dorsal hump reduction are to alter to the dorsum to comply with the patient's desires and the previously described aesthetic "ideals" while preventing further deformity. Particularly, one must maintain mucosal integrity, ensure against future midvault collapse, maintain internal nasal valve support and patency, preserve or reconstitute the keystone region to prevent an "inverted V" deformity, and prevent an open roof deformity without creating too wide a dorsum. Each of these considerations will be discussed as follows.

The surgeon should have an idea before making an incision how much dorsum to remove. Intraoperatively, subjective judgment by the surgeon is ultimately a critical element. There are also tools that can aid in the process, including presurgical digital photographic morphing, 3-dimensional analysis, physical modeling, and simple photographic analysis. It is the authors' practice to hang full-page, preoperative patient photographs on the wall of the operating room, as well as lateral view morphed projection for intraoperative reference, as local anesthesia and edema have a tendency to blunt one's intraoperative assessment.

SURGICAL TECHNIQUE
Authors' Technique for Open Approach

In the senior author's (J.R.M) practice, the open approach is used in 80% of cases. The skin of the nasal tip is elevated bluntly using a cotton-tipped applicator in combination with fine, sharp scissors. Over the domes, the sub-perichondrial plane is elevated to the supratip region. The Pitanguy ligament is isolated and divided, as are the scroll ligaments; these may be reapproximated at conclusion. The sub-perichondrial plane is continued over the cartilaginous dorsum. At the caudal edge of the nasal bones, this is elevated in continuity with the subperiosteal plane (**Fig. 7**).

Bone First? Or Cartilage First?

The dorsal hump has cartilaginous and osseous components. The question arises as to which of

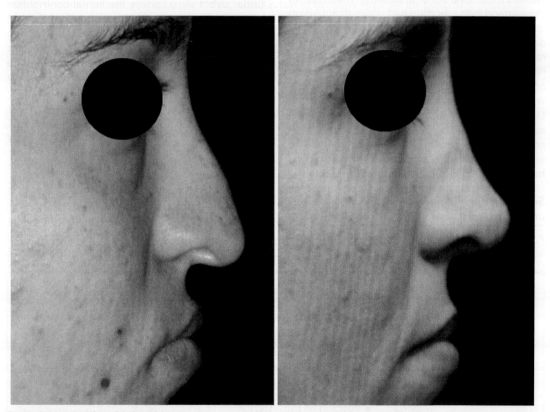

Fig. 5. Patient with mild dorsal hump that is exacerbated by a ptotic nasal tip (*left*). Hump reduction before achieving tip support resulted in a slight over-reduction of the dorsum and exaggerated supratip break once the tip was raised to an optimal position (*right*).

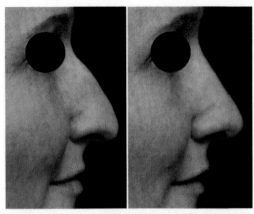

Fig. 6. Patient with an over-projected dorsum with a moderate dorsal hump that is exacerbated by a ptotic nasal tip (*left*). Judicious hump reduction with concurrent tip elevation and de-projection resulted in a pleasing dorsal profile (*right*).

these should be reduced first. In a traditional component reduction, the cartilaginous dorsum is reduced first as noted later in this article. However, some surgeons, including the senior author herein, perform the osseous reduction first. This is typically done using a powered instrument such as a diamond bur or piezotome, which allows the surgeon with precision and under direct vision to take down the osseous hump, leaving the underline upper lateral cartilages fully intact. The result in this sequence is a completely cartilaginous keystone (**Fig. 8**). It permits total preservation of the upper lateral cartilages, which are useful when closing the midvault later in the operation. Up to a moderate-sized hump, the sequence is easily accomplished. With the largest humps, it is sometimes not possible to see over the top to accomplish this technique, so the cartilaginous hump should be addressed first.

Separation of the Cartilaginous Components and Mucosa

As the tip is retracted inferiorly, the anterior septal angle is identified. The anterior septal angle is the gateway to the dorsum, indicating the position of the caudal edge of the upper lateral cartilage. The caudal septum is lightly scored to permit identification and then elevation of the submucoperichondrial plane. Using a blunt elevator, the entire right side of the septum is elevated extending inferiorly along the maxillary crest, posteriorly to the perpendicular plate, and anteriorly along the junction of the upper lateral cartilages with the dorsal aspect of the septum. At this site, the ligamentous attachments of the upper lateral cartilage to the septum are identified. Using a sharp scissor, the upper lateral cartilage is then separated from the septum (**Fig. 9**). On the left side, the upper lateral cartilage is again identified, and elevation of the mucoperichondrium is again carried out but to a more limited extent. The upper lateral cartilage is freed from the septum on the left, but the elevation only is done such that it would permit the component reduction of the septal hump and allow placement of either spreader graft or spreader flaps (**Fig. 10**). Otherwise, mucosal attachments remain intact to the septum.

Reduction of the Cartilaginous Septum

Under direct visualization, the septal contribution to the hump is reduced. Based on the plan set forth before operation and on analysis, the septum is marked to indicate the extent of reduction. It is important that the leading edge of the dorsum be a clean edge. Therefore, resection is done with a straight and sharp instrument. The use of a Number 11 blade with the tip broken off will allow for the creation of a straight edge. Sharp straight or angled scissors similarly provide the necessary means (**Fig. 11**). It is important to note that alterations in the quadrangular cartilage (cartilaginous septum), including dorsal and caudal reductions, be performed before septoplasty or septal cartilage harvest. When septal cartilage is removed, a dorsal and caudal "L" strut of 10 to 15 mm should be maintained to support the dorsum. If septal cartilage harvest is performed before reductive

Table 1
Considerations at preoperative examination

Frontal View	Lateral View	Palpation
• Straightness of the dorsum • Dorsal aesthetic lines • Width of the bony pyramid and middle third	• Position of the radix • Nasofrontal angle • Shape of the dorsum and degree of over-projection • Position of the anterior septal angle • Degree of tip ptosis	• Nasal bone height and width • Upper lateral cartilage strength, width • Thickness of skin/soft tissue envelope

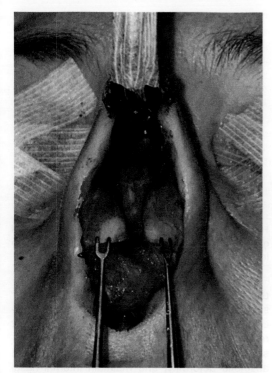

Fig. 7. Complete exposure of the nasal dorsum is paramount to obtaining adequate reduction. Exposure should extend from the tip to the bony radix.

modifications, the dimensions of the resulting L-strut will be reduced and can result in future saddle-nose deformity and/or midvault collapse.

Bony Reduction

Osseous reduction may be done with a variety of instruments, and it is not the intent herein to advocate for a particular method. Small to moderate humps may be addressed fairly easily with a series of graded Fomon rasps. Traditional use

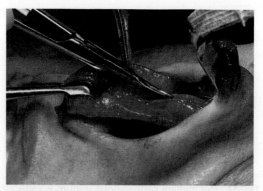

Fig. 9. The upper lateral cartilage is sharply separated from the cartilaginous septum.

of double-side guarded osteotome is an option in any instance, but particularly for large osseous humps. Powered instruments such as diamond bur or piezotome require relatively more subperiosteal exposure, but facilitate a gradual and controlled reduction (**Fig. 12**). Bony reduction should be judicious; over-resection of nasal bones is difficult to correct. In addition, extreme care must be taken to preserve the keystone region. It is important to avoid disrupting the attachments of the upper lateral cartilage with the nasal bones. This can result in the loss of support for the cartilaginous midvault as well as a visible concavity at the junction of bone and cartilage. Midvault reconstruction with spreader flaps or grafts may not be able to eliminate the contour deformity that can result from upper lateral detachment. In the authors' opinion, it is this particular problem that provides the strongest incentive for consideration of "dorsal preservation" techniques.[17] With any technique, it is also important to fully retract and protect the nasal soft tissue during bony reduction.

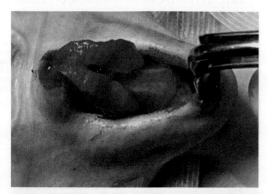

Fig. 8. Reduction of the osseous component of the dorsal hump first allows for preservation of the cartilaginous keystone region.

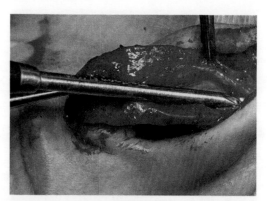

Fig. 10. The mucoperichondrium is elevated off the cartilaginous septum to allow room for the use of spreader grafts or spreader flaps.

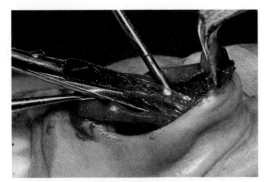

Fig. 11. The midline cartilaginous septum is reduced sharply.

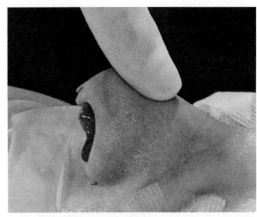

Fig. 13. Manual palpation with a saline-moistened gloved finger should be performed frequently to identify contour irregularities.

Frequent Verification

The nasal skin and soft tissue should be redraped over the dorsum frequently to verify dorsal height, shape, and contour. The dorsum should be manually palpated with a saline-moistened gloved finger to identify contour irregularities (**Fig. 13**). Operative edema or a thick skin and soft tissue envelope may hide abnormalities that cannot be appreciated visually on the operating table, but become increasingly apparent weeks to months after surgery.

Reduction of the Upper Lateral Cartilages

Following dorsal hump reduction by a component technique, excess upper lateral cartilage will be present to a variable extent depending on the size of the dorsal hump. If direct repair of the midvault or spreader graft reconstruction is to be performed, there may be such redundancy that is necessary to trim excess upper lateral cartilage (**Fig. 14**).

Midvault Reconstruction

Any dorsal reduction necessitates reconstruction of the nasal midvault. As compared with en bloc

dorsal resection, component reduction allows for several available options that can be catered specifically to each patient. The goals of midvault reconstruction are to restore nasal stability, preserve the dorsal aesthetic lines, prevent nasal aesthetic deformity, and maintain internal nasal valve competence. Typically, reconstruction is performed by 1 of 3 common techniques: (1) primary closure of the upper lateral cartilages, (2) placement of spreader grafts, or (3) placement of turnover (or spreader or auto-spreader) flaps. In each instance, the upper lateral cartilages and grafts or flaps, if present, are secured to the midline nasal septum. The literature is replete with indications for each technique, and these are discussed later herein.[18–20]

Osteotomies

Are osteotomies universally required following dorsal hump reduction? It depends on 3 factors: the size of the hump, the aesthetic width of the upper third, and the presence of a visible or palpable

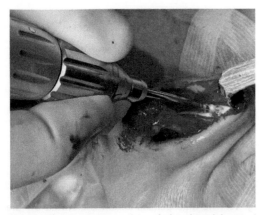

Fig. 12. The osseous portion of the dorsal hump is judiciously reduced with a powered diamond burr.

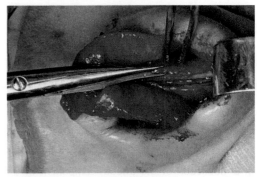

Fig. 14. Judicious trimming of the upper lateral cartilage is performed as needed.

open roof. The first of these, size, bears relevance because resection of a large hump will likely result in either or both of the subsequent factors. A dorsal hump is narrower at its apex than it is at its base. Therefore, the perceptible width of the dorsum becomes wider after the hump is removed (**Fig. 15**). The predicted width of the upper third must be considered in the plan. A patient with a large hump who is comfortable with the appearance of dorsal width may be dissatisfied if that proportionality changes. In such case, osteotomy and infracture intend to preserve width proportions. An open roof in the past (in true Joseph method) meant that composite resection including mucosa resulted in communication with the nasal cavity itself under the skin (see **Fig. 1**). Nowadays, the mucosa is preserved, therefore there is no true "open roof," as it had been originally coined; but there can be a visible and palpable open space where the bone was resected.

After reduction of a small dorsal hump, infracture is not needed if there is little to no osseous defect (no open roof) and if the width of the upper third is aesthetically acceptable. If the osseous defect is large enough that it cannot be repaired to a smooth contour with spreader grafts or flaps and/or if the upper third is wider than desired, then osteotomies and medialization of the nasal bones are necessary. Classically, lateral osteotomies can be performed in the "low-low," "low-high," or "high-low-high" fashion (**Fig. 16**). These classifications are termed according to their starting and ending positions on the bony nasal sidewall. Low refers to a lateral position closer to the facial plane, and high refers to a more medial position, higher on the lateral nasal wall. These can be performed from intranasal, transcutaneous, or even buccal sulcus approaches.

A low-low osteotomy starts at the base of the piriform aperture and ends lateral to the

nasomaxillary suture line. This technique mobilizes a larger segment of nasal bone and is used when trying to correct a large open roof deformity or when trying to narrow a very wide bony pyramid. It is also helpful to use when a patient has small nasal bones, as a high technique may not provide enough bone sufficient to close the defect. A low-high osteotomy is used when trying to close a small or medium open roof, or in a patient with large nasal bones, where there is ample nasal bone to sufficiently close the defect. A high-low-high osteotomy was introduced in 1970 by Webster and colleagues,[21] and is one of the most commonly performed osteotomies today. This starts in a slightly high position initially, and flares laterally to the maxillary groove along the middle of the osteotomy before returning to a high position just inferior to the nasofrontal suture. In all of the techniques, the mid-portion of the osteotomy (most of it) is relatively low—close to the facial plane—to avoid having a visible or palpable step off. The high-low-high technique leaves a triangle of bone inferiorly and anteriorly termed "Webster's Triangle" (see **Fig. 16**), which carries the presumed benefit of supporting the upper lateral cartilages. It also avoids medialization of the anterior head of the inferior turbinate, resulting in narrowing of the airway, although this point has been debated. In each of these techniques, it is important to not carry the osteotomy too far superiorly into the frontal bone, or a "rocker deformity" will result. This occurs after the osteotomy extends too far cephalically onto the frontal process of the nasal bones; when the nasal bones are medialized, and the superior portion of the bony segment is cantilevered or rocked laterally, creating bony contour deformity along the nasal root (**Box 1**).

DISCUSSION
Midvault Reconstruction

Following dorsal hump reduction, adequate midvault reconstruction is crucial to optimizing functional and aesthetic outcome. Inadequate support of the middle third of the nose can result in midvault collapse with saddle-nose deformity, inverted V deformity, dorsal asymmetries, contour abnormalities, and functional airway obstruction. Reduction rhinoplasty, by nature, decreases the cross-sectional area of the nasal airway and can narrow the internal nasal valve (INV). The normal angle of the apex of the INV (formed by the upper lateral cartilage and the midline nasal septum) ranges from 10 to 15°, and this can be inadvertently narrowed when resecuring the upper lateral cartilages back to the septum.[22,23] Early reports in

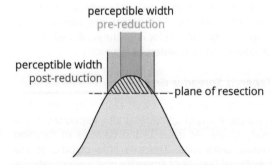

Fig. 15. Because the dorsal hump is narrower at its apex than at its base, it's perceptible width increases after hump removal. (Illustrated by Lauren Halligan, CMI; copyright Duke University; with permission under a CC BY-ND 4.0 license.)

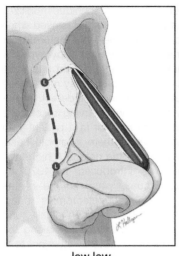 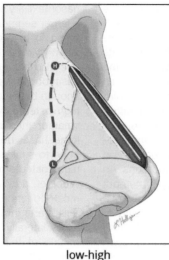 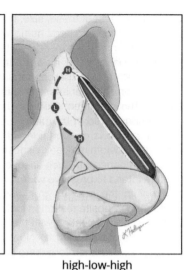

| low-low | low-high | high-low-high |

Fig. 16. Lateral osteotomies are made in 1 of 3 classic fashions: low-low, low-high, or high-low-high. The latter preserves the Webster Triangle, a small triangle of anteriorly projecting bone that helps support the upper lateral cartilages (*far right, shaded purple*). (Illustrated by Lauren Halligan, CMI; copyright Duke University; with permission under a CC BY-ND 4.0 license.)

the literature suggested that subjective airway impairment was present in as many as 10% of cosmetic rhinoplasty patients, with acoustic rhinometry measurements showing internal nasal valve area decreases of up to 25% after rhinoplasty.[24,25]

Box 1
Steps to dorsal reduction (external approach)

1. Elevate skin and soft tissue envelope to expose the lower lateral cartilages, upper lateral cartilages, and nasal bones up to the radix.

2. Sharply separate the upper lateral cartilages from the cartilaginous septum. Elevate mucoperichondrium on either side of the septum to the extent necessary for septal harvest/septoplasty and midvault repair with spreader grafts or flaps when needed.

3. Reduce the cartilaginous septum; this should be done before septal harvest.

4. Reduce the nasal bones.

5. Replace the skin and soft tissue envelope frequently and palpate with a saline-moistened gloved finger to verify a smooth dorsum and prevent contour abnormalities.

6. Reconstruct the midvault; use of spreader grafts or spreader flaps where indicated to avoid narrowing the dorsum and internal nasal valves.

7. Perform osteotomies with infracture to optimize the width of the upper third and to correct open roof deformity.

Spreader Grafts

As a remedy to many of the short-term and long-term sequelae of surgery of the nasal dorsum, the spreader graft was first introduced by Sheen[26] in 1984 and has since become one of the most common surgical techniques for midvault reconstruction (**Fig. 17**). The spreader graft is adaptable and versatile. Sheen[26] advised that certain anatomic conditions predisposed to midvault collapse after dorsal reduction: short nasal bones, weak upper lateral cartilages, thin skin, or combinations of these. Although his original work addressed sequelae, spreader grafts were later popularized in primary surgery as well. Primary applications have included prophylactic midvault support, correction of dorsal angulation, nasal lengthening, support for a fractured dorsal L-strut, or correction of unilateral asymmetry.

Tapered Spreader Grafts

There has been a renewed discussion regarding the indications of spreader grafts, especially in primary cases. At issue is the balance of function versus aesthetics. There is little dispute in the functional benefit of spreader grafts when valvular support is needed[27,28]; however, it has been argued that spreader grafts can create excess width in the middle third and can create sharp and overtly straight dorsal aesthetic lines. To

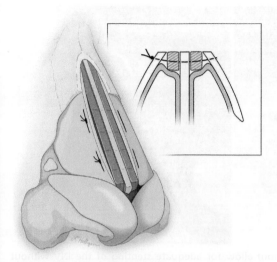

Fig. 17. Cartilage spreader grafts are placed between the medial upper lateral cartilage and the cartilaginous septum. (Illustrated by Lauren Halligan, CMI; copyright Duke University; with permission under a CC BY-ND 4.0 license.)

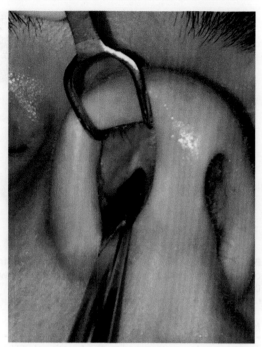

Fig. 18. The INV is bordered by the caudal edge of the upper lateral cartilage, the nasal septum, and the anterior portion of the inferior turbinate.

address aesthetic concerns, certain modifications have been described.[29–31] Tapered spreader grafts address width sequelae. Most septal cartilage specimens are thickest near their articulation with the perpendicular plate and are thinner caudally. Spreader grafts are designed on the longest dimension of the specimen, and therefore will have a gradation of thickness. The internal valve angle is formed by the junction of the upper lateral cartilage and the septum (**Fig. 18**).

However, the valve angle is not the INV. The INV is a cross-section, the site of minimal cross-sectional area; this flow-limiting cross-section lies at the caudal limit of the upper lateral cartilage as depicted. It does not extend the length of the midvault. Therefore, the thickest portion of a spreader graft should lie at the INV, where it is externally hidden beneath the supratip. The graft then tapers superiorly to the nasal bones. In this way, excessive widening of the midvault can be avoided (**Fig. 19**).

Recessed Spreader Grafts

Recessed spreader grafts are depicted in **Fig. 20**. These grafts are placed approximately 2 mm below the leading edge of the dorsal septum. The grafts are secured first to the septum on either side. The upper lateral cartilages are then placed on slight tension as they are pulled over the edge of the spreader graft and secured in the midline to the septum. The spreader graft acts as a

fulcrum, and the resulting tension acts to resist inward movement as a consequence of negative pressure generated in deep inspiration. For patients with weak or redundant upper lateral cartilage, this offers a mechanical advantage. In combination with graft tapering, this modification softens the contours of the dorsal edges to further facilitate creation of smooth dorsal aesthetic lines.

Auto-Spreader Flaps

Spreader flaps were designed to use the excess upper lateral cartilage for the purpose of repairing the midvault with greater support than would be provided by direct repair. The turnover auto-spreader flap technique was first described by Fomon in 1950,[32] but was re-introduced in 1992 by Wood,[33] and described further by Oneal and Burkowitz[34] shortly thereafter. Spreader flaps use the excess from the upper lateral cartilages to fold over and give the surgeon the opportunity to close the midvault with control over the width and internal aperture (**Fig. 21**). A primary advantage of the spreader flap over the spreader graft is that it obviates the need to harvest septal cartilage. It restores the continuity of the midvault with a natural contour. It is indicated in patients with dorsal hump reductions that result in an excess of upper lateral cartilage of at least 2 mm in order to perform the inward fold.

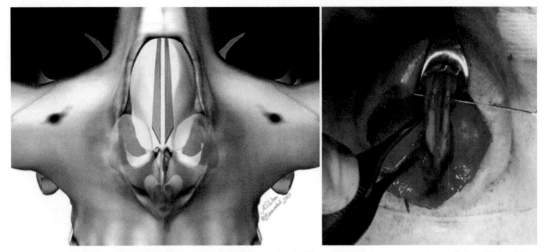

Fig. 19. Tapered spreader grafts (*green* in *left* illustration) allow for adequate stenting of the INV without creating overly straight dorsal aesthetic lines or too wide a dorsum (*right*). (*Courtesy of* Jeffrey R. Marcus, MD, Durham, NC [left illustration].)

Indications for Spreader Grafts Versus Flaps

There is controversy regarding the functional utility of spreader flaps for maintaining patency of the internal valve. Several investigators have attempted to demonstrate functional superiority of flaps or grafts, but all studies to date have failed to do so.[19,35,36] However, there are instances in which either spreader grafts or spreader flaps are presumed to have an advantage. For example, spreader grafts are, on average, thicker than spreader flaps. The width of the cartilaginous portion of the nasal septum near the base, from where most spreader grafts are taken, ranges from 2 to 3 mm on average.[37] The upper lateral cartilages, on the other hand, are usually no

more than 0.5 mm thick, although some investigators have suggested modifications to functionally "thicken" a turnover spreader flap.[38] Spreader grafts are used more frequently in instances of dorsal angulation, where the thicker, stronger graft can better withstand the forces of a curved septum, not to mention submucous septal resection (and hence available graft material) is frequently indicated as well. Spreader grafts, therefore, tend to be used with most dorsal asymmetries, including those involving concave upper lateral cartilages or even a deviated tip. Similarly, thin or weak upper lateral cartilages with inspiratory collapse and resulting functional obstruction often necessitate the thicker graft as well.

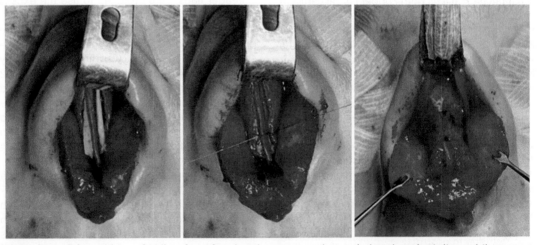

Fig. 20. Recessed spreader grafts allow for softer dorsal contours and smooth dorsal aesthetic lines while preventing too wide a dorsum.

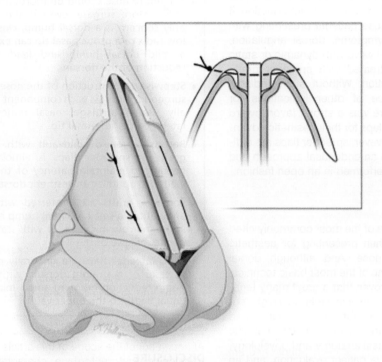

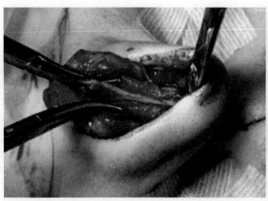 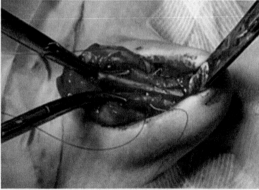

Fig. 21. After being detached from the septum, the medial upper lateral cartilages can be used as auto-spreader flaps (*above*). The upper lateral cartilages are turned inward (*bottom left*) and are then secured to the cartilaginous septum (*bottom right*). (Top image illustrated by Lauren Halligan, CMI; copyright Duke University; with permission under a CC BY-ND 4.0 license.)

Table 2 Considerations for use of spreader grafts versus spreader flaps	
Spreader Grafts	**Spreader Flaps**
• Dorsal angulation • Small dorsal hump (<2 mm) reduction with narrow midvault • Dynamic valve collapse (internal nasal valve [INV] collapse during inspiratory effort) • Static valve collapse (narrow INV resulting in obstruction unrelated to breathing cycle)	• Straight dorsum • Large dorsal hump (>2 mm) reduction • Midvault equal in width to upper vault following osteotomies

In a 2020 consensus paper regarding the repair of the midvault following dorsal hump reduction, it was advised that those patients presenting with nasal obstructive symptoms, dorsal angulation, and a narrow internal valve with dynamic or static valve collapse be treated with spreader grafts following the reduction. Without such findings, and in the absence of other indications for spreader grafts, there was a strong favor toward the use of spreader flaps for their aesthetic advantage (**Table 2**).[18] However, spreader flaps are difficult to perform from an endonasal approach and are almost always performed in an open fashion.

SUMMARY

A dorsal hump is one of the most commonly cited patient concerns when presenting for aesthetic evaluation of the nose. And although dorsal hump reduction is one of the most basic technical goals, history has proven that a great many technical nuances exist explaining a relatively high secondary revision rate. Effective dorsal hump reduction requires an appreciation for aesthetic ideals, mastery of nasal anatomy and physiology, thorough preoperative patient evaluation, and an understanding of each surgical maneuver as well as its secondary effects on the nose. These must be anticipated and addressed at the time of the index operation to prevent untoward sequelae that can be very distressing to patients. Component dorsal hump reduction allows for a tailored approach to each individual nose, where each maneuver can be performed with precision and control. Adequate reconstruction of the midvault is paramount to preventing many of the undesirable effects of rhinoplasty, including further aesthetic and functional deformities. The last several decades have far expanded the options for reconstruction of the midvault, including spreader grafts and spreader flaps, each with many modifications that can be catered to every type of nose. Comprehensive understanding of these concepts will allow for effective dorsal reduction that results in great patient and surgeon satisfaction.

CLINICS CARE POINTS

- Although the surgical approach to dorsal hump reduction should be catered to each patient's desired aesthetic or functional result, there is a well-established canon of aesthetic ideals that can be used to guide a surgeon's plan.

- The entire nose should be thoroughly evaluated before surgery, even if the patient's only concern is a dorsal hump; classically, a low radix or a ptotic nasal tip can exacerbate a mild dorsal hump and lead to over-reduction of the dorsum.

- Stepwise deconstruction of the nose allows a surgeon to address each component individually: septal cartilage, nasal bones, upper lateral cartilages, nasal tip.

- Reconstruction of midvault with spreader grafts or spreader flaps is almost always needed to maintain patency of the INV as well as to optimize an aesthetic dorsal profile.

- Spreader grafts are preferred with dorsal angulation, a small (<2 mm) hump reduction with a narrow midvault, or with static or dynamic collapse of the INV.

- Auto-spreader flaps are generally preferred in cases of a straight dorsum with a large hump reduction (>2 mm) and a midvault of equal width to the upper vault.

DISCLOSURE

J.R. Marcus receives royalties for intellectual property from Stryker for the SmartLock Hybrid MMF and royalties from Thieme Medical Publishing. The other authors have no other financial interest to declare in relation to the content of this article.

REFERENCES

1. Lee MR, Unger JG, Rohrich RJ. Management of the nasal dorsum in rhinoplasty: a systematic review of the literature regarding technique, outcomes, and complications. Plast Reconstr Surg 2011;128(5):538e–50e.

2. Eisenberg I. A history of rhinoplasty. S Afr Med J 1982;62(9):286–92.

3. Barrett DM, Casanueva F, Wang T. Understanding approaches to the dorsal hump. Facial Plast Surg 2017;33(2):125–32.

4. Straatsma BR, Straatsma CR. The anatomical relationship of the lateral nasal cartilage to the nasal bone and the cartilaginous nasal septum. Plast Reconstr Surg (1946) 1951;8(6):433–55.

5. Rees TD. Aesthetic plastic surgery. Philadelphia (PA): Saunders; 1980.

6. McKinney P, Johnson P, Walloch J. Anatomy of the nasal hump. Plast Reconstr Surg 1986;77(3):404–5.

7. Sheen JH. Aesthetic rhinoplasty. St. Louis (MO): Mosby; 1978.

8. Toriumi DM. Structure approach in rhinoplasty. Facial Plast Surg Clin North Am 2005;13(1):93–113.

9. Rohrich RJ, Muzaffar AR, Janis JE. Component dorsal hump reduction: the importance of maintaining dorsal aesthetic lines in rhinoplasty. Plast Reconstr Surg 2004;114(5):1298–308. discussion 309–12].

10. Aiach G, Laxenaire A, Vendroux J. Deepening the nasofrontal angle. Aesthetic Plast Surg 2002; 26(Suppl 1):S5.

11. Momoh AO, Hatef DA, Griffin A, et al. Rhinoplasty: the African American patient. Semin Plast Surg 2009;23(3):223–31.

12. Suhk J, Park J, Nguyen AH. Nasal analysis and anatomy: anthropometric proportional assessment in Asians-aesthetic balance from forehead to Chin, part I. Semin Plast Surg 2015;29(4):219–25.

13. Leong SC, White PS. A comparison of aesthetic proportions between the healthy Caucasian nose and the aesthetic ideal. J Plast Reconstr Aesthet Surg 2006;59(3):248–52.

14. Kassir R, Venkataram A, Malek A, et al. Non-Surgical Rhinoplasty: The Ascending Technique and a 14-Year Retrospective Study of 2130 Cases. Aesthetic Plast Surg 2021;45(3):1154–68.

15. Williams LC, Kidwai SM, Mehta K, et al. Nonsurgical rhinoplasty: a systematic review of technique, outcomes, and complications. Plast Reconstr Surg 2020;146(1):41–51.

16. Fattahi T, Sabooree S. New concepts in dorsal hump reduction. Oral Maxillofac Surg Clin North Am 2021; 33(1):31–7.

17. Saban Y, Daniel RK, Polselli R, et al. Dorsal preservation: the push down technique reassessed. Aesthet Surg J 2018;38(2):117–31.

18. Avashia YJ, Marshall AP, Allori AC, et al. Decision-making in middle vault reconstruction following dorsal hump reduction in primary rhinoplasty. Plast Reconstr Surg 2020;145(6):1389–401.

19. Rudy S, Moubayed SP, Most SP. Midvault reconstruction in primary rhinoplasty. Facial Plast Surg 2017;33(2):133–8.

20. Kovacevic M, Riedel F, Göksel A, et al. Options for middle vault and dorsum restoration after hump removal in primary rhinoplasty. Facial Plast Surg 2016;32(04):374–83.

21. Webster RC, Davidson TM, Smith RC. Curved lateral osteotomy for airway protection in rhinoplasty. Arch Otolaryngol 1977;103(8):454–8.

22. Ballert JA, Park SS. Functional considerations in revision rhinoplasty. Facial Plast Surg 2008;24(3): 348–57.

23. Kasperbauer JL, Kern EB. Nasal valve physiology. Implications in nasal surgery. Otolaryngol Clin North Am 1987;20(4):699–719.

24. Beekhuis GJ. Nasal obstruction after rhinoplasty: etiology, and techniques for correction. Laryngoscope 1976;86(4):540–8.

25. Grymer LF. Reduction rhinoplasty and nasal patency: change in the cross-sectional area of the nose evaluated by acoustic rhinometry. Laryngoscope 1995;105(4 Pt 1):429–31.

26. Sheen JH. Spreader graft: a method of reconstructing the roof of the middle nasal vault following rhinoplasty. Plast Reconstr Surg 1984;73(2):230–9.

27. Coan BS, Neff E, Mukundan SJ, et al. Validation of a cadaveric model for comprehensive physiologic and anatomic evaluation of rhinoplastic techniques. Plast Reconstr Surg 2009;124(6):2107–17.

28. Boccieri A, Macro C, Pascali M. The use of spreader grafts in primary rhinoplasty. Ann Plast Surg 2005; 55(2):127–31.

29. Rohrich RJ, Hollier LH. Use of spreader grafts in the external approach to rhinoplasty. Clin Plast Surg 1996;23(2):255–62.

30. Acartürk S, Gencel E. The spreader-splay graft combination: a treatment approach for the osseocartilaginous vault deformities following rhinoplasty. Ann Plast Surg 2003;27(4):275–80.

31. Grigoryants V, Baroni A. The use of short spreader grafts in rhinoplasty for patients with thick nasal skin. Ann Plast Surg 2013;37(3):516–20.

32. Fomon S, Gilbert JG, Caron AL, et al. Collapsed ALA: pathologic physiology and management. Arch Otolaryngol 1950;51(4):465–84.

33. Wood WG. Using the upper lateral cartilage as a spreader graft. Presented at the American Society of Plastic Surgeons Meeting. Washington DC, November, 1992.

34. Oneal RM, Berkowitz RL. Upper lateral cartilage spreader flaps in rhinoplasty. Aesthet Surg J 1998; 18(5):370–1.

35. Saedi B, Amaly A, Gharavis V, et al. Spreader flaps do not change early functional outcomes in reduction rhinoplasty: a randomized control trial. Am J Rhinol Allergy 2014;28(1):70–4.

36. Yoo S, Most SP. Nasal airway preservation using the autospreader technique: analysis of outcomes using a disease-specific quality-of-life instrument. Arch Facial Plast Surg 2011;13(4):231–3.

37. Hwang K, Huan F, Kim DJ. Mapping thickness of nasal septal cartilage. J Craniofac Surg 2010; 21(1):243–4.

38. Gruber RP, Park E, Newman J, et al. The spreader flap in primary rhinoplasty. Plast Reconstr Surg 2007;119(6):1903–10.

Combining Open Structural and Dorsal Preservation Rhinoplasty

Priyesh N. Patel, MD[a], Sam P. Most, MD[b],*

KEYWORDS

- Dorsal preservation rhinoplasty • Dorsal hump • Structural preservation

KEY POINTS

- The theoretic functional and cosmetic benefits of dorsal preservation surgery are based on the en bloc treatment of the nasal vault and this can be combined with open structural methods.
- The push-down and let-down are the 2 primary techniques used to manage the osseous nasal vault in dorsal preservation rhinoplasty (DPR), with the latter involving additional resection of a wedge of lateral bone.
- The let-down technique may be superior to the push-down with regard to nasal valve dimensions, but does not seem to be better than Joseph hump reduction with midvault reconstruction in cadaveric studies.
- A variety of techniques can be used to manage the septum in DPR, each largely differentiated by the location of septal cartilage resection.
- Partial preservation techniques have been described with success.
- Dorsal hump recurrence in DPR can be limited by scoring of any remaining cartilage, multiple suture fixation, using the let-down rather than the push-down for larger humps, and performing a lateral keystone dissection.
- Robust patient-reported outcomes and comparative studies are needed to confirm the functional and aesthetic benefits of different DPR techniques.

INTRODUCTION

Preservation rhinoplasty has received significant global interest over the last several years. In 2018, Daniel[1] published an editorial questioning the destructive methodology of the pervasive Joseph cannon of reduction rhinoplasty, urging the need for a rhinoplasty revolution: one that supports preservation rather than resection. Fundamentally, preservation rhinoplasty involves minimal disruption of the soft tissue envelope and nasal ligaments with a subperichondrial

dissection, in addition to limited lateral crural resection.[1–4] Although the former component is receiving increased support in light of detailed anatomic dissection and functional implications, the latter has already been widely incorporated into many rhinoplasty practices secondary to known aesthetic and functional implications of over-resected lateral crural cartilage.[3–5] Another component of preservation rhinoplasty pertains to the en bloc lowering of the dorsum with conservation of the nasal keystone, also known as dorsal preservation rhinoplasty (DPR). DPR can be

[a] Division of Facial Plastic and Reconstructive Surgery, Department of Otolaryngology, Vanderbilt University Medical Center, 1215 21st Ave S (Suite 7209), Nashville, TN 37232, USA; [b] Division of Facial Plastic and Reconstructive Surgery, Stanford University School of Medicine, 801 Welch Road, Stanford, CA 94304, USA
* Corresponding author.
E-mail address: smost@stanford.edu

Clin Plastic Surg 49 (2022) 97–109
https://doi.org/10.1016/j.cps.2021.07.006

applied in combination with or independently of other preservation techniques and is the focus of this article.

ORIGINS AND DESCRIPTION OF DORSAL PRESERVATION RHINOPLASTY

A thorough history of DPR was recently described.[6] In 1899, J. Goodale,[7,8] an otolaryngologist from the United States, reported on the use of lateral and root osteotomies with mobilization of an intact nasal vault to lower the nasal dorsum in a patient with a bony-cartilaginous hump. In this technique, which has become known as the push-down (PD) technique (**Fig. 1**), once the sidewalls and root of the bony vault have been mobilized, lowering of the dorsum occurs with resection of a subdorsal segment of cartilage and ethmoid bone. The nasal sidewalls are displaced into the nasal cavity to accommodate the decreased dorsal height. In 1914, O. Lothrop[9] similarly described using a subdorsal cartilage resection, resection of a wedge of ethmoid bone, and both lateral and transverse osteotomies to allow descent of the dorsum. However, he also described lateral wedge-shaped resections of bone at the sidewalls. In this technique, which has become known as the let-down (LD) procedure (**Fig. 2**), the lateral aspects of the bony vault rest on (rather than resting within) the maxilla.[10–12] The PD technique can be performed with a lateral ostectomy of bone (thereby thinning the lateral nasal wall).[13] When the walls are pushed into the nasal cavity, there is thereby a lower chance of resulting narrowing of the airway.

The original descriptions by Goodale[7,8] and Lothrop[9] are the mainstay of managing the bony nasal vault in preservation rhinoplasty. However, Mobilization of the bone, is only 1 requisite of dorsal lowering. The other involves some form of septal resection that allows the overlying nasal architecture to descend. The fusion of the perichondrium of the cartilaginous vault with the periosteum of the nasal bones over the dorsum is flexible.[14] In addition, the septal cartilage extends subdorsally under the nasal bones such that the bony cap sits above cartilage and not septal bone. As such, when a portion of the cartilaginous septum is removed, the dorsum (including the bony portion) descends. Also, the flexibility of the dorsum allows the convexity associated with a hump to be reduced during its decent.[15] Importantly, this process results in not only a lowering effect of the dorsum but also increased rotation at the anterior aspect of the septum and the nasal tip.

MODIFICATIONS OF PRESERVATION RHINOPLASTY: APPROACHES TO THE SEPTUM

Although the management of the bony vault has remained largely consistent in descriptions of dorsal preservation surgery (PD or LD), variations in the management of the septum have been developed (**Fig. 3**). Although many European and American surgeons had contributed to preservation concepts in the 1900s (Sebileau, Dufourmentel, Maurel, Huizing, Willemont, Wayoff, Pirsig, Cottle, Hinderer, Drumheller, Barelli),[16–25] the following is dedicated to highlighting key modifications that exist in the management of the septum.

Subdorsal Resection

Original descriptions by Lothrop,[9] Goodale,[7,8] and Maurel involved primarily an immediate subdorsal resection of cartilage (see **Fig. 3**A).[24] These techniques have been more recently championed by preservation rhinoplasty surgeons including Gola and Saban.[9,15,26,27] In this technique, an incision is made immediately under the dorsum, following the contour of the dorsal hump, and a second cut is made lower, corresponding with the desired dorsal height. The intervening cartilage, as well as a small amount of subdorsal ethmoid bone, is resected. Once the bony vault is mobilized, the dorsum is lowered and anchored to the underlying stable septal cartilage.

Inferior Strip

In 1926, Sebileau and Dufourmentel published on a method that involved resection of an inferior strip of bone and cartilage (see **Fig. 3**B).[23] Similar to the subdorsal resection, this method was able to accomplish resection of the 3 nasal pillars (both lateral walls and septum) to lower the nasal dorsum. Again, the amount of excised cartilage represents the degree of dorsal height reduction. One criticism of this method is the greater difficulty in stabilizing the septum to the maxillary crest.

Cottle and Septum Pyramidal Adjustment and Repositioning Method

In 1946, M. Cottle from the United States had modified both the subdorsal and inferior septal resection, creating a fusion between the two (see **Fig. 3**C).[25,28] He separated the cartilaginous septum from the ethmoid plate and resected a segment of ethmoid bone superiorly. Although bone was resected superiorly, a strip of cartilage was excised inferiorly at the maxillary spine to allow for lowering of the dorsum. This technique also required a complete vertical split between

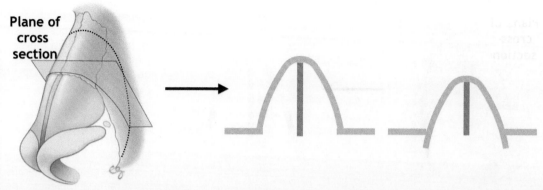

Fig. 1. PD technique. The PD technique involves lateral and root osteotomies (*dotted line*), followed by resection of a segment of the septum. This technique allows en bloc lowering of the nasal pyramid, with the nasal sidewalls being displaced into the nasal cavity to accommodate the decreased dorsal height.

the bony and cartilaginous septum. This method was also championed by Dewes, who used the term septum pyramidal adjustment and repositioning (SPAR) to describe a dorsal conserving approach that involved a resection of a small amount of ethmoid bone, removal of a small vertical strip of cartilage in the posterior portion of the quadrangular cartilage, and removal of a portion of the inferior septum/maxillary crest.[29] Similar to the inferior strip method, this technique requires anchoring of the cartilage to the maxillary crest.

Intermediate Septal Resection/Intermediate Split

In 1999, Ishida and colleagues[30] described a septal strip excision that is performed closer to the midaspect of the cartilaginous septum (rather than subdorsal or at the maxillary crest) (see **Fig. 3**D). In this technique, the septal resection extends from the caudal border of the septum to the perpendicular plate at the level of the transverse osteotomy. In the original description of this method by Ishida and colleagues,[30] the nasal bones were managed with resection using an osteotome or rasp. Because the bony vault is resected and the key stone is violated, this technique differs from traditional dorsal preservation techniques. However, the location of septal cartilage excision is an important evolution of preservation techniques. Compared with inferior cartilaginous resections, this method affords the ability to anchor the superior septal cartilage to lower cartilage with suture techniques, thereby better stabilizing the dorsal position. In a more recent description of the intermediate strip preservation method (Vitruvian man split maneuver), Neves and colleagues[31] describe how a vertical chondrotomy at the prominent point of the hump

allows the dorsum to be flexed, thereby reducing the profile convexity.

Split Tetris Concept

The split tetris concept, described by Neves and colleagues,[32,33] represents a modification of the intermediate septal resection, and shares features with the Cottle/SPAR methods (see **Fig. 3**E). In this technique, a 5-mm to 8-mm tetris block is designed in the septum between the W point (caudal edge of the upper lateral cartilages) and the most prominent aspect of the dorsal hump. Under this segment, a trapezoid segment of cartilage, corresponding with the amount of hump to be reduced, is resected. Superiorly, in a subdorsal fashion, a posterior triangular wedge of cartilage (and sometimes bone) is resected to the level of the transverse osteotomy. The combination of a high posterior resection and lower anterior cartilage resection shares features with the Cottle technique. An incision into the tetris block at its midaspect helps facilitate dorsal flexion (split tetris). A segment of the anterior tetris block may have to be resected to allow room for this flexion. Suture techniques are then used to stabilize the dorsal position. Kovacevic and colleagues[40] described a similar modification to the Cottle technique, although, rather than a rectangular subdorsal block, a triangular cartilaginous wedge is maintained (see **Fig. 3**F).[3,34,35]

Modified Subdorsal Strip Method

Most and coworkers have reported on a modified subdorsal resection in which a high septal resection is performed (see **Fig. 3**G).[36,37] This method shares features with the tetris method. In this technique, a 3-mm to 5-mm subdorsal strut of cartilage is preserved. This length is more than the

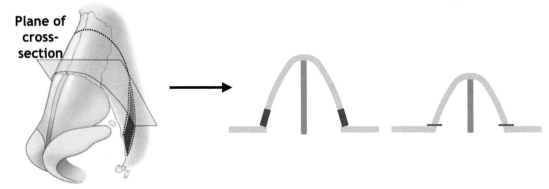

Fig. 2. LD technique. The LD technique involves lateral and root osteotomies (*dotted line*), followed by resection of a wedge-shaped portion of bone at the sidewalls (*magenta*) and a segment of the septum. This technique allows en bloc lowering of the nasal pyramid, with the nasal sidewalls resting on the maxilla (rather than within it).

subdorsal strip method and less than the intermediate strip method. The high dorsal cut is started posterior to the anterior septal angle, allowing the preservation of a 1-cm to 1.5-cm caudal strut. This strut can be trimmed secondarily or left in the original more projected location to allow for adjustment of the tripod complex. If the caudal strut has to be removed (eg, anterior septal reconstruction), keeping a subdorsal strut of cartilage allows the new caudal strut to be stabilized to the dorsum.[38,39] One or 2 vertical incisions are made into the subdorsal cartilage at a location that corresponds to the apex of the dorsal hump, thereby facilitating flexion of the overlying dorsum similar to the split tetris method. Suture techniques are then used to stabilize the dorsal position. In this technique, along with others that preserve lower portions of the septum, additional septum can be removed for obstructive reasons or harvested for grafting needs. Kovacevic and colleagues[40] similarly reported on a technique that involves preserving a triangular subdorsal strip of cartilage (measuring 2–3 mm).[3,34,40] A triangular resection is performed to minimize the amount of inadvertent radix lowering. This cut extends to the height of the dorsal hump and close to where the cartilaginous septum meets the ethmoid plate, followed by resection of a small amount of ethmoid bone. In addition, the preservation of some subdorsal cartilage is thought to limit the risk of scar contracture that can deform the middle vault over time.[34]

MODIFICATIONS OF PRESERVATION RHINOPLASTY: APPROACHES TO THE OSSEOCARTILAGINOUS COMPLEX

Although complete preservation of the junction between the upper lateral cartilages, septum, and nasal bones is a hallmark of traditional preservation rhinoplasty, certain modifications have been developed that represent partial preservation concepts.[35]

As mentioned earlier, Ishida and colleagues[30] described a midseptal cartilage resection to lower the dorsum while preserving the attachment of the upper lateral cartilage to the septum. However, the nasal bones are separated from the upper lateral cartilage and the osseous hump is treated independently with the use of osteotomes or rasps. As such, this technique preserves only the middle third of the nose. A modification of this technique has been described in which the continuity between the bony cap and cartilaginous dorsum is left intact.[41] This technique involves separation of the upper lateral cartilages from the nasal bones, disarticulation of the entire septal bony-cartilaginous junction, resection of septal cartilage (either high, mid, or low), and osteotomies along the dorsal aesthetic lines that meet in the midline and encompass the bony cap. This technique results in a mobile complex involving the septum and dorsum (including the bony cap), which allows lowering of a dorsal hump. Subsequent modification of the remaining bony vault is then performed (eg, rasping), followed by lateral osteotomies to medialize the nasal bones. By preserving the dorsal cartilage–bony cap junction, this technique more closely resembles traditional dorsal preservation descriptions. Importantly, this technique allows for preservation methods to be applied in the setting of larger humps or more distorted bony architecture.

Ferreira and colleagues[42] have also reported on a middle-third preservation technique (spare roof technique) in which the midline upper lateral cartilage–septal cartilage junction is preserved. Subdorsal cartilage is removed to allow the middle third and a portion of the dorsal hump to be

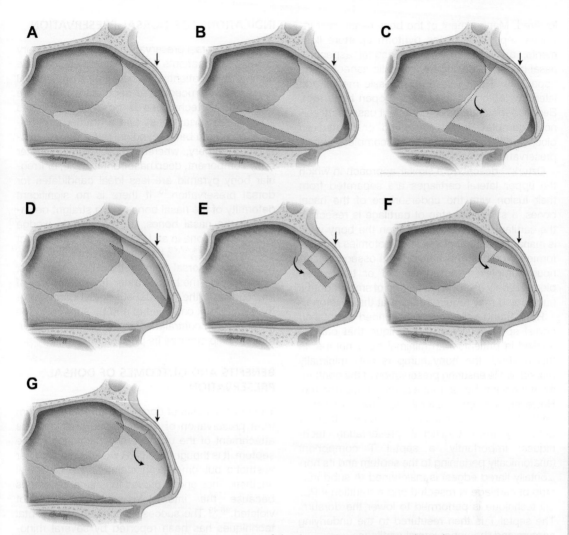

Fig. 3. Approaches to the septum in DPR. Lowering of the dorsum in preservation rhinoplasty requires resection of the septum. Several approaches have been described and are shown here, with dotted lines representing cuts and shaded gray areas representing septal resection. (*A*) Subdorsal resection: championed by Lothrop, Goodale, Maurel, Gola, and Saban, this technique involves an incision made immediately under the dorsum, following the contour of the dorsal hump. A second cut is made lower, corresponding with the desired dorsal height. The intervening cartilage, as well as a small amount of subdorsal ethmoid bone, is resected. (*B*) Inferior strip: first described by Sebileau and Dufourmentel, this method involves resection of inferior cartilage at the maxillary crest. (*C*) Cottle and septum pyramidal adjustment and repositioning (SPAR) method: in these techniques, the cartilaginous septum is separated from the ethmoid plate. A segment of ethmoid bone is resected superiorly and cartilage is excised inferiorly at the maxillary crest. This technique requires anchoring of the cartilage to the maxillary crest. The curved arrow indicates the anterior displacement of cartilage with descent. (*D*) Intermediate septal resection/intermediate split/Vitruvian method: first described by Ishida and colleagues,[30,41] this involves a septal strip excision that is performed closer to the midaspect of the cartilaginous septum and extends to the caudal border of the septum. A vertical chondrotomy (Vitruvian method) at the prominent point of the hump would allow for the dorsum to be flexed, thereby reducing the profile convexity. (*E*) Split tetris concept: in this technique, a 5-mm to 8-mm tetris block is designed in the septum, under which a trapezoid segment of cartilage is resected. Superiorly, in a subdorsal fashion, a posterior triangular wedge of cartilage (and sometimes bone) is resected. An incision into the tetris block at its midaspect helps facilitate dorsal flexion. A segment of the anterior tetris block may have to be resected to allow room for this flexion. (*F*) Kovacevic modification to Cottle technique: this technique shares features with the tetris concept. Rather than a rectangular subdorsal block, a triangular cartilaginous wedge is maintained. (*G*) Modified subdorsal strip method (MSSM): in this technique, a 3-mm to 5-mm subdorsal strut of cartilage is preserved (more than the subdorsal strip method and less than the intermediate strip method). The high dorsal cut is started posterior to the anterior septal angle,

lowered. Management of the bony nasal vault involves separation of the pyriform aperture ligaments, an ostectomy of the caudal aspect of nasal bones (exposing the cephalic aspect of the upper lateral cartilages), and classic medial and lateral osteotomies to close the open bony roof. Because the entirety of the dorsal osseocartilaginous complex is not preserved or treated en bloc, it differs from traditional complete dorsal preservation techniques.

Ozturk[43] described a similar approach in which the upper lateral cartilages are separated from their fusion with the undersurface of the nasal bones, a subdorsal strip of cartilage is resected, the cartilage is lowered, and then the bony vault is managed with rasping. No osteotomies are performed. Again, in this method, the osseocartilaginous complex is not preserved or treated en bloc. It is only useful in the setting of smaller dorsal humps and may require grafting at the keystone.

Robotti and colleagues[44] described a modified dorsal split preservation technique that can be applied in patients with minimal bony humps. In this method, the bony hump is only minimally rasped, while ensuring preservation of the continuity of the nasal bones to the cartilaginous dorsum. However, the upper lateral cartilages are separated from the cartilaginous septum, thereby departing from traditional preservation techniques. Importantly, a septal T component (anatomically pertaining to the septum and its horizontally flared edges) is maintained. A subdorsal strip of cartilage is resected and a traditional PD/LD technique is performed to lower the dorsum. The septal T is then resutured to the underlying septum and the upper lateral cartilages.

Tas[45] also described a modified method that shares features with the description by Robotti and colleagues[44] and Ishida and colleagues.[41] In his dorsal roof technique, the bony-cartilaginous junction is left intact (similar to Ishida and colleagues'[41] description), but the upper lateral cartilages are dissected off the septum (thereby similar to the septal T). However, medial osteotomies (at the dorsal aesthetic lines) and a radix osteotomy are also performed such that the entire bony-cartilaginous dorsum descends into the nose for elimination of the dorsal hump. Subsequently, lateral and transverse osteotomies are performed to narrow the dorsum and eliminate the space created by descent of the midaspect of the bony vault.

INDICATIONS FOR DORSAL PRESERVATION

In general, dorsal preservation is limited to primary cases and in patients with a moderately kyphotic hump.[11,36] In patients who have had a prior dorsal preservation procedure, a secondary procedure using similar techniques is possible.[46] Patients with shorter nasal bones and a greater cartilaginous hump are better candidates for dorsal preservation surgery, whereas those with a greater bony component, deep nasofrontal angle, or irregular bony pyramid are less ideal candidates for dorsal preservation.[15] If there is no significant deformity of the nasal bones but a straight deviation of the nasal bones, an asymmetric wedge resection of bone in an LD procedure can correct this deviation.[24,47,48] If doing this when using the modified subdorsal strip method (MSSM), tetris, or Kovacevic methods, rather than resection of any cartilage, the residual subdorsal cartilage or the tetris block can overlap and be sutured to the lower septum contralateral to the side of the deviation to help stabilize its position.[33]

BENEFITS AND OUTCOMES OF DORSAL PRESERVATION

Theoretic benefits of dorsal hump reduction stem from preservation of the keystone area and the attachment of the upper lateral cartilages to the septum. It is thought that DPR would yield superior aesthetic outcomes with maintenance of dorsal aesthetic lines and improved functional outcomes because the internal nasal valve is not violated.[36,49] The success of preservation septal techniques has been reported by several rhinoplasty surgeons, although studies with objective measures of success and studies comparing outcomes with Joseph hump reduction are limited.[50]

Saban and colleagues[15] have described excellent results in a series of 320 patients who underwent a subdorsal resection technique with endoscopic visualization. Of these patients, 30 were given the Nasal Obstruction Symptom Evaluation (NOSE) questionnaire, and 90% of these patients reported improvements. The same technique has been used by Gola[51] (n = 1000) and Tuncel and Aydogdu[46] (n = 520) with reports of great functional and aesthetic outcomes, but without any objective or patient-subjective measures.

The authors have reported improved patient postoperative Standardized Cosmesis and Health

allowing for the preservation of a 1-cm to 1.5-cm caudal strut. One or 2 vertical incisions can be made into the subdorsal cartilage at a location that corresponds to the apex of the dorsal hump, thereby facilitating flexion of the overlying dorsum. Downward arrows indicate lowering of dorsum; curved arrows indicate an anterior rotation with descent of the dorsum.

Nasal Outcomes Survey (SCHNOS; O = obstructive, C = cosmetic) scores and visual analog scale (VAS; F = functional, C = cosmetic) scores in patients undergoing the MSSM.[36,37] In the patients who underwent a combined functional and cosmetic operation, the SCHNOS and VAS scores improved postoperatively for all functional and aesthetic domains (P<.001). For patients who underwent cosmetic operations alone, the VAS-C and SCHNOS-C significantly improved postoperatively. The VAS-F and SCHNOS-O did not change significantly in this group. In a cadaveric radiologic study, these authors showed that the internal nasal valve dimensions/angle did not change in the LD technique or Joseph hump resection with midvault reconstruction, but did decrease with the PD technique.[52] This finding is likely secondary to the medialization of the nasal sidewall into the nasal cavity with the PD technique. Importantly, it does not support a significant functional benefit of the LD relative to standard hump resection if appropriate midvault reconstruction is performed.

In a report of 100 patients undergoing some form of preservation surgery, Kosins[53] reports success in 31 patients undergoing dorsal preservation with 1-year follow-up (6 required radix grafts to maintain radix position and 3 had a very mild residual hump not requiring revision). Atolini and colleagues[54] reported on the SPAR method in 153 patients with good success (13 requiring revisions for small residual humps). Kovacevic and colleagues[40] also reported success with less than 10% revision rates in 205 patients undergoing the subdorsal triangular resection and subdorsal Cottle modification methods.[40] In these studies, no patient-subjective or patient-objective measure is used.

Ishida and colleagues[41] reported minimal complications in 48 patients undergoing the cartilage PD technique with bony cap preservation (1 with displacement of the bony cap, and 1 with a mild hump recurrence). Tas[45] reported success with the dorsal roof technique in 52 patients using the rhinoplasty outcomes evaluation questionnaire, with 44 patients completing the survey at 1 year and showing positive functional and aesthetic results. The same questionnaire was used to show success in the modified cartilaginous PD maneuver by Ozturk[43] in 62 patients. In 41 patients, Robotti and colleagues[44] showed favorable outcomes with a natural-looking profile based on surgeon assessment at a mean follow-up of 6 months after the dorsal split preservation technique. Ishida and colleagues[30] described satisfactory functional and aesthetic results in a series of 120 patients undergoing the midseptal cartilage strip resection

technique. No patient assessment tool is used in this study.

Santos and colleagues,[55] in a cohort of 100 patients who underwent the spare roof technique, found there was an improvement in aesthetic and functional scores postoperatively. At 12 months postoperatively, mean aesthetic VAS scores showed a significant improvement from 3.67 to 8.44 (P<.001), and mean aesthetic scores from the Utrecht Questionnaire for Outcome Assessment in Aesthetic Rhinoplasty also showed improvement (13.9–7.08, P<.001). Mean functional VAS scores were improved at 12 months postoperatively. In a randomized prospective study of 250 patients, aesthetic and functional VAS scores were better in the patients undergoing a spare roof technique compared with component dorsal hump resection.[56] Although this technique is a middle-third-only preservation technique, it suggests that preservation of the internal nasal valve has superior functional results, in contrast with the aforementioned cadaveric study suggesting equivalent nasal valve dimensions with the LD and conventional hump reductions with a well-reconstructed middle vault.[52]

CHALLENGES AND LIMITATIONS OF DORSAL PRESERVATION

Perhaps one of the greatest limitations of preservation surgery is the recurrence of a dorsal hump.[46,57] The rate of hump recurrence with preservation surgery ranges between 3.4% and 12%.[15,30,46,53,54] Several techniques have been advocated to minimize the recurrence of humps: (1) scoring of any remaining subdorsal cartilage to improve cartilage flexion, (2) multiple-site suture fixation oriented in both craniocaudal and posterior-anterior dimensions, (3) using the LD procedure rather than the PD for larger humps, and (4) performing a lateral keystone dissection with separation of the upper lateral cartilages from the nasal bones (termed the ballerina maneuver by Goksel and Saban[58] or the lateral wall split maneuver by Neves and colleagues[33]).[46,57] Regardless of these techniques, the risk of hump recurrence will be higher than excisional techniques.

Another consideration is the possibility of excessive inferior displacement of the upper nasal vault, yielding a step at the radix or the appearance of a shorter nose. Because the entire nasal vault is mobilized, excessive resection of the cartilage or bone underlying the nasal bones can cause the radix to drop (rather than the intended flexion at this site). Methods to limit this include a conservative resection of septal cartilage/bone, a triangular subdorsal wedge resection as opposed to a rectangle, or a longitudinal cut into the ethmoid (rather than resection if the radix position does not require lowering).[32,34,36,59] In addition, if the transverse osteotomy is made in an oblique fashion, it allows for more of a hinge movement at this site.[59] If a step does occur, a radix graft using soft tissue or morselized cartilage may be necessary for camouflage.

In the event of excessive downward pressure onto the ethmoid bone after the transverse osteotomy is made, there is a possibility of this force propagating inferiorly and posteriorly.[34] This can result in disruption of the cribriform plate and subsequent cerebrospinal fluid leak. Therefore, careful and complete osteotomies need to be performed, and ethmoid bone should be carefully resected to the level of the transverse osteotomy

to prevent the need for excessive downward pressure.

STRUCTURAL AND PRESERVATION RHINOPLASTY

The surge in interest in DPR is evident in the plethora of nearly simultaneous modifications and innovations in how to treat the septum. Part of the reason for this increased interest is the adoption of dorsal preservation methods as a component of open structural rhinoplasty. The senior author has adopted this structural/preservation approach in rhinoplasty practice (**Figs. 4–6**).[36,37] **The components of preservation rhinoplasty have been described by Kosins and Daniel[2] as preservation of the (1) dorsum, (2)**

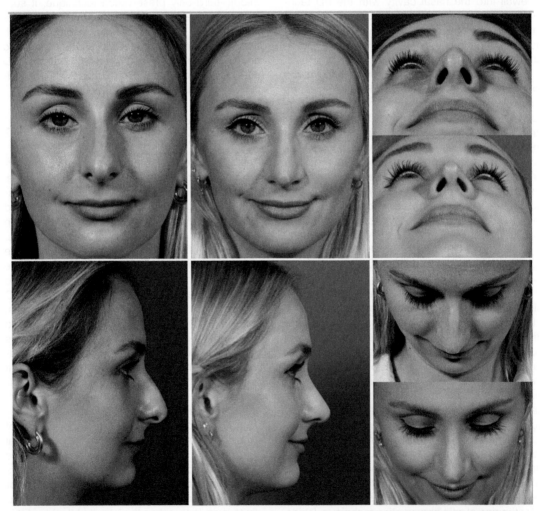

Fig. 4. Structural/preservation rhinoplasty. This patient underwent dorsal reduction with osseocartilaginous dorsal preservation (MSSM), and tip treatment with the following structural methods: mini–lateral-crural-strut grafting for tip narrowing and stabilization tongue in groove to reset the columella/tip/lobule profile, and alar-spanning sutures.

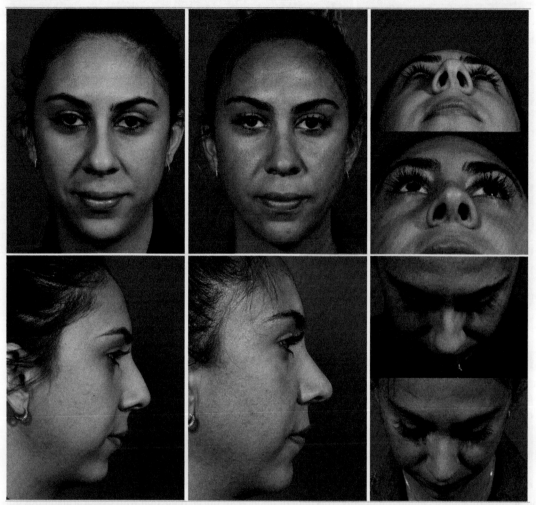

Fig. 5. Structural/preservation rhinoplasty. This patient underwent dorsal reduction with osseocartilaginous dorsal preservation (MSSM), tip treatment with the following structural methods: minimal cephalic trim (2 mm) with mini–lateral-crural-strut grafting to narrow the tip, stabilize, and to straighten lower lateral cartilages, a unilateral right-spreader graft, tongue in groove, and alar-spanning sutures.

ala, and (3) soft tissue skin envelope. Preservation of the integrity of the alar cartilage has been part of our open-structure rhinoplasty practice for more than a decade.[60–63] **Thus, integration of dorsal preservation into our open-structure rhinoplasty practice was the next logical step. Components of structural/preservation rhinoplasty (Fig. 7) are:**

1. External (open) approach to the nose with structural methods for reconstruction of tip support in all. This approach includes use of septal extension grafts, tongue in groove, and columellar struts, as preferred.

2. Alar preservation (minimal to no resection of the alar cartilage, with augmentation when required), including lateral crural tensioning, cephalic cartilage turn-in flaps, lateral crural strut, or mini–lateral crural strut grafts for strengthening weak cartilages.

3. Preservation of the osseocartilaginous vault, as described earlier.

As can be seen from **Fig. 7**, the authors envision DPR as simply another method to be incorporated into traditional structural rhinoplasty methods. **Figs. 4–6** show representative examples of patients undergoing structural preservation techniques.

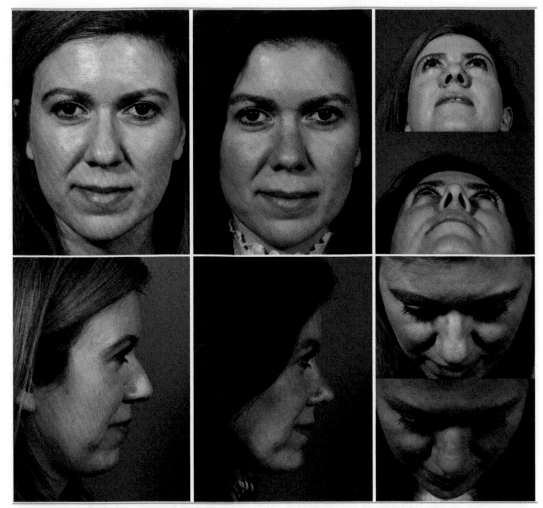

Fig. 6. Structural/preservation rhinoplasty. This patient underwent dorsal reduction with osseocartilaginous dorsal preservation (MSSM), tip treatment with the following structural methods: bilateral alar preservation hinge-flaps, tongue in groove, and alar-spanning sutures.

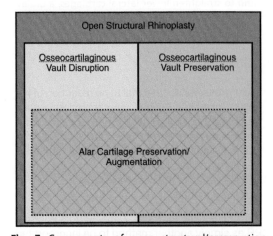

Fig. 7. Components of open structural/preservation rhinoplasty include modifications of the nasal tip and ala cartilage preservation and/or augmentation. These modifications can occur in the context of either preservation or resection of the osseocartilaginous vault.

SUMMARY

Trends in rhinoplasty have tended toward preservation and manipulation versus resection. Preservation of the alar cartilages was promoted at the turn of the twenty-first century and has been accepted into open structural rhinoplasty practice by many. Incorporation of dorsal preservation into open structural approaches is the next logical step. Although preservation rhinoplasty has been largely used in the setting of endonasal operations, its successes using open approaches have been made evident.[36] Open structural modifications to the nasal tip with preservation management of the dorsum (structural preservation) allows for the use of tip-altering techniques that are commonly used by rhinoplasty surgeons. In preservation techniques that maintain a caudal strut of cartilage (eg, tetris concept or MSSM method), there is the possibility of using this segment to adjust the tip projection and rotation (similar to caudal septal extension grafts). Modifications to septal resections in DPR that maintain the integrity of the lower septum also allow cartilage harvesting, which can be used for grafting or for alleviation of obstructive deviations.[49] Partial dorsal preservation techniques (eg, middle-third cartilage preservation techniques) also allow for an intermediate step between complete dorsal preservation and structural techniques, expanding the indications for preservation rhinoplasty.[35,64] The use of piezo electric saws is also aiding surgeons in making precise osteotomies, alleviating some of the anxiety that surrounds preservation techniques.[58,65] With the resurgence of DPR, the refinement of current techniques, the development of others, and continued research into the functional and aesthetic implications of this technique are to be expected.

CLINICS CARE POINTS

- If a rhinoplasty patient has a nice dorsal contour on preoperative frontal view, the use of preservation techniques to maintain dorsal aesthetic lines should be considered.
- If selecting a preservation technique, the LD technique may be superior to the PD technique in managing larger dorsal humps and preventing functional sequalae.
- Although a variety of techniques can be used to successfully manage the septum in DPR, those techniques that require anchoring the septum to the maxillary spine may be more challenging.
- Certain septal resections in DPR preserve the caudal strut, allowing it to be used for modification of tip positioning.
- To minimize the risk of dorsal hump recurrence in DPR, surgeons should consider scoring of any remaining subdorsal cartilage, multiple suture fixation, and performing a lateral keystone dissection.

REFERENCES

1. Daniel RK. The preservation rhinoplasty: a new rhinoplasty revolution. Aesthet Surg J 2018;38(2):228–9.
2. Kosins AM, Daniel RK. Decision making in preservation rhinoplasty: a 100 case series with one-year follow-up. Aesthet Surg J 2020;40(1):34–48.
3. Cakir B, Saban Y, Daniel RK, et al. Preservation rhinoplasty book. Istanbul: Septum Publishing; 2018.
4. Daniel RK, Palhazi P. The nasal ligaments and tip support in rhinoplasty: an anatomical study. Aesthet Surg J 2018;38(4):357–68.
5. Surowitz JB, Most SP. Complications of rhinoplasty. Facial Plast Surg Clin North Am 2013;21(4):639–51.
6. Kern EB. History of dorsal preservation surgery: seeking our historical godfather(s) for the "Push Down" and "Let Down" operations. Facial Plast Surg Clin North Am 2021;29(1):1–14.
7. Goodale JL. A new method for the operative correction of exaggerated roman nose. Boston Med Surg J 1899;140:112.
8. Goodale JL. The correction of old lateral displacements of the nasal bones. Boston Med Surg J 1901;145:538–9.
9. Lothrop O. An operation for correcting the aquiline nasal deformity; the use of new instrument; report of a case. Boston Med Surg J 1914;170:835–7.
10. Lopez-Ulloa F. Let down technique. 2011. Available at: https://www.rhinoplastyarchive.com/articles/let-down-technique. Accessed December 12, 2019.
11. Montes-Bracchini JJ. Nasal profile hump reduction using the let-down technique. Facial Plast Surg 2019;35(5):486–91.
12. Montes-Bracchini JJ. Preservation rhinoplasty (let-down technique) for endonasal dorsal reduction. Facial Plast Surg Clin North Am 2021;29(1):59–66.
13. Ozturk G. Push down technique with ostectomy. Ann Chir Plast Esthet 2021;66(4):329–37.
14. Palhazi P, Daniel RK, Kosins AM. The osseocartilaginous vault of the nose: anatomy and surgical observations. Aesthet Surg J 2015;35(3):242–51.
15. Saban Y, Daniel RK, Polselli R, et al. Dorsal preservation: the push down technique reassessed. Aesthet Surg J 2018;38(2):117–31.
16. Huizing EH. Push-down of the external nasal pyramid by resection of wedges. Rhinology 1975;13(4):185–90.
17. Wayoff M, Perrin C. [Global mobilization of the nasal pyramid according to Cottle's technic: its possibilities in functional nose surgery]. Acta Otorhinolaryngol Belg 1968;22(6):675–80.
18. Pirsig W, Konigs D. Wedge resection in rhinosurgery: a review of the literature and long-term results in a hundred cases. Rhinology 1988;26(2):77–88.
19. Willemot J, Vrebos J, Pollet J. [Plastic surgery and otorhinolaryngology]. Acta Otorhinolaryngol Belg 1967;21(5):463–732.
20. Barelli PA. Long term evaluation of "push down" procedures. Rhinology 1975;13(1):25–32.
21. Drumheller GW. The push down operation and septal surgery. Boston: Little, Brown, and Company; 1973.
22. Hinderer KH. Fundamentals of anatomy and surgery of the nose. Ann Arbor (MI): Aesculapius Publishing Co; 1971.

23. Sebileau P, Dufourmentel L. Correction chirurgicale des difformités congénitales et acquises de la pyramide nasale. Paris: Arnette; 1926. p. 104–5.

24. Maurel G. Chirurgie maxilla-faciale. Paris: Le François; 1940. p. 1127–33.

25. Cottle MH, Loring RM. Corrective surgery of the external nasal pyramid and the nasal septum for restoration of normal physiology. Ill Med J 1946;90: 119–35.

26. Gola R, Nerini A, Laurent-Fyon C, et al. [Conservative rhinoplasty of the nasal canopy]. Ann Chir Plast Esthet 1989;34(6):465–75.

27. Saban Y, Braccini F, Polselli R. [Rhinoplasty: morphodynamic anatomy of rhinoplasty. Interest of conservative rhinoplasty]. Rev Laryngol Otol Rhinol (Bord) 2006;127(1–2):15–22.

28. Friedman O, Ulloa FL, Kern EB. Preservation rhinoplasty: the endonasal cottle push-down/let-down approach. Facial Plast Surg Clin North Am 2021; 29(1):67–75.

29. Ferraz M, Zappelini CEM, Carvalho GM, et al. Cirurgia conservadora do dorso nasal – a filosofia do reposicionamento e ajuste do septo piramidal (S.P.A.R.). Rev Bras Cir Cabeça Pescoço 2013;42:124–30.

30. Ishida J, Ishida LC, Ishida LH, et al. Treatment of the nasal hump with preservation of the cartilaginous framework. Plast Reconstr Surg 1999;103(6): 1729–33 [discussion: 1734–5].

31. Neves JC, Arancibia Tagle D, Dewes W, et al. The split preservation rhinoplasty: "the Vitruvian Man split maneuver". Eur J Plast Surg 2020;43:323–33.

32. Neves JC, Arancibia Tagle D, Dewes W, et al. The segmental preservation rhinoplasty: the split tetris concept. Facial Plast Surg 2021;37(1):36–44.

33. Neves JC, Tagle DA, Dewes W, et al. A segmental approach in dorsal preservation rhinoplasty: the tetris concept. Facial Plast Surg Clin North Am 2021; 29(1):85–99.

34. Toriumi DM, Kovacevic M. Dorsal preservation rhinoplasty: measures to prevent suboptimal outcomes. Facial Plast Surg Clin North Am 2021; 29(1):141–53.

35. Kosins AM. Expanding indications for dorsal preservation rhinoplasty with cartilage conversion techniques. Aesthet Surg J 2021;41(2):174–84.

36. Patel PN, Abdelwahab M, Most SP. A review and modification of dorsal preservation rhinoplasty techniques. Facial Plast Surg Aesthet Med 2020;22(2): 71–9.

37. Patel PN, Abdelwahab M, Most SP. Dorsal preservation rhinoplasty: method and outcomes of the modified subdorsal strip method. Facial Plast Surg Clin North Am 2021;29(1):29–37.

38. Spataro E, Olds C, Nuyen B, et al. Comparison of primary and secondary anterior septal reconstruction: a cohort study. Facial Plast Surg 2019;35(1): 65–7.

39. Surowitz J, Lee MK, Most SP. Anterior septal reconstruction for treatment of severe caudal septal deviation: clinical severity and outcomes. Otolaryngol Head Neck Surg 2015;153(1):27–33.

40. Kovacevic M, Buttler E, Haack S, et al. [Dorsal preservation septorhinoplasty]. HNO 2020. [Epub ahead of print].

41. Ishida LC, Ishida J, Ishida LH, et al. Nasal hump treatment with cartilaginous push-down and preservation of the bony cap. Aesthet Surg J 2020;40(11): 1168–78.

42. Ferreira MG, Monteiro D, Reis C, et al. Spare roof technique: a middle third new technique. Facial Plast Surg 2016;32(1):111–6.

43. Ozturk G. Push-down technique without osteotomy: a new approach. Aesthet Plast Surg 2020;44(3): 891–901.

44. Robotti E, Chauke-Malinga NY, Leone F. A modified dorsal split preservation technique for nasal humps with minor bony component: a preliminary report. Aesthet Plast Surg 2019;43(5):1257–68.

45. Tas S. Dorsal roof technique for dorsum preservation in rhinoplasty. Aesthet Surg J 2020;40(3): 263–75.

46. Tuncel U, Aydogdu O. The probable reasons for dorsal hump problems following let-down/push-down rhinoplasty and solution proposals. Plast Reconstr Surg 2019;144(3):378e–85e.

47. Ozucer B, Cam OH. The effectiveness of asymmetric dorsal preservation for correction of i-shaped crooked nose deformity in comparison to conventional technique. Facial Plast Surg Aesthet Med 2020;22(4):286–93.

48. East C. Preservation rhinoplasty and the crooked nose. Facial Plast Surg Clin North Am 2021;29(1): 123–30.

49. Patel PN, Abdelwahab M, Most SP. Combined functional and preservation rhinoplasty. Facial Plast Surg Clin North Am 2021;29(1):113–21.

50. Levin M, Ziai H, Roskies M. Patient satisfaction following structural versus preservation rhinoplasty: a systematic review. Facial Plast Surg 2020;36(5): 670–8.

51. Gola R. Functional and esthetic rhinoplasty. Aesthet Plast Surg 2003;27(5):390–6.

52. Abdelwahab MA, Neves CA, Patel PN, et al. Impact of dorsal preservation rhinoplasty versus dorsal hump resection on the internal nasal valve: a quantitative radiological study. Aesthet Plast Surg 2020; 44(3):879–87.

53. Kosins AM, Daniel RK. Decision making in preservation rhinoplasty: a 100 case series with one-year follow-up. Aesthet Surg J 2019;40(1):34–48.

54. Atolini NJ, Lunelli V, Lang GP, et al. Septum pyramidal adjustment and repositioning - a conservative and effective rhinoplasty technique. Braz J Otorhinolaryngol 2019;85(2):176–82.

55. Santos M, Rego AR, Coutinho M, et al. Spare roof technique in reduction rhinoplasty: prospective study of the first one hundred patients. Laryngoscope 2019;129(12):2702–6.

56. Ferreira MG, Santos M, Carmo DOE, et al. Spare roof technique versus component dorsal hump reduction: a randomized prospective study in 250 primary rhinoplasties, aesthetic and functional outcomes. Aesthet Surg J 2021;41(3):288–300.

57. Tuncel U, Aydogdu IO, Kurt A. Reducing dorsal hump recurrence following push down-let down rhinoplasty. Aesthet Surg J 2021;41(4):428–37.

58. Goksel A, Saban Y. Open piezo preservation rhinoplasty: a case report of the new rhinoplasty approach. Facial Plast Surg 2019;35(1):113–8.

59. Sadri A, East C, Badia L, et al. Dorsal preservation rhinoplasty: core beam computed tomography analysis of the nasal vault, septum, and skull base-its role in surgical planning. Facial Plast Surg 2020; 36(3):329–34.

60. Murakami CS, Barrera JE, Most SP. Preserving structural integrity of the alar cartilage in aesthetic rhinoplasty using a cephalic turn-in flap. Arch Facial Plast Surg 2009;11(2):126–8.

61. Sazgar AA, Most SP. Stabilization of nasal tip support in nasal tip reduction surgery. Otolaryngol Head Neck Surg 2011;145(6):932–4.

62. Sazgar AA, Woodard C, Most SP. Preservation of the nasal valve area with a lateral crural hinged flap: a cadaveric study. Aesthet Plast Surg 2012;36(2): 244–7.

63. Tellioglu AT, Cimen K. Turn-in folding of the cephalic portion of the lateral crus to support the alar rim in rhinoplasty. Aesthet Plast Surg 2007;31(3):306–10.

64. Kosins AM. Incorporating dorsal preservation rhinoplasty into your practice. Facial Plast Surg Clin North Am 2021;29(1):101–11.

65. Goksel A, Patel PN, Most SP. Piezoelectric osteotomies in dorsal preservation rhinoplasty. Facial Plast Surg Clin North Am 2021;29(1):77–84.

Treatment of the Crooked Nose

Sarah R. Akkina, MD, MS[a,b,*], Sam P. Most, MD[b]

KEYWORDS

- Crooked nose • Nasal asymmetry • Nasal deviation • Nasal deformity • Dorsal preservation

KEY POINTS

- There are favorable and unfavorable facial skeletal and dorsal septal configurations that can aid or hinder surgical outcomes.
- Both structural and camouflage techniques can be used for surgical correction.
- Classifying the type of deviation between the bony third, the middle third, and the base third/tip allows the surgeon to tailor intervention in each of these areas.
- Dorsal preservation offers a method to approach the crooked nose without the drawbacks of conventional hump reduction and osteotomies.
- Patient-reported outcome measures are a fundamental means to measure operative success.

INTRODUCTION

The crooked nose is a challenging esthetic and functional problem. The term "crooked nose," also referred to as the twisted, deviated, or asymmetric nose, has come to represent deviations of the nasal dorsum and pyramid from the facial midline (Fig. 1). While deviations can be congenital, they can also be the result of trauma and surgical interventions gone awry. In addition to the displeasing appearance, significant nasal airway compromise can result from nasal deviation. Correction must focus on a balance of esthetics and function, with the most successful outcomes tailored to addressing each of the deviated components in kind.

HISTORY

Correction of the crooked nose has been a recognized challenge throughout history. The earliest known nasal surgeons were thought to have originated in India with Sushruta in 1000 to 800 BC and focused on nasal reconstruction for severe trauma, infection, or tumors.[1] However, the

discovery of aseptic technique and therefore safer surgeries by Joseph Lister in the 1840s marked a shift toward nasal surgery undertaken for more esthetically unfavorable deviations.[1–3] In this context, corrective techniques were able to proliferate and evolve. Through the late 19th century, the primary approach to correct deviations of the nasal septum was to fracture the septum and maintain midline position with intranasal tubes left for months.[4,5] While successful for bony deviations, cartilaginous deflections did not correct as easily and tended to return to the former position. Morris Asch, a New York surgeon based at the Nye York Eye and Ear Infirmary and the Manhattan Eye and Ear Hospital, addressed this issue by pioneering the development of special forceps designed specifically for reducing the cartilaginous segment of the nasal septum.[6] His technique used blunt force trauma to disrupt intrinsic cartilage memory and attachments of the cartilaginous septum, but stipulated this only be used for cartilaginous deviation to reduce the danger of uncontrolled fractures into the perpendicular plate of the ethmoid or vomer. As this did not address the

[a] Department of Otolaryngology Head & Neck Surgery, University of Washington, 1959 Northeast Pacific Street, Campus Box 356515, Seattle, WA 98105, USA; [b] Division of Facial Plastic and Reconstructive Surgery, Department of Otolaryngology–Head & Neck Surgery, Stanford University School of Medicine, 801 Welch Road, Palo Alto, CA 94305, USA
* Corresponding author. Division of Facial Plastic and Reconstructive Surgery, Department of Otolaryngology–Head & Neck Surgery, Stanford University School of Medicine, 801 Welch Road, Palo Alto, CA 94305, USA
E-mail address: sakkina@stanford.edu

Clin Plastic Surg 49 (2022) 111–121
https://doi.org/10.1016/j.cps.2021.07.007

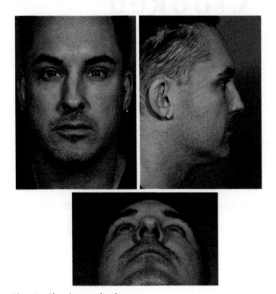

Fig. 1. Classic crooked nose.

additional factors responsible for cartilaginous deformities, patients did not have lasting improvement. Other surgeons of the era, including Robert Krieg and Gustav Killian, started to explore complete excision of the entire deflected cartilaginous septal segment with later refinement into removing only deviated segments with mucosal preservation.[7] Submucosal techniques progressed further, championed by Otto Freer in his seminal paper of 1912 in which he described developing submucous resections and a more full exploration into the causes of septal deflections.[8] However, Freer advocated removal of the entire septal cartilage and blamed resulting dorsal saddling on cicatricial forces of healing.[5] Later work by George Killian showed the structural importance of retaining caudal and dorsal aspects of septal cartilage, and proceeding surgeons including Maurice Cottle, Jacques Joseph, and Jack Sheen continued to progress the field with techniques focused on realignment and preservation.[5,9] Today, with a much more in-depth understanding of how each nasal component contributes to deviation, modern techniques continue to focus on correction of the crooked nose through targeted realignment of deviated components.

BACKGROUND ASSESSMENT

As in any patient assessment, evaluation of the crooked nose patient must first begin with a thorough history. Particular areas of focus for the crooked nose include history of trauma, prior surgeries, and any functional concerns including nasal

congestion and/or obstruction. After taking a complete patient history, the surgeon must perform a thorough examination and accurately define the components of the nose and their contribution to the nasal deviation to tailor interventions accordingly (**Table 1**). This includes evaluation of the external lining or skin envelope, the nasal skeleton or bony-cartilaginous framework, and the mucosa. The contribution of the mucosa to the deviation may be minor, but the mucosa should be respected during the surgical approach for optimal healing. In addition, evaluation of the nasal airway must be documented. This includes evaluation of the septum, internal valve, and any lateral wall insufficiency in zones 1 or 2. Furthermore, as recommended by a multidisciplinary rhinoplasty workgroup, a comprehensive patient-reported outcome measure (PROM) is administered.[10] A recommended PROM is the Standardized Cosmesis Health Nasal Outcomes Survey (SCHNOS) as it captures both functional and cosmetic domains (**Table 2**).[11]

The foundation of the bony-cartilaginous pyramid must also be evaluated, including the entirety of the midface structure. Occult midface asymmetry (OMA) is a common contributor to the appearance of nasal deviation, and this must be identified and discussed with the patient as surgical corrections to the nose will not address the OMA (**Fig. 2**).[12,13] In one prior study, as many as 97% of patients referred for consideration of esthetic rhinoplasty had significant degrees of facial asymmetry, with the greatest variation at the midline to ala distance.[13] Of this group, only 38% of patients were considered asymmetrical through subjective assessment, showing that differences may be subtle and still affect ultimate postoperative outcomes.[13]

Structural contributors to the crooked nose can be further examined in terms of extrinsic and intrinsic forces.[14–16] Extrinsic forces include attachments between the bony pyramid and the upper and lower lateral cartilages as well as the septum. Intrinsic forces represent the structure inherent to the cartilages themselves. The actions of both types of forces can be significantly influenced by trauma or surgery. To account for each of these factors in the surgical approach, the nose can be subdivided into thirds. The upper third represents mainly bony deviations, the middle third represents deviations of the upper lateral cartilage and corresponding septum, and the lower third represents deviations of the lower lateral cartilages and caudal septum. The septal cartilage itself can be subdivided into 6 different basic types of deformity: septal tilt deformity, C-shaped anteroposterior deviation, localized deviations or large spurs, S-shaped anteroposterior

Table 1
Components of the nasal evaluation and associated surgical methods for correction

Nasal Component	Surgical Method
Upper Third	Osteotomies Dorsal preservation (letdown, pushdown) Onlay grafts
Middle Third	Upper lateral cartilage fibrous attachment release Spreader grafts Extended spreader grafts Septal extension graft Clocking or septal rotation stitch Onlay grafts
Lower Third	Internal cartilage tension release Septoplasty Full extracorporeal septoplasty Anterior septal reconstruction Septal extension graft Anterior nasal spine cartilage release and trim Columellar strut graft Augmentation of nasal base Onlay grafts

Table 2
Standardized cosmesis health nasal outcomes survey (SCHNOS)

	Over the Past Month, How Much of a Problem Was the Following:	No Problem					Extreme Problem
1.	Having a blocked or obstructed nose	0	1	2	3	4	5
2.	Getting air through my nose during exercise	0	1	2	3	4	5
3.	Having a congested nose	0	1	2	3	4	5
4.	Breathing through my nose during sleep	0	1	2	3	4	5
5.	Decreased mood and self-esteem due to my nose	0	1	2	3	4	5
6.	The shape of my nasal tip	0	1	2	3	4	5
7.	The straightness of my nose	0	1	2	3	4	5
8.	The shape of my nose from the side	0	1	2	3	4	5
9.	How well my nose suits my face	0	1	2	3	4	5
10.	The overall symmetry of my nose	0	1	2	3	4	5

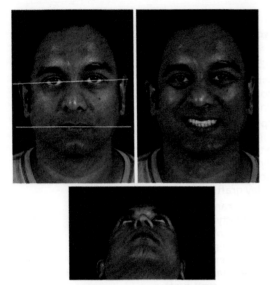

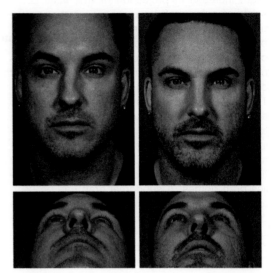

Fig. 3. Before and after sequential "open book" osteotomies for a crooked nose.

Fig. 2. Occult midface asymmetry. Notice that lines drawn through the oral commissures and the lateral canthi are not parallel (*top left*). The smiling photo reveals similar relationship between lateral canthi and occlusal plane. The base view shows mid-face hypoplasia on the right.

deformity, C-shaped cephalocaudal deformity, and S-shaped anteroposterior deformity.[17] Once the area of deviation is identified, operative approaches can include structural techniques and camouflage techniques. The technique chosen should be proportionate to the deviations identified.

DISCUSSION: SURGICAL TREATMENT
Approach to the Upper Nasal Third

Surgical approaches to the upper nasal third typically include addressing the nasal bones as a primary component of deviation. Osteotomies are the main technique used to correct bony deviations in this area. The primary considerations for addressing the bony vault are anomalies of (1) the direction of the nasal bones, (2) the width of the bony base, and (3) the shape of the nasal bones (ie, concave vs convex). The type of osteotomies to be used will vary based on these factors, and can be undertaken via an external or endonasal approach. While in standard rhinoplasty (ie, to close an open roof) a medial to lateral order is used so as not to destabilize medial segments and risk comminuted fracturing, a different approach is required in the setting of a crooked bony vault. In this case, sequential osteotomies from the concave to the convex side in open-book fashion may allow for progressive shifting of the bony deviation in a more controlled fashion

(**Fig. 3**).[5,18] For instrumentation, standard osteotomes can be used in which case instruments maintained in sharp condition are ideal for maximal precision. Alternatively, new technology advancement has led to the use of piezosurgery for osteotomies. In this method, bone is cut with micrometric ultrasonic piezoelectric waves through various frequencies and energies, resulting in reduced nasal mucosal damage and comminuted fractures.[19,20] An additional advantage of the piezo instrument is that the bony vault can be contoured precisely, even after bones are mobilized. However, additional subperiosteal elevation must be performed before piezo instrumentation osteotomies to allow for the larger instrumentation (**Fig. 4**).

Onlay grafts can also be used to create a more symmetric appearance. Such grafts have only an esthetic effect, and do not alter the underlying structural integrity of the nose though also, therefore, do not improve function when used in isolation. Onlay grafting can be used alone or in combination with structural techniques. The most common graft materials used are autologous grafts, with many surgeons favoring septal, conchal, or rib cartilage. As onlay grafts do confer a greater possibility of visibility, distortion, and absorption, there is a growing trend toward diced cartilage use as a means to provide both reduced visibility and easier molding. The senior author's preferred methods include morselized cartilage or diced cartilage with or without fibrin glue (**Fig. 5**).[21] Deep temporalis fascia grafts have also been used to envelope diced cartilage and reduce resorption with decent success.[22] While

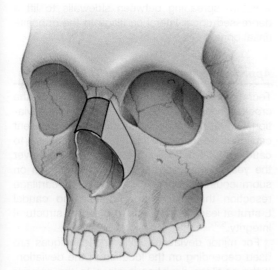

Fig. 4. Limit of subperiosteal elevation for traditional osteotomy (*magenta*) and additional exposure for use of piezo instrumentation for osteotomies (*green*).

there has been concern raised for the long-term results with smaller cartilage fragments, outcomes studies have shown that resorption of diced cartilage and unfavorable appearance is rare.[23] Synthetic graft materials can also be used and include porous polyethylene, acellular dermis, and expanded polytetrafluoroethylene. These graft materials do have higher complication rates of infection and extrusion, therefore are generally not preferred to autologous materials.[24] Onlay techniques can also be used for camouflage of deformities in the middle and lower nasal third.

Approach to the Middle Nasal Third or Middle Vault

Middle vault deviation correction techniques aim to straighten a crooked dorsal septum and/or the upper lateral cartilages. The first step of this process is usually to separate fibrous attachments between the upper lateral cartilages and the dorsal septum. This release can relax asymmetric tension, allow trimming of asymmetric dorsal cartilage projection, and give space for the positioning of spreader grafts. Autologous cartilage is the preferred material for spreader grafts, although the use of other graft material such as porous polyethylene has also been described.[25–27] Either unilateral or bilateral spreader grafts can be used, with placement of thicker spreader grafts (4 mm) on the concave side of curvature to provide support and straightening (**Fig. 6**).[24] Spreader grafts serve a dual purpose in providing stability and widening the internal nasal valve for patients with concomitant nasal obstruction. They also typically widen the nasal dorsum, which may or may not be esthetically advantageous to the patient. If nasal deviation continues through the middle vault into the tip, an extended spreader graft can be used to help further straighten the distal nasal dorsum. A septal extension graft can also be used alone or in combination for a similar purpose.[28]

The clocking or septal rotation suture is a further refined method to straighten dorsal septal deviation.[17] An asymmetric horizontal mattress suture is placed between the upper lateral cartilage and the septal cartilage at the point of deviation (**Fig. 7**). Different placements of the suture can

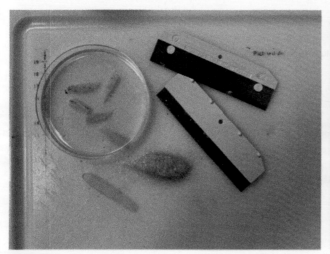
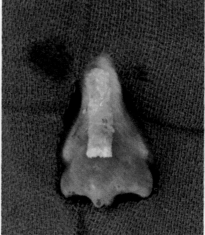

Fig. 5. Diced rib cartilage. Left panel, preparation of the graft. This can be molded into a semicircular cylinder using a 3 cc syringe and fibrin glue (not shown). On the right panel, the graft is placed on the nasal dorsum externally before placement in the nose. This is typically the last step in a rhinoplasty.

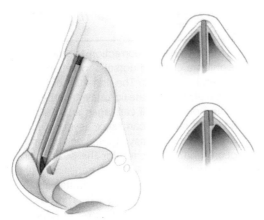

Fig. 6. A left-sided unilateral spreader graft to correct a left midvault deficiency.

affect the degree of septal rotation, lending great adaptability to this technique in addressing deviation.[29] Another advantage is that this rotation stitch does not widen the middle vault. This technique can be easily combined with other deviation correction techniques. Other suture placement techniques have been described to resuspend the middle vault and improve deviations, including a suture between the nasal bones and the upper later cartilage with a unilateral spreader graft and a suture spreading between sidewalls to lift a depressed upper lateral cartilage to the opposite nasal bone.[30,31]

Approach to the Lower Nasal Third

Techniques used in the lower aspect of the crooked nose must address base and tip deviation. Caudal septal deviation is the most prevalent cause of deviation in this area. Approaches to caudal septal deflection have varied widely over the years, with classical techniques focused on submucous septoplasty with deviated cartilage resection that maintains a dorsal and caudal L-strut at least 10 mm wide to preserve structural integrity.[5,32]

For minor deviations, different techniques are used depending on the location of the deviation. If the cartilage deviation is close to the anterior nasal spine, release of the septal cartilage at this point and trimming the residual excess can address the bulk of deviation, followed by reattachment to the periosteum to secure the cartilage in the straightened position.[24] For caudal margin deviations, the columella can be bolstered with a columellar strut graft.[24,33] Releasing of internal cartilage tension alone has been another method used to improve cartilage deviation, including

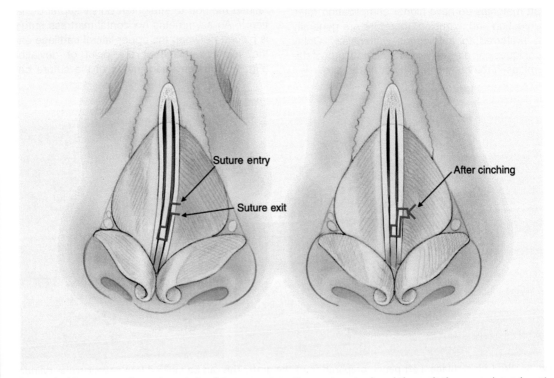

Fig. 7. Clocking or septal rotation stitch of Guyuron. A mattress suture is placed through the upper lateral cartilage at points superior to the corresponding points in the septum on the side of the desired deflection.

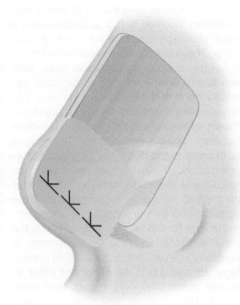
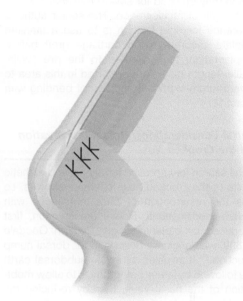

Fig. 8. Schematic representation of septal extension graft (SEG, *left*) and anterior septal reconstruction (ASR, *right*).

cartilage scoring, cross-hatching, and wedging. However, in isolation, this technique can lead to recurrence of deviation.

For more significant cases of caudal deviation, a septal extension graft may be placed on the side opposite the deviation to "reset" the midline, and has been shown to have minimal to no impact on the nasal airway (**Fig. 8**).[34] However, for the severely crooked nose, intrinsic and extrinsic cartilage forces may not be overcome with this technique. Modern approaches have become more aggressive in removing the entirety of the anterior septum to replace it with straight and structurally sound cartilage. The extracorporeal septoplasty technique involves exposure and removal of the entire native septum en bloc, reconstruction of the septum to straighten deviations which can include interrupted sutures, release of tension lines, and rasping, and finally reimplantation of the septum.[35,36] A major drawback of this technique is destabilizing the keystone region, which led to a variety of modifications of the standard extracorporeal septoplasty.[37–39] The senior author's preferred method, the anterior septal reconstruction, addresses this by modifying the septal resection such that the dorsal septal cartilage of the keystone area is retained (see **Fig. 8; Fig. 9**).[35,40]

Resetting the nasal base is critical in maintaining a straight caudal septum and nasal dorsum. If the nasal base is significantly deficient, premaxilla augmentation can be very useful, and can be

performed unilaterally to create a more symmetric foundation to the nose.[41,42] The preferred graft material for this is autologous tissue, usually septal or costal cartilage, but allograft or alloplast may be used. On rare occasions, rigid caudal septal

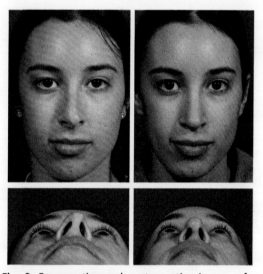

Fig. 9. Preoperative and postoperative images of a revision rhinoplasty patient with a twisted lower 1/3. The repair consisted of anterior septal reconstruction, bilateral spreader grafts, right-sided mini-lateral-crural-strut graft, and a midvault clocking suture. A thin morselized septal cartilage camouflage graft was used on the tip as well.

fixation may be used for severe deviations with a greater risk of recalcitrance. The senior author's preference for rigid fixation is to use a titanium miniplate secured to the cartilage graft before reimplantation, then secured to the premaxilla. Smaller-length plates are preferred in this area to prevent future exposure and risk of bending with impact.[43]

Special Considerations: Dorsal Preservation and the Crooked Nose

As the search for improved functional and esthetic results to the crooked nose dilemma evolves, so does the resurrection of past techniques with modern modifications. Dorsal preservation, first introduced by otolaryngologist Joseph Goodale in 1899, was originally described for dorsal hump reduction.[44] It involves removing subdorsal cartilage followed by lateral osteotomies to allow mobilization of the nasal vault, thereby reducing the dorsal hump as the dorsum relaxes to rest on the trimmed nasal septum. While the technique has evolved, mainstays of practice continue to include maintenance of the osseocartilaginous dorsum without violating the bony-cartilaginous interface.[45] In doing so, the keystone region is not violated and its stability can be maintained. Modifications have arisen in regards to areas of septal cartilage removed.[46–50] To combat poor

visualization with other methods, the senior author's preferred modified septal technique uses a high-septal resection but leaves 3-5 mm of subdorsal strut. These same dorsal preservation techniques can be used for the crooked nose, with variations based on the location of deviated aspects of the bony and cartilaginous dorsum. For an asymmetric bony pyramid, the dorsal preservation letdown technique can be used with inclusion of secondary lateral osteotomies to remove wedges of asymmetric bone. For I-shaped deformities characterized by a longer nasal bone on the contralateral deviation side and a shorter bone on the ipsilateral side, a combination of the letdown technique for the longer side and push-down technique for the shorter side (in which the osteotomy is made and the bony pyramid is "pushed down") can accomplish a suitable correction (**Figs. 10** and **11**).[51] An important pitfall to avoid is that dorsal preservation may itself result in a dorsal let down with an unplanned axis deviation of the dorsum. This must be addressed through additional deviation correction with correction of anterior septal angle position when needed.

MEASURING OUTCOMES

Given the operative challenge the crooked nose presents, having appropriate quantifiable methods

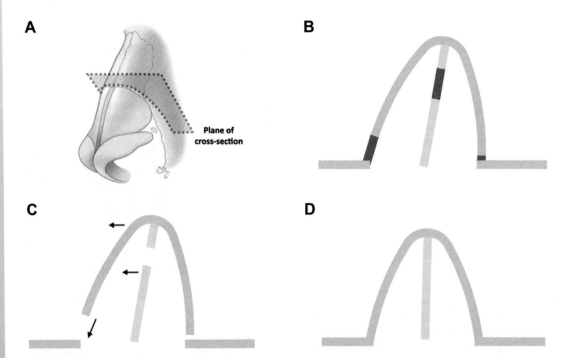

Fig. 10. Sequence for asymmetric let-down dorsal preservation. (*A*) Level of cross-section. (*B*) Areas of bony cuts and septal resection are shown in red. (*C*) Arrows demonstrate rotation of osseocartilaginous vault. (*D*) Final position of vault.

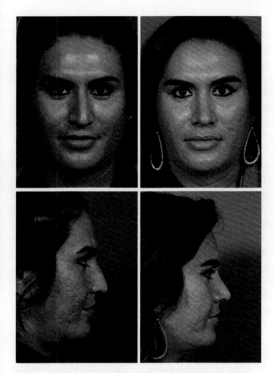

Fig. 11. Before and after sequential asymmetric let-down dorsal preservation for a crooked nose.

to measure surgical success are critical. There are currently multiple validated PROMs that have become more widely used in recent years. While the nasal obstruction symptom valuation scale (NOSE) has the most prevalent use, it focuses on nasal obstructive symptoms alone.[52] Conversely, the FACE-Q(R) and rhinoplasty outcomes evaluation tools focus on nasal cosmesis without reporting functional outcomes.[53–55] The SCHNOS was thus developed to combine both functional and cosmetic concerns into one self-reported questionnaire.[11] The SCHNOS has most recently been used to evaluate outcomes of facial asymmetry on the crooked nose as well as severe caudal septal deviation repair via modified extracorporeal endonasal septoplasty.[56,57] As approaches to correct the crooked nose continue to evolve, the successes and failures must be measured using these tools to finally obtain the ultimate goal: long-lasting patient satisfaction.

SUMMARY

While the crooked nose is a functional and esthetic challenge, numerous methods have been developed to address each aspect of deviation. As new methods like modified dorsal preservation evolve, we must continue to quantify operative success through PROMs to keep moving the field forward and achieve improved patient satisfaction.

CLINICS CARE POINTS

- Facial asymmetry may contribute to the appearance of the crooked nose and must be discussed with patients preoperative to reduce postoperative dissatisfaction
- Deviations of the upper nasal third are primarily addressed through osteotomies, which can be external or endonasal, medial to lateral or sequential, and use traditional osteotomies or new technology including piezosurgery
- Deviations of the middle nasal third or middle vault are generally corrected through removing attachments between the upper lateral cartilage and the septum, spreader grafts, extended spreader grafts, septal extension grafts, and clocking sutures
- Deviations of the lower nasal third typically require addressing the caudal septum through removing cartilage deviations either through standard septoplasty techniques or advanced techniques including extracorporeal and modified extracorporeal septoplasty with anterior septal reconstruction
- The nasal base may require either augmentation or rigid fixation to retain straightness and optimal esthetic outcomes
- Dorsal preservation with its modern modifications represents a newer method to address the crooked nose without disrupting the keystone region
- Patient-reported outcome tools are considered standard methods to measure success in rhinoplasty, both functionally and esthetically

DISCLOSURE

The authors have nothing to disclose.

REFERENCES

1. Champaneria MC, Workman AD, Gupta SC. Sushruta: father of plastic surgery. Ann Plast Surg 2014;73(1):2–7.
2. Clemons BJ. The first modern operating room in America. Aorn J 2000;71(1):164–8, 170.
3. Toledo-Pereyra LH, Toledo MM. A critical study of Lister's work on antiseptic surgery. Am J Surg 1976;131(6):736–44.

4. Freshwater MF. A critical comparison of Davis' principles of plastic surgery with Gillies' plastic surgery of the face. J Plast Reconstr Aesthet Surg 2011; 64(1):17–26.

5. Stepnick D, Guyuron B. Surgical treatment of the crooked nose. Clin Plast Surg 2010;37(2):313–25.

6. Asch M. Treatment of nasal stenosis due to deflective septum with and without thickening of the convex side. Laryngoscope 1899;6:340–61.

7. Mann W. Nasal surgery in German speaking countries around the turn of the century. Rhinology 1991;29(1):79–84.

8. Freer O. The anatomy of deflections of the nasal septum. presented at: Trans 34th Annual Meeting Amer Laryngol Assoc; 1912; Atlantic City, September 21, 1912.

9. Behrbohm H, Briedigkeit W, Kaschke O. Jacques Joseph: father of modern facial plastic surgery. Arch Facial Plast Surg 2008;10(5):300–3.

10. Manahan MA, Fedok F, Davidson C, et al. Evidence-based performance measures for rhinoplasty: a multidisciplinary performance measure Set. Plast Reconstr Surg 2021;147(2):222e–30e.

11. Moubayed SP, Ioannidis JPA, Saltychev M, et al. The 10-Item Standardized cosmesis and health nasal outcomes Survey (SCHNOS) for functional and cosmetic rhinoplasty. JAMA Facial Plast Surg 2018;20(1):37–42.

12. Hafezi F, Naghibzadeh B, Nouhi A, et al. Asymmetric facial growth and deviated nose: a new concept. Ann Plast Surg 2010;64(1):47–51.

13. Chatrath P, De Cordova J, Nouraei SA, et al. Objective assessment of facial asymmetry in rhinoplasty patients. Arch Facial Plast Surg 2007;9(3):184–7.

14. Rohrich RJ, Gunter JP, Deuber MA, et al. The deviated nose: optimizing results using a simplified classification and algorithmic approach. Plast Reconstr Surg 2002;110(6):1509–23 [discussion: 1524–5].

15. Ahmad J, Rohrich RJ. The crooked nose. Clin Plast Surg 2016;43(1):99–113.

16. Byrd HS, Salomon J, Flood J. Correction of the crooked nose. Plast Reconstr Surg 1998;102(6):2148–57.

17. Guyuron B, Uzzo CD, Scull H. A practical classification of septonasal deviation and an effective guide to septal surgery. Plast Reconstr Surg 1999;104(7): 2202–9 [discussion: 2210–2].

18. Most SP, Murakami CS, Larrabee WF. Surgery of the bony nasal vault. In: Facial Plastic and reconstructive surgery. 3rd edition. New York: Thieme Medical Publishers; 2009. p. 547–53.

19. Kurt Yazar S, Serin M, Rakici IT, et al. Comparison of piezosurgery, percutaneous osteotomy, and endonasal continuous osteotomy techniques with a caprine skull model. J Plast Reconstr Aesthet Surg 2019;72(1):107–13.

20. Göksel A, Patel PN, Most SP. Piezoelectric osteotomies in dorsal preservation rhinoplasty. Facial Plast Surg Clin North Am 2021;29(1):77–84.

21. Tasman AJ. Dorsal augmentation-diced cartilage techniques: the diced cartilage glue graft. Facial Plast Surg 2017;33(2):179–88.

22. Calvert J, Kwon E. Techniques for diced cartilage with deep temporalis fascia graft. Facial Plast Surg Clin North Am 2015;23(1):73–80.

23. Ledo TO, Ramos HHA, Buba CM, et al. Outcome of free diced cartilage grafts in rhinoplasty: a Systematic Review. Facial Plast Surg 2020. https://doi.org/10.1055/s-0040-1714664.

24. Shipchandler TZ, Papel ID. The crooked nose. Facial Plast Surg 2011;27(2):203–12.

25. Mendelsohn M. Straightening the crooked middle third of the nose: using porous polyethylene extended spreader grafts. Arch Facial Plast Surg 2005;7(2):74–80.

26. Gürlek A, Ersoz-Ozturk A, Celik M, et al. Correction of the crooked nose using custom-made high-density porous polyethylene extended spreader grafts. Aesthet Plast Surg 2006;30(2):141–9.

27. Boccieri A, Macro C, Pascali M. The use of spreader grafts in primary rhinoplasty. Ann Plast Surg 2005; 55(2):127–31.

28. Chen YY, Kim SA, Jang YJ. Centering a deviated nose by caudal septal extension graft and unilaterally extended spreader grafts. Ann Otol Rhinol Laryngol 2020;129(5):448–55.

29. Keeler JA, Moubayed SP, Most SP. Straightening the crooked middle vault with the clocking stitch: an Anatomic study. JAMA Facial Plast Surg 2017; 19(3):240–1.

30. Dayan SH, Shah AR. A suture suspension technique for improved repair of a crooked nose deformity. Ear Nose Throat J 2004;83(11):743–4.

31. Pontius AT, Leach JL Jr. New techniques for management of the crooked nose. Arch Facial Plast Surg 2004;6(4):263–6.

32. Wexler MR. Surgical repair of the caudal end of the septum. Laryngoscope 1977;87(3):304–9.

33. Suh MK. Correction of the deviated tip and columella in crooked nose. Arch Plast Surg 2020;47(6): 495–504.

34. Patel PN, Abdelwahab M, Shukla ND, et al. Functional outcomes of septal extension grafting in aesthetic rhinoplasty: a Cohort Analysis. Facial Plast Surg Aesthet Med 2020. https://doi.org/10.1089/fpsam.2020.0304.

35. Most SP, Rudy SF. Septoplasty: basic and advanced techniques. Facial Plast Surg Clin North Am 2017; 25(2):161–9.

36. McGrath M, Bell E, Locketz GD, et al. Review and update on extracorporeal septoplasty. Curr Opin Otolaryngol Head Neck Surg 2019;27(1):1–6.

37. Asher SA, Kakodkar AS, Toriumi DM. Long-term outcomes of Subtotal septal reconstruction in rhinoplasty. JAMA Facial Plast Surg 2018;20(1):50–6.

38. Loyo M, Markey JD, Gerecci D, et al. Technical refinements and outcomes of the modified anterior

septal Transplant. JAMA Facial Plast Surg 2018; 20(1):31–6.

39. Wilson MA, Mobley SR. Extracorporeal septoplasty: complications and new techniques. Arch Facial Plast Surg 2011;13(2):85–90.

40. Most SP. Anterior septal reconstruction: outcomes after a modified extracorporeal septoplasty technique. Arch Facial Plast Surg 2006;8(3):202–7.

41. Fanous N, Yoskovitch A. Premaxillary augmentation: adjunct to rhinoplasty. Plast Reconstr Surg 2000; 106(3):707–12.

42. Yamani VR, Ghosh S, Tirunagari S. Nasal correction in nasomaxillary hypoplasia (Binder's syndrome): an optimised classification and treatment. Indian J Plast Surg 2016;49(3):314–21.

43. Patel PN, Kandathil CK, Most SP. Outcomes of combined anterior septal reconstruction and dorsal hump reduction. Laryngoscope 2020;130(12): E803–10.

44. Goodale J. A new method for the operative correction of exaggerated roman nose. Boston Med Surg J 1899;140:112.

45. Lee J, Abdul-Hamed S, Kazei D, et al. The first Descriptions of dorsal preservation rhinoplasty in the 19th and early- to mid-20th Centuries and Relevance Today. Ear Nose Throat J 2020. https://doi.org/10.1177/0145561320925572. 145561320925572.

46. Gola R, Nerini A, Laurent-Fyon C, et al. [Conservative rhinoplasty of the nasal canopy]. Ann Chir Plast Esthet 1989;34(6):465–75. Rhinoplastie conservatrice de l'auvent nasal.

47. Saban Y, Braccini F, Polselli R. [Rhinoplasty: morphodynamic anatomy of rhinoplasty. Interest of conservative rhinoplasty]. Rev Laryngol Otol Rhinol (Bord) 2006;127(1–2):15–22. La rhinoplastie : anatomie morpho-dynamique de la rhinoplastie. Intérêt de la rhinoplastie "conservatrice".

48. Saban Y, Daniel RK, Polselli R, et al. Dorsal preservation: the push down technique Reassessed. Aesthet Surg J 2018;38(2):117–31.

49. Patel PN, Abdelwahab M, Most SP. A Review and modification of dorsal preservation rhinoplasty techniques. Facial Plast Surg Aesthet Med 2020;22(2): 71–9.

50. East C. Preservation rhinoplasty and the crooked nose. Facial Plast Surg Clin North Am 2021;29(1): 123–30.

51. Özücer B, Çam OH. The Effectiveness of asymmetric dorsal preservation for correction of I-shaped crooked nose deformity in comparison to conventional technique. Facial Plast Surg Aesthet Med 2020;22(4):286–93.

52. Stewart MG, Witsell DL, Smith TL, et al. Development and validation of the nasal obstruction symptom evaluation (NOSE) scale. Otolaryngol Head Neck Surg 2004;130(2):157–63.

53. Schwitzer JA, Sher SR, Fan KL, et al. Assessing patient-reported satisfaction with appearance and quality of life following rhinoplasty using the FACE-Q Appraisal scales. Plast Reconstr Surg 2015; 135(5):830e–7e.

54. Klassen AF, Cano SJ, Schwitzer JA, et al. FACE-Q scales for health-related quality of life, early life impact, satisfaction with outcomes, and decision to have treatment: development and validation. Plast Reconstr Surg 2015;135(2):375–86.

55. Alsarraf R, Larrabee WF Jr, Anderson S, et al. Measuring cosmetic facial plastic surgery outcomes: a pilot study. Arch Facial Plast Surg 2001; 3(3):198–201.

56. Dasdar S, Kianfar N, Sadeghi M, et al. The impact of facial asymmetry on the surgical outcome of crooked nose: a case Control study. Aesthet Surg J 2020. https://doi.org/10.1093/asj/sjaa405.

57. Sözen T, Dizdar D, Göksel A. Awareness of facial asymmetry and its impact on postoperative satisfaction of rhinoplasty patient. Aesthet Plast Surg 2020. https://doi.org/10.1007/s00266-020-01968-9.

Cleft Rhinoplasty

Cristen E. Olds, MD[a], Jonathan M. Sykes, MD[a,b],*

KEYWORDS

- Cleft rhinoplasty • Cleft nasal deformity • Cleft • Primary cleft rhinoplasty
- Definitive cleft rhinoplasty • Cleft lip • Cleft lip management

KEY POINTS

- All patients with a cleft lip deformity have an associated nasal deformity that ranges in severity.
- A thorough understanding of the anatomy of the cleft nose aids the surgeon in selecting proper techniques for repair.
- Advantages of early surgical intervention include minimizing the deformity as the child grows and lessening asymmetry to facilitate optimal nasal growth.
- Analysis and performance of orthognathic surgery should be done prior to secondary cleft rhinoplasty to optimize the overall result.
- Goals of secondary rhinoplasty include relief of nasal obstruction, creation of symmetry and definition of the nasal base and tip, and management of nasal scarring and webbing.
- Septal reconstruction in the cleft nose is a key maneuver in cleft rhinoplasty.

INTRODUCTION

The nasal deformity associated with congenital cleft lip is a complex defect that results in significant aesthetic and functional problems. The defect involves all tissue layers, including the bony platform of the nose, the mucosal lining, the cartilaginous infrastructure, and the soft tissue envelope. The extent of the nasal deformity varies with the degree of lip abnormality; it may be unilateral or bilateral and subtle or complete.[1]

All patients with a cleft lip deformity have an associated deformity of the nose that ranges in severity. In many patients with congenital clefts, the secondary nasal deformity is minimal. The appearance of the nose in some patients with clefts, however, often is the feature that is the most noticeable to the observer. The variability of the secondary cleft nasal deformity is related to the nature of the original deformity, the results of all surgeries performed on the lip and nose, and the growth and scarring of the nose. In addition, patients with clefts have significantly increased rates of nasal obstruction, obstructive sleep apnea, and functional nasal problems.[2–4] Patients with bilateral cleft lip and palate have significantly reduced cross-sectional nasal airway area, creating more severe nasal obstruction in this population than among patients with unilateral cleft lip and palate (or cleft palate alone).[5]

The goals of comprehensive management of the cleft nasal deformity include minimizing functional problems and normalization of the appearance of the nose. This requires the surgeon to have an understanding of the pathophysiology of clefting and the 3-dimensional nature of the cleft nasal deformity. This article discusses the pathophysiology of the cleft lip nasal deformity and the timing of surgical repair and highlights a selection of techniques currently used to address the deformity.

ANATOMY AND PATHOPHYSIOLOGY OF THE CLEFT NASAL DEFORMITY

Unilateral and bilateral cleft lip deformities have well-described characteristic nasal defects

---

[a] Roxbury Institute, 450 N Roxbury Drive, #400, Beverly Hills, CA 90210, USA; [b] Facial Plastic and Reconstructive Surgery, UC Davis Medical Center, Sacramento, CA, USA
* Corresponding author. 5 Medical Plaza Drive, Suite 100, Roseville, CA 95661.
E-mail address: jmsykes@ucdavis.edu

Clin Plastic Surg 49 (2022) 123–136
https://doi.org/10.1016/j.cps.2021.08.002

(**Table 1**).[6] Understanding the pathophysiology of the cleft nasal deformity aids the surgeon in choice of techniques to address these deformities.

Cleft lip and palate deformities are the most common congenital orofacial deformities, with an estimated frequency of 1 in 700 worldwide.[7] Cleft deformities result from a failure of the fusion of the median nasal processes with the maxillary processes (formed by the first pharyngeal arch). The paired median nasal processes fuse to form the premaxilla, philtrum, columella, and nasal tip during normal development. The bilateral maxillary processes form the lateral aspects of the upper lip.[8,9]

In complete, unilateral cleft lip patients, the maxilla on the cleft side is deficient. Due to this deficiency, the alar base on the cleft side does not fuse in the midline and is positioned more posterior, lateral, and inferior than the alar base on the noncleft side (**Fig. 1**).[10] As a result of deficient skeletal base, the lateral crus of the lower lateral cartilage (LLC) on the cleft side is lengthened and the medial crura is shortened in relation to the LLC on the noncleft side, although the degree of cartilaginous deformation can be significant, but there generally is no hypoplasia of the cartilage itself.[11] The attachment of the upper lateral cartilage to the LLC is affected by the change in position of the LLC, which effectively weakens the scroll region.[12] Furthermore, there can be retrusion of the nasal bone on the cleft side, malposition of the medial maxilla, and lateral displacement of the medial canthus. The septum is attached to the noncleft maxilla inferiorly by the nasolabial musculature, and asymmetric traction on the caudal septum causes it to be deviated to the noncleft side with dorsal bowing toward the cleft side (**Figs. 2 and 3**).[13] The internal nasal valve on the cleft side is compromised due to the dorsal bowing of the septum, malpositioned LLC and nasal bone retrusion. All of these underlying structural abnormalities cause deviation of the nasal tip toward the noncleft side and flattening of the dome on the cleft side.[11]

In complete, bilateral cleft lip patients, the maxilla is deficient bilaterally, which allows the prolabium to have unopposed anterior growth.[14] The alar bases are displaced in a posterior, lateral, and inferior position compared with development without clefting. The deficient skeletal base leads to longer lateral crura of the LLCs bilaterally and short, splayed medial crura of the LLCs. This creates an under-projected, broad, and flat nasal tip.[15] The columella is shortened due to the malposition of the prolabium and the shortening of the medial crura, and the shorter columella makes the broad, snubbed nasal tip even more pronounced (**Fig. 4**).

The characteristic unilateral and bilateral cleft nasal deformities can appear along a spectrum of severity—in patients with incomplete cleft lips, these nasal deformities are less pronounced.[16] Even though the defects may be subtle, it can be determined how the anatomic structures will be positioned based on these characteristic changes from their normal relationships, and this

Table 1
Anatomic characteristics of the unilateral cleft lip nasal deformity

Anatomic Site	Associated Deformity
Nasal tip	Deviation of tip and columella toward noncleft side Long lateral crus and short medial crus of LLC with domal blunting Deprojected, widened tip on cleft side
Alar base and sill	Wide alar base on cleft side Cleft side alar base positioned laterally, inferiorly, and posteriorly Cleft nostril horizontally oriented Nasal floor and sill may be absent on cleft side Maxillary deficiency underlying alar base on cleft side
Septum	Caudal septum deviated toward noncleft side Cartilaginous and bony septum toward cleft side
Upper lateral cartilage	Weak scroll region on cleft side Interval valve collapse on cleft side
Internal nasal valve	Compromised by septal deviation and collapse of upper lateral cartilage
Bony pyramid	Wide bony dorsum

Adapted from Chapter 69: Cleft Lip Rhinoplasty. In: Papel I et al., eds. Facial Plastic and Reconstructive Surgery. 4th ed. Thieme Publishers; 2016:897; with permission.

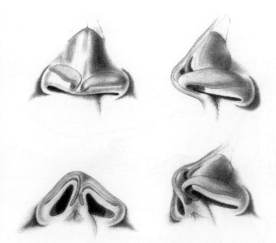

Fig. 1. Multiple views (Anteroposterior - upper left; lateral - upper right; basal - lower left; oblique - lower right) of a left unilateral cleft lip nasal deformity, with characteristic inferior, posterior, and lateral displacement of the alar base and horizontally oriented nostril on the cleft side. (*From* Sykes JM Senders CW, Wang TD, Cook TA. Use of the open approach for repair of secondary cleft lip nasal deformity. *Fac Plast Surg N* Am 1993; 1: 111-.126; with permission.)

understanding used to normalize both form and function.

TIMING OF THE CLEFT NASAL REPAIR

The ideal repair of a cleft nasal deformity is performed in 2 stages (**Table 2**). Major septal work has been suggested to have a negative impact on nasal growth, so major septal and cartilaginous dissection should not be performed until the patient has completed facial growth, because

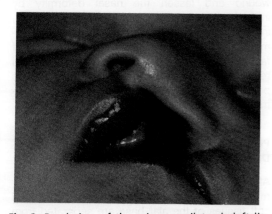

Fig. 2. Basal view of the primary unilateral cleft lip and nasal deformity, demonstrating deviation of the columella toward the noncleft side as well as widening and malposition of the cleft side alar base with horizontal orientation of the cleft side nostril.

the septum functions as a growth center of the face.[17,18] For this reason, definitive repair of the cleft nasal deformity must be delayed. Primary surgery can be performed at an early age, however, without inhibiting nasal growth because there is no resection of the cartilaginous and bony septum.

Primary cleft rhinoplasty generally is performed at the time of the cleft lip repair at the age of 3 months to 6 months. In the newborn, however, the extent of the skeletal and alar base asymmetry should be analyzed in order to plan the primary rhinoplasty. This allows the surgeon to utilize the lip incisions to address the nasal ala and LLC and allows avoidance of additional general anesthetic events in the child's first year of life. Primary rhinoplasty addresses dome asymmetry and repositions the nasal and alar base, allowing for functional and aesthetic improvement without jeopardizing nasal and facial growth.

The secondary (definitive) procedure is performed once a patient has reached facial skeletal maturity. In girls, this generally is performed at approximately 15 years to 17 years of age (or approximately 2 years after menarche) and in boys at approximately 16 years to 18 years of age.[11] At this time, major septal reconstruction can be performed, in addition to definitive rhinoplasty. Often, auricular or costal cartilage as well as resected septal cartilage is required to provide adequate structural support.

PRIMARY RHINOPLASTY

Historically, controversy has existed as to whether primary cleft tip rhinoplasty had a positive influence on the eventual appearance the nose in patients with clefts. Experimental work by Sarnat and Wexler,[18] Bernstein,[19] and other investigators had demonstrated growth retardation of the nose and midface following aggressive resection of the nasal septum and mucoperichondrium. The concern on the part of surgeons reluctant to perform early surgery on the nose in cleft patients was that surgery at an early age contributes to nasal growth inhibition. No experimental or clinical studies have ever proved, however, that minor manipulations (without resection) of the nasal tip or nasal base interfere with future nasal growth.[19]

For these reasons, most contemporary surgeons perform alteration in the nose at the time of lip repair. The purpose of primary rhinoplasty is to close the anterior nasal floor and sill; to relocate the posteriorly, inferiorly, and laterally displaced alar base; and to bring early symmetry to the nasal base and tip.[11,20]

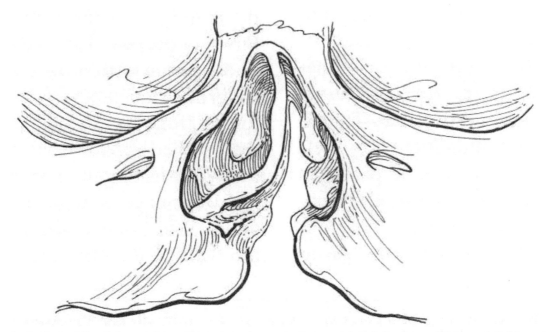

Fig. 3. Coronal illustration of the caudal septum, demonstrating caudal deviation toward the noncleft side and more posterior deviation toward the cleft side. (*From* Jablon JH, Sykes JM. Nasal airway problems in the cleft lip population. *Fac Plast Surg Clin N Am* 1999; 7: 391-403; with permission.)

THE ROLE OF PRESURGICAL NASOALVEOLAR MOLDING

Presurgical nasoalveolar molding (PNAM) is an important adjunct, especially among patients with broad can be used in patients with wide or

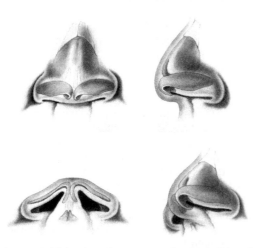

Fig. 4. Multiple views (anteroposterior, lateral, basal, and oblique) of a bilateral cleft lip nasal deformity, with characteristic broad, under-projected nasal tip with bilaterally wide, malpositioned alar bases. (*From* Sykes JM Senders CW, Wang TD, Cook TA. Use of the open approach for repair of secondary cleft lip nasal deformity. *Fac Plast Surg N Am* 1993; 1: 111-126; with permission.)

very asymmetric clefts to (1) reposition the malaligned alveolar segments, (2) narrow the cleft gap, (3) improve nasal tip symmetry in unilateral clefts, (4) elongate the columella, and (5) expand the nasal soft tissues in bilateral clefts. PNAM utilizes a custom, removable intraoral alveolar molding device with nasal molding prongs, which is adjusted every 7 days to 14 days. This requires a motivated family (who understand the treatment goals) and a dedicated orthodontist. If used properly, PNAM can lessen the tension across the lip wound and lessen the nasal deformity by increasing symmetry of the nasal tip cartilages, increasing tip projection, and elongating the columella as well as encouraging a normal trajectory of facial growth in the time between birth and surgical repair (**Fig. 5**).[21,22] Primary rhinoplasty then can be performed to improve nasal appearance and optimize nasal growth.

PRIMARY CLEFT RHINOPLASTY—TECHNICAL DETAILS

After the cleft lip incisions are made and the primary lip dissection is completed, the muscle and soft tissues of the alar base are separated from their maxillary attachments. The malpositioned alar base is freed by creating an internal alotomy at the head of the inferior turbinate. If adequate soft tissue dissection of the alar base is performed,

Table 2
Timing and goals of cleft rhinoplasty

Rhinoplasty Subtype	Timing	Goals
Primary	3–6 mo of age, concurrent with lip repair	Closure of nasal floor and sill Reorientation of LLC Septal realignment without excision
Intermediate	Between primary and secondary repair (typically 1–14 y of age)	Stabilize the nasal base Lengthen the columella Fine-tune tip symmetry
Secondary (definitive)	Completion of nasal and midface growth (14 y of age in girls, 16 in boys)	Restore nasal airway through septal reconstruction Address nasal valve scarring/webbing Restore symmetry of nasal tip and base Augment maxilla at alar base

Adapted from Chapter 69: Cleft Lip Rhinoplasty. In: Papel I et al., eds. Facial Plastic and Reconstructive Surgery. 4th ed. Thieme Publishers; 2016:901; with permission.

the cleft alar base can be repositioned (during closure) in the optimal 3-dimensional position. During the initial cleft lip repair, the alar base should be reconstructed in a manner that mirrors the noncleft alar base.[23]

The cleft side LLC then is dissected from its cutaneous attachments by creating a medial and a lateral tunnel. These subcutaneous tunnels are connected and allow the cleft LLC to be repositioned into a more symmetric fashion.[24] Care is taken to not violate the vestibular skin, avoiding the complication of secondary adhesions and nasal valve stenosis.

Next comes closure of the nasal floor and sill. This closure is started first with reapproximation of the musculature of the nasal base, including the transverse nasal muscle. The skin of the nasal sill is then closed with 5-0 chromic catgut suture, with particular attention paid to creating symmetry between the cleft nasal sill and the noncleft side. It is important to not narrow the sill excessively, because a nasal base that is too wide is easy to

narrow during a secondary procedure, whereas an excessively narrow sill is difficult to widen.

The final component of primary cleft rhinoplasty is to alter the cleft nasal tip into a more projected, symmetric position. After the nasal sill is reestablished and the lip is repaired in a layered fashion, the cleft LLC is repositioned to create a narrowed, projected nasal tip.[25] This is achieved with internal mattress sutures or tie-over external bolsters (**Figs. 6** and **7**).[24] A new dome is created with a lengthened medial crus and a shortened lateral crus. If nasal bolsters are used, they are removed in 7 days to 10 days. The resulting nasal tip is more symmetric, defined, and projected.

INTERMEDIATE CLEFT RHINOPLASTY

Intermediate rhinoplasty in patients with congenital clefting of the lip is defined as any nasal surgery performed between the time of initial lip repair and the time of definitive rhinoplasty (when the patient reaches facial skeletal maturity) but is most

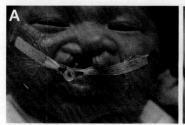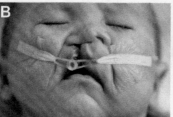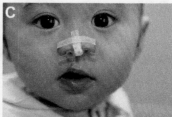

Fig. 5. PNAM. (*A*) Child with right complete cleft lip and palate at the beginning of PNAM. (*B*) Narrowed cleft gap, lip defect, and improved lip and nasal base symmetry at the conclusion of this child's PNAM course. (*C*) Postoperative image, directly after repair of cleft lip with concurrent cleft rhinoplasty.

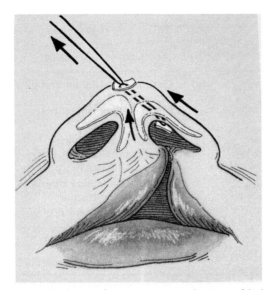

Fig. 6. Basal view demonstrating application of bolsters to reposition the cleft LLC; bolsters will remain in place for 7 days to 10 days postoperatively. Note force vectors on the LLC (*black arrows*). (*From* Sykes, JM Senders CW. Surgery of the cleft lip nasal deformity. *Oper Tech Otolaryngol Head Neck Surg* 1990; 1: 219-224; with permission.)

commonly performed before a child enters school (age 4–6 years).[26] The use of intermediate rhinoplasty in patients with unilateral cleft nasal deformities has decreased as surgeons have become more adept at primary rhinoplasty. Many patients with bilateral clefts, however, have significant deformities during adolescence, and intermediate rhinoplasty may be used to attain improved nasal symmetry and tip projection (as well as address nasal webbing that may have resulted from primary rhinoplasty), may be performed concurrently with revision lip surgery, and minimizes the social stigmata associated with clefting.[27]

The goals of intermediate cleft rhinoplasty vary according to the needs of the patient. Children with unilateral cleft nasal deformities that were not addressed at the time of initial lip repair can be good candidates for tip rhinoplasty as adolescents. In patients with bilateral clefts and significant under-projection of the nasal tip, columellar lengthening may be indicated during childhood. Lastly, if a child is suffering social ridicule, rhinoplasty may be performed to minimize the existing deformity.[28]

Intermediate rhinoplasty usually involves recruitment of upper lip skin into the columella in patients who require additional tip projection. In unilateral cases, extra skin is provided with either a midline V-to-Y advancement, or with an asymmetric V-to-Y advancement, which utilizes the cleft scar for advancement into the columellar base. After undermining the nasal tip skin with either an endonasal tip delivery approach or a modified external rhinoplasty, an interdomal suture may be utilized to augment nasal tip projection, provide tip definition, and improve nasal tip symmetry.

During most intermediate rhinoplasties, limited undermining of the nasal soft tissues is performed because this minimizes postoperative scarring. In most cases, intermediate rhinoplasty is not the final nasal procedure, and a more definitive nasal procedure with septal reconstruction and cartilage grafting of deficient areas is performed after full facial growth has been attained. Philosophically,

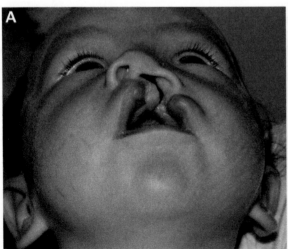
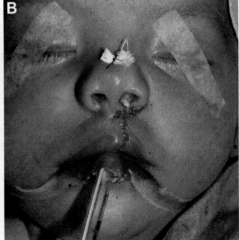

Fig. 7. Primary cleft rhinoplasty, concurrent with lip repair. (*A*) Preoperative deformity. (*B*) Completed lip repair and primary rhinoplasty; note the use of a bolster to reposition the dome of the left lower cartilage. The bolster suture is tightened until trace blanching of the skin is noted.

the surgeon should realize that the patient will grow and the adolescent nose will change and should attempt to minimize the intermediate deformity without creating excess scarring. The intermediate cleft rhinoplasty, therefore, usually does not include aggressive septal reconstruction, osteotomies, or significant cartilage grafting.

ORTHOGNATHIC SURGERY

In cleft patients with significant dentofacial deformities, surgery to correct skeletal abnormalities and to optimize dental occlusion often necessary; this should be performed prior to definitive (secondary) cleft rhinoplasty. When performed, orthognathic surgery has the advantage of maximizing the skeletal profile and improving the crossbite and underjet that commonly accompany oral clefting. Studies have shown that it is the cleft palatoplasty (usually performed at approximately 12 months of age) that is responsible for restriction of maxillary growth in an anterior-posterior and a transverse dimension.[29] Palatoplasty often results in maxillary hypoplasia (with resultant underjet) and transverse maxillary width restriction (with resulting buccal crossbite) due to mild, sustained posterior traction on the palate.

Skeletal correction of the hypoplastic cleft maxilla requires advancement, and often transverse widening, of the maxilla. This procedure usually is performed in conjunction with an orthodontist. In most instances, 12 months to 18 months of preoperative orthodontic treatment is necessary to align the dental arches. This can minimize the occlusal deformity and often decreases the amount of movement necessary during orthognathic surgery. It may require dental extractions to accommodate tooth movements and eliminate crowding.

There are 2 basic approaches that can be used to correct the dentofacial and skeletal deformities associated with congenital clefting. The first approach is conventional orthognathic surgery, including maxillary advancement and widening with or without mandibular setback. The other approach is to perform a standard Le Fort I maxillary osteotomy and placement of distraction osteogenesis (DO) devices (**Fig. 8**).

If conventional orthognathic surgery is planned, treatment of both the maxilla and mandible often is required for adequate skeletal correction.[29] The maxilla often is scarred from prior palatal surgery, precluding a large advancement to adequately correct the underjet. Operating on both jaws allows the surgeon to split the difference and maximize the skeletal relationship and correct the class III occlusion.

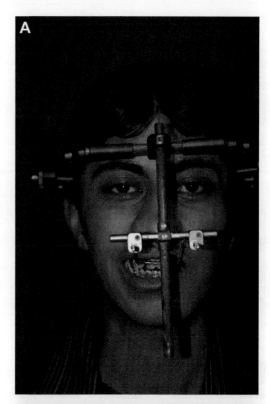

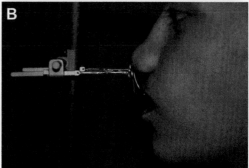

Fig. 8. (*A*) Frontal and (*B*) lateral views of an adolescent patient status post Le Fort I osteotomy, undergoing midface advancement via RED.

DO utilizes either an internal distractor or a rigid external distractor (RED) device. Use of DO allows the surgeon to progressively advance the maxilla after Le Fort I osteotomies are created (**Fig. 9**). This method often is necessary to correct significant cleft jaw discrepancies, in which maxillary advancement is inhibited by palatal scarring and the possible presence of a pharyngeal flap. Pharyngeal flaps often are required on cleft patients to correct the velopharyngeal incompetence that often is associated with repaired cleft palates and acts as a rubber band on the posterior palate, inhibiting full anterior repositioning of the maxilla. After completing the maxillary osteomy and

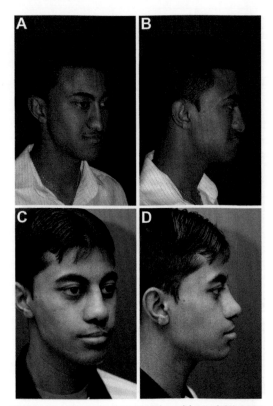

Fig. 9. Preoperative oblique (*A*) and lateral (*B*) views of an adolescent patient with a secondary cleft nasal deformity, class III malocclusion and midface hypoplasia. Posteroperative oblique (*C*) and lateral (*D*) views. The patient underwent Le Fort I osteotomies and midface advancement via RED, followed by definitive cleft septorhinoplasty with use of autologous costal cartilage grafting.

placing the distraction device, a waiting (latency) period allows sufficient postoperative healing before distraction begins. The maxilla then is distracted over a 4-week to 6-week period prior to consolidation. Distraction grows both bone and soft tissue and improves the skeletal base that supports the nose.

SECONDARY (DEFINITIVE) CLEFT RHINOPLASTY

The extent of the secondary nasal deformity varies according to the extent of the original lip and nose defect, any surgery performed, and the specific trajectory of the patient's nasal growth. Definitive nasal surgery is performed after full nasal growth (completion of facial growth at ages 15–17 in girls and ages 16–18 in boys).[11]

SURGICAL APPROACH

The approach to secondary cleft septorhinoplasty varies according to the requirements of the

reconstruction. The authors generally prefer an external approach with or without an alotomy on the cleft side for maximal exposure of nasal structures. The incision for the open approach has numerous configurations that reflect specific aspects of the reconstruction. The traditional inverted-V incision can be modified to recruit upper lip skin to the columella with a V-to-Y closure, or the incision can be made asymmetrically onto the nasal skin on the cleft side to recruit this skin inward to address a superiomedial alar web (**Fig. 10**).[30] Finally, an evolution of techniques has been described related to the recruitment of tissue from the lip repair with a sliding chondrocutaneous flap.[31] This flap provides additional tissue to augment the vestibular lining and reduce the alar-columellar web, and, when it is combined with open rhinoplasty, the chondrocutaneous flap can permit tip stability and refinement.

SEPTAL RECONSTRUCTION

Repair of the cleft nasal septum is a crucial aspect of cleft nasal reconstruction, which typically is challenging. The pathophysiology of the septal deformity includes the deficient bony maxilla and the abnormal pull of the aberrant and hypoplastic orbicularis oris muscles. In the unilateral cleft deformity, the deficient premaxilla and the palatal cleft cause the septum to deviate to the cleft side. Anteriorly, the asymmetric unopposed pull of the orbicularis muscles and the deficient bony maxilla causes the septum to deviate to the noncleft side.[13] The septal deformity associated with unilateral clefts is characteristic and always present; the extent of the deformity, however, is variable and related to the extent of the original cleft deformity. The nasal septum in the bilateral cleft lip deformity is usually midline, being deviated caudally to the less involved side if asymmetry exists.

Repair of the cleft septum is the foundation of the rhinoplasty. Complete septal reconstruction requires adequate exposure and complete breakdown of the ligamentous attachments, which contribute to the septal deviation. The septum can be accessed through a separate hemitransfixion incision or directly through the open approach. Adequate caudal and dorsal struts should be preserved while deviations in the cartilage and bone are corrected. To return the caudal septum to the midline, the surgeon often must remove a strip of cartilage inferiorly, allowing the septum to swing over the nasal spine. This position can be maintained by suturing the cartilage to the spine with a 5-0 long-acting absorbable monofilament suture.

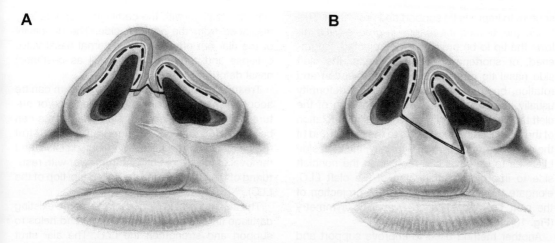

Fig. 10. (*A*) Basal view of a left secondary cleft lip deformity demonstrating the modification of the standard external rhinoplasty incision. (*B*) Basal view demonstrating a modified Bardach incision; closure of the incision in a V-to-Y fashion will advance additional skin and soft tissue from the upper lip to the columella, therefore lengthening it. (*From* Sykes JM Senders CW, Wang TD, Cook TA. Use of the open approach for repair of secondary cleft lip nasal deformity. *Fac Plast Surg N* Am 1993; 1: 111-126; with permission.)

If the septal support is not sufficient after resection of the deviated segments, reconstruction with cartilage grafts is needed to maintain adequate central segment support. Septal support can be achieved with a variety of grafting methods. The septum can be splinted and supported with a cartilaginous septal extension graft. The septal extension graft can be sutured to the caudal end of the existing septum in an end-to-end or an end-to side technique. The important concept is that at the conclusion of grafting and repositioning of the septum, that the caudal aspect of the septum is straight and well supported. Extended spreader grafts also be can used to aid in support of the caudal and dorsal septum, and they can improve the cross-sectional airway of the internal nasal valve as well as help correct dorsal external deviations (**Fig. 11**).[32]

In patients who have severe nasal septal deviation (in which resection, repositioning, and cartilage grafting are inadequate), complete removal and reshaping of the nasal septum may be required. This technique, termed *extracorporeal septoplasty*, involves explantation of the septal cartilage, reshaping of this cartilage on the operative field (out of the patient), and reimplantation of the septum with fixation both caudally and dorsally.[33] Often, this technique is combined with cartilage grafting for support and strength of the reimplanted septum. Regardless of the technique used, at the end of the septoplasty, the septum should be straight to maximize the cleft airway, and well supported, to allow the tip to be resuspended adequately.

TREATMENT OF THE NASAL TIP

The nasal tip in patients with congenital clefting of the lip is poorly supported. In the unilateral deformity, the tip is asymmetric secondary to the short medial crus on the cleft side. In the bilateral deformity, the tip usually is under-projected and the columella is short. Tip techniques, therefore, are designed to improve tip symmetry and to improve definition and projection.

After the nasal septum is straightened and supported, the nasal tip can be resuspended on the

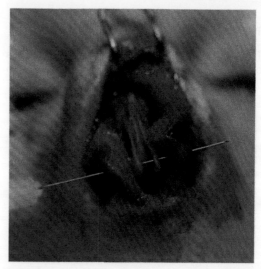

Fig. 11. Intraoperative view of extended spreader graft placement. Note use of a hypodermic needle to stabilize the grafts as they are sutured into place.

septum to improve tip support and projection. This technique, termed the *tongue-in-groove* (*TIG*), allows the tip to be projected, deprojected, lengthened, or shortened.[34] In most clefts, the cleft side nasal tip requires increased projection and rotation, because the secondary nasal deformity usually has under-projection and hooding of the cleft tip. The TIG technique involves suture fixation of the medial crura of the LLCs to the caudal end of the nasal septum (**Fig. 12**). Typically, the cleft side LLC has to be advanced more than the noncleft side to improve the flattening of the cleft LLC, elongate the medial crura, increase projection of the cleft tip, and enhance overall tip symmetry (**Fig. 13**).

Another method used to improve support and projection is the columellar strut cartilage graft. The columellar strut graft is a sturdy piece of cartilage that is placcde between the medial crura of the LLCs. The medial crura can be advanced on this graft and suture fixated to enhance projection and support.

A final maneuver, which can be used to increase tip projection and symmetry, is vertical division of the LLCs (**Fig. 14**). On the cleft side, this maneuver usually is performed lateral to the existing dome. Division of the cartilages lateral to the dome increases the medial crural element and increases projection of the nasal tip. After division is performed, the cartilages are reconstituted with suture. After the central tip segment is supported with 1 of these maneuvers, a cartilaginous tip graft can be added to camouflage irregularities and improve tip definition. These tip grafts typically are suture fixated with permanent or absorbable monofilament suture.

TREATMENT OF THE CLEFT ALAR RIM

The cleft side lateral crus of the LLC usually is concave. This concavity often is associated with

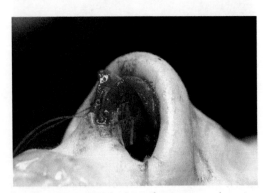

Fig. 12. Intraoperative view of TIG suture placement and columellar strut graft.

alar malposition, with the cartilage often inferiorly displaced from the noncleft side. The concavity of the alar rim often causes external nasal valve collapse and a functional (as well as aesthetic) nasal deformity.

Treatment of the malpositioned alar rim can be accomplished with cartilage grafting and/or suture repositioning. The cleft side lateral crus can be supported with (1) alar rim graft, (2) alar strut graft, (3) alar turn-in flap, and (4) excision and removal of the entire LLC and turn over with resuturing of the segment (the so-called flip-flop of the LLC).[35-38]

The alar rim graft is placed inferior to the existing cartilage (in a nonanatomic position) and helps to support and strengthen the LLC. The alar strut graft, if used, is placed on the deep surface of the LLC, with the graft sutured to the undersurface of the cartilage. The lateral extent of this graft typically is placed in a soft tissue pocket at the piriform aperture. Both of these grafts aid in elevating the level of the alar rim and repositioning the rim laterally.

The LLC turn-in flap utilizes the cephalic portion of the LLC. In most rhinoplasty procedures, the cephalic portion of the LLC is resected and discarded. In the turn-in flap technique, this previously resected cartilage is transposed on a pedicle and sutured to the undersurface of the remaining LLC, in order to strengthen and support the LLC and to flatten the preexisting concavity. The flip-flop technique involves dissecting the lateral crura of the LLC off of the underlying vestibular skin, excising this portion, turning it over, and resuturing it to the vestibular lining. This changes the shape of the alar rim from concave to convex. All these maneuvers are designed to strengthen and reposition the malformed alar rim cartilage. If there still is significant malposition of the cleft LLC after these maneuvers are completed, the LLC can be sutured to the upper lateral cartilage to securely reposition the alar rim more superiorly (**Fig. 15**).

TREATMENT OF THE ALAR BASE

The alar base often is asymmetric and abnormal in shape, with alar base depression on the cleft side a common finding on examination. The etiology of this deformity is related to the congenitally deficient skeletal nasal base and to any surgery performed prior to the definitive rhinoplasty. In many cases, the insertion of the lateral alar rim (the alar-facial junction) is malpositioned as a result of the original cleft lip repair. A small malposition during the cleft lip repair can result in a larger disparity with growth. For this reason, the

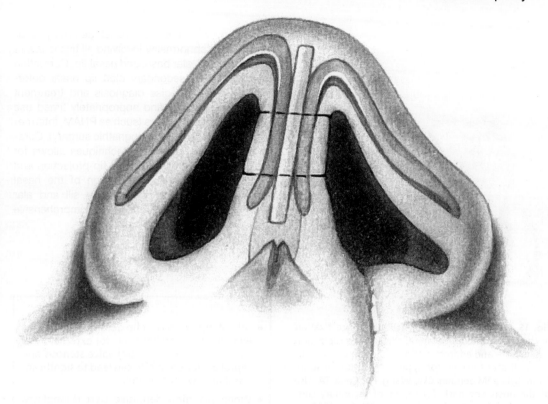

Fig. 13. Basal view depicting the placement of the cartilaginous columellar strut and asymmetric advancement of the LLCs onto the strut to improve tip symmetry. (*From* Sykes JM Senders CW, Wang TD, Cook TA. Use of the open approach for repair of secondary cleft lip nasal deformity. *Fac Plast Surg N* Am 1993; 1: 111-126; with permission.)

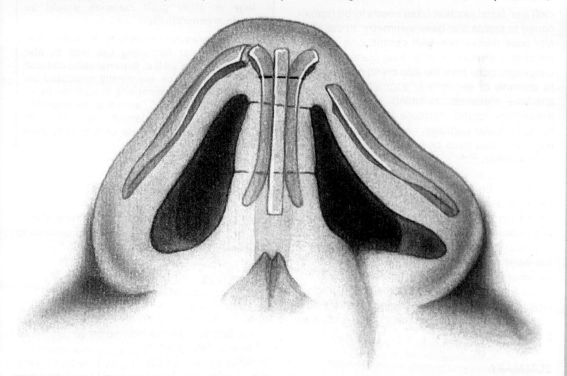

Fig. 14. Basal view depicting asymmetric division of the LLCs to increase tip projection and symmetry. (*From* Sykes JM Senders CW, Wang TD, Cook TA. Use of the open approach for repair of secondary cleft lip nasal deformity. *Fac Plast Surg N* Am 1993; 1: 111-126; with permission.)

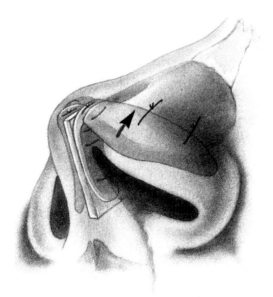

Fig. 15. Oblique view demonstrating suture fixation of the LLC to the upper lateral cartilage to reposition the alar rim and address vestibular hooding. Black arrow indicates force vector applied by suture fixation. (*From* Sykes JM Senders CW, Wang TD, Cook TA. Use of the open approach for repair of secondary cleft lip nasal deformity. *Fac Plast Surg N* Am 1993; 1: 111-126; with permission.)

cleft alar-facial junction often needs to be repositioned to create alar base symmetry. In cases of alar base malposition with contributing skeletal deficiency, alveolar bone grafting (generally using cancellous bone from the iliac crest) may be used to primarily or secondarily augment this region; alternate materials, including homologous or autologous costal cartilage grafts, vomerine bone, auricular cartilage, and various alloplastic materials, also have been used to perform this augmentation.[39–41]

Another common secondary deformity that is a result of the original cleft lip repair is a lack of complete closure of the sill of the nose. This defect occurs when the superior portion of the orbicularis oris muscle is incompletely closed. This causes a lack of symmetry of the alar base at the level of the nasal sill. This deformity often is obvious to the observer and creates a noticeable abnormal shape to the inferior aspect of the nostril. Reconstruction of this requires reopening of the superior aspect of the lip and realignment of the orbicularis muscle.

SUMMARY

The anatomic characteristics of the unilateral and bilateral cleft lip nasal deformities have been well described, with the cleft nasal deformity a 3-dimensional abnormality involving all tissue layers of the nasal sill, alar base, and nasal tip. Correction of primary and secondary cleft lip nasal deformities requires precise diagnosis and treatment as well as judicious and appropriately timed use of adjunctive procedures (such as PNAM, intermediate rhinoplasty, and orthognathic surgery). Careful use of cleft rhinoplasty techniques allows for maximal improvement in nasal tip projection and symmetry as well as optimization of the nasal airway. Management of the nasal sill and alar base also must be addressed for comprehensive management of the cleft nose.

CLINICS CARE POINTS

- All patients with cleft lip deformity should be evaluated comprehensively for external nasal deformity as well as nasal valve stenosis and septal deviation, which can lead to significant nasal airway obstruction.
- When planning definitive cleft rhinoplasty, evaluate for maxillary deficiency contributing to alar base malposition; plans for augmentation with autologous or homologous cartilage or other graft materials should be made preoperatively.
- During definitive rhinoplasty, be aware that cleft side alar flattening can lead to alar malposition as well as external valve collapse (which should be specifically evaluated on preoperative examination); in addition to repositioning the LLC, attention to strengthening the lower lateral crus (through cartilage grafting or use of a turn-in flap) should be considered.

DISCLOSURE

The authors have no commercial of financial conflicts of interest and have no funding sources to disclose.

REFERENCES

1. Sykes JM, Senders CW. Pathologic anatomy of cleft lip, palate, and nasal deformities. In: Meyers AD, editor. Biological basis of facial plastic surgery. 1st ed. Thieme; 1993. p. 57–71.
2. Sykes JM, Senders CW. Surgery of the cleft lip nasal deformity. Oper Tech Otolaryngol Head Neck Surg 1990;1(4). https://doi.org/10.1016/S1043-1810(10)80061-2.

3. Fernandes MD, Salgueiro AGNS, Bighetti EJB, et al. Symptoms of obstructive sleep apnea, nasal obstruction, and enuresis in children with nonsyndromic cleft lip and palate: a prevalence study. Cleft Palate Craniofac J 2019;56(3). https://doi.org/10.1177/1055665618776074.

4. Sobol DL, Allori AC, Carlson AR, et al. Nasal airway dysfunction in children with cleft lip and cleft palate. Plast Reconstr Surg 2016;138(6). https://doi.org/10.1097/PRS.0000000000002772.

5. Fukushiro AP, Kiemle Trindade IE. Nasal airway dimensions of adults with cleft lip and palate: differences among cleft types. Cleft Palate Craniofac J 2005;42(4). https://doi.org/10.1597/03-081.1.

6. Huffman W, Lierle DM. Studies on the pathologic anatomy of the unilateral harelip nose. Plast Reconstr Surg 1949;4(3). https://doi.org/10.1097/00006534-194905000-00001.

7. Bernheim N, Georges M, Malevez C, et al. Embryology and epidemiology of cleft lip and palate. B-ENT 2006;2(S4):11–9.

8. Enlow D. Facial growth. 3rd edition. W.B. Saunders; 1990.

9. Capone R, Sykes J. Evaluation and management of cleft lip and palate disorders. In: Papel I, editor. Facial plastic and reconstructive surgery. 3rd ed. Thieme; 2009. p. 1059–60.

10. Sykes JM, Jang YJu. Cleft lip rhinoplasty. Facial Plast Surg Clin North Am 2009;17(1). https://doi.org/10.1016/j.fsc.2008.10.002.

11. Stenström SJ. The alar cartilage and the nasal deformity in unilateral cleft lip. Plast Reconstr Surg 1966;38(3). https://doi.org/10.1097/00006534-196609000-00007.

12. Crockett D, Bumstead R. Nasal airway, otologic, and audiologic problems associated with cleft lip and palate. In: Bardach J, Morris H, editors. Multidisciplinary management of cleft lip and palate. WB Saunders; 1990.

13. Jablon JH, Sykes JM. Nasal airway problems in the cleft lip population. Facial Plast Surg Clinic North Am 1999;7:391–404.

14. Hopper R, Cutting C, Grayson B. Cleft lip and palate. In: Thorne C, editor. Grabb and Smith's plastic surgery. 6th edition. Lippincott Williams & Wilkins; 2009. 1082-undefined.

15. Coleman J, Sykes JM. Cleft lip rhinoplasty. In: Papel I, editor. Facial plastic and reconstructive surgery. 3rd edition. Thieme; 2009. 1082-undefined.

16. Allori AC, Mulliken JB, Meara JG, et al. Classification of cleft lip/palate: then and now. Cleft Palate Craniofac J 2017;54(2). https://doi.org/10.1597/14-080.

17. Sarnat BG, Wexler MR. Growth of the face and jaws after resection of the septal cartilage in the rabbit. Am J Anat 1966;118(3). https://doi.org/10.1002/aja.1001180306.

18. Bernstein L. Early submucous resection of nasal septal cartilage: a pilot study in canine pups. Arch Otolaryngol Head Neck Surg 1973;97(3). https://doi.org/10.1001/archotol.1973.00780010281012.

19. Mccomb HK, Coghlan BA. Primary repair of the unilateral cleft lip nose: completion of a Longitudinal study. Cleft Palate Craniofac J 1996;33(1). https://doi.org/10.1597/1545-1569_1996_033_0023_protuc_2.3.co_2.

20. Gudis DA, Patel KG. Update on primary cleft lip rhinoplasty. Curr Opin Otolaryngol Head Neck Surg 2014;22(4). https://doi.org/10.1097/MOO.0000000000000066.

21. Grayson BH, Maull D. Nasoalveolar molding for infants born with clefts of the lip, alveolus, and palate. Clin Plast Surg 2004;31(2). https://doi.org/10.1016/S0094-1298(03)00140-8.

22. Attiguppe P, Karuna Y, Yavagal C, et al. Presurgical nasoalveolar molding: a boon to facilitate the surgical repair in infants with cleft lip and palate. Contemp Clin Dentistry 2016;7(4). https://doi.org/10.4103/0976-237X.194104.

23. Sykes J, Senders C. Surgical treatment of the unilateral cleft nasal deformity at the time of lip repair. Facial Plast Surg Clin North Am 1995;3(1):69–77.

24. Shih CW, Sykes JM. Correction of the cleft-lip nasal deformity. Facial Plast Surg 2002;18(4). https://doi.org/10.1055/s-2002-36493.

25. Mulliken JB, Martínez-Pérez D. The principle of rotation advancement for repair of unilateral complete cleft lip and nasal deformity: technical variations and analysis of results. Plast Reconstr Surg 1999;104(5). https://doi.org/10.1097/00006534-199910000-00003.

26. Kaufman Y, Buchanan E, Wolfswinkel E, et al. Cleft nasal deformity and rhinoplasty. Semin Plast Surg 2013;26(04). https://doi.org/10.1055/s-0033-1333886.

27. Gary C, Sykes JM. Intermediate and definitive cleft rhinoplasty. Facial Plast Surg Clin North Am 2016;24(4). https://doi.org/10.1016/j.fsc.2016.06.017.

28. Sykes J, Senders C. Surgical management of the cleft lip nasal deformity. Curr Opin Otolaryngol Head Neck Surg 2008;16(4):339–46.

29. Ross RB. Treatment variables affecting facial growth in complete unilateral cleft lip and palate. Cleft Palate J 1987;24(1):5–77.

30. Sykes J, Senders C, Wang T, et al. Use of the open approach for repair of secondary cleft lip nasal deformity. Fac Plast Surg North Am 1993;1:111–26.

31. Wang TD, Madorsky SJ. Secondary rhinoplasty in nasal deformity associated with the unilateral cleft lip. Arch Facial Plast Surg 1999;1(1). https://doi.org/10.1001/archfaci.1.1.40.

32. Haack J, Papel ID. Caudal septal deviation. Otolaryngol Clin North Am 2009;42(3). https://doi.org/10.1016/j.otc.2009.03.005.

33. Most SP. Anterior septal reconstruction. Arch Facial Plast Surg 2006;8(3). https://doi.org/10.1001/archfaci.8.3.202.

34. Kridel RWH, Scott BA, Foda HMT. The tongue-in-groove technique in septorhinoplasty. Arch Facial Plast Surg 1999;1(4). https://doi.org/10.1001/archfaci.1.4.246.

35. Rohrich RJ, Raniere J, Ha RY. The alar contour graft: correction and prevention of alar rim deformities in rhinoplasty. Plast Reconstr Surg 2002;109(7). https://doi.org/10.1097/00006534-200206000-00050.

36. Gunter JP, Friedman RM. Lateral crural strut graft: technique and clinical applications in rhinoplasty. Plast Reconstr Surg 1997;99(4). https://doi.org/10.1097/00006534-199704000-00001.

37. Murakami CS, Barrera JE, Most SP. Preserving structural integrity of the alar cartilage in aesthetic rhinoplasty using a cephalic turn-in flap. Arch Facial Plast Surg 2009;11(2). https://doi.org/10.1001/archfacial.2008.524.

38. Ballert J, Park S. Functional rhinoplasty: treatment of the dysfunctional nasal sidewall. Facial Plast Surg 2006;22(1). https://doi.org/10.1055/s-2006-939952.

39. Chen H, Chen C-Y, Fang Q-Q, et al. Computed tomography–assisted auricular cartilage graft for depression of the alar base in secondary unilateral cleft lip repair: a preliminary report. Cleft Palate Craniofac J 2019;56(1). https://doi.org/10.1177/1055665618770306.

40. Cuzalina A, Tamim A. Cleft lip and palate patient rhinoplasty. In: Contemporary rhinoplasty. IntechOpen; 2019. https://doi.org/10.5772/intechopen.82116.

41. Elfeki B, Elhussiny Khater AM, Bahaa El-Din AM, et al. Alar base augmentation using vomerine bone graft in patients with cleft lip nasal deformity. Ann Plast Surg 2020;85(5). https://doi.org/10.1097/SAP.0000000000002432.

Dorsal Augmentation

Grace J. Graw, MD[a],[*], Jay W. Calvert, MD[b]

KEYWORDS

- Rhinoplasty • Nasal dorsum • Deficient dorsum • Dorsal augmentation • Autologous
- Diced cartilage with deep temporalis fascia graft • Allogeneic • Synthetic

KEY POINTS

- A thorough facial analysis, keeping in mind the preservation of overall nasofacial harmony, is key in achieving desired outcomes.
- A variety of dorsal augmentation techniques, including both autologous and nonautologous (ie, allogeneic and synthetic) sources, exists for the management of the deficient nasal dorsum.
- Selection of an optimal graft source depends on the degree of dorsal augmentation required (ie, soft tissue only, soft tissue and structural support, and so forth.).
- The authors believe autologous graft sources to be the gold standard for dorsal augmentation because of their decreased immunoreactivity, native semblance, and reliability.
- Although autologous graft sources are thought to be advantageous in eventual outcomes of nasal dorsal augmentation, some surgeons may choose nonautologous sources because of their off-the-shelf availability, ease of use, and avoidance of donor-site morbidity.

  Video content accompanies this article at http://www.plasticsurgery.theclinics.com.

INTRODUCTION/HISTORY/DEFINITIONS/BACKGROUND

Dorsal augmentation is an essential technique in every rhinoplasty specialist's armamentarium, both in primary and revision rhinoplasties. Etiologies contributing to deficiency of the nasal dorsum can be intrinsic or acquired. A low dorsal height is a prevalent characteristic in Asian and black ethnicities. As such, these patient populations often request dorsal augmentation to improve their esthetic appearance. A deficient osseocartilaginous framework can also be caused by infection, trauma, and previous rhinoplasty.[1] In revision cases, patients often present due to prior overresection of the nasal dorsum, in addition to irregular contour deformities secondary to discernible grafts or structural elements underneath the skin envelope.[2] Oftentimes, dorsal augmentation is sought after in these cases, to treat both the esthetic appearance and structural function of the nose.

To achieve dorsal augmentation, a variety of sources, of autologous, allogeneic, and synthetic origin, has been used over time and commonly debated. Autologous options include cartilage (ie, septal, conchal, costal), bone (ie, calvarium, rib, iliac crest), osseocartilage (rib), diced cartilage with fascia (DC-F), fascia, perichondrial, and dermofat grafts. Allogeneic sources include allograft costal cartilage, allograft bone, and AlloDerm grafts, and synthetic sources include silicone implants and expanded tetrafluoroethylene (ePTFE). See **Box 1** for a full overview of each category. Of note, autologous and allogeneic options are almost exclusively used in Western countries, whereas synthetic materials dominate as the source of augmentation in Asian countries.[3,4]

A myriad of factors, including nasal analysis, surgical approach, and execution, contributes to

[a] Private Practice, Graw Beauty | Dr. Grace, 1515 EL Camino Real, Palo Alto, CA 94306, USA; [b] Division of Plastic and Reconstructive Surgery, University of Southern California, 465 North Roxbury Drive, Suite 1001, Beverly Hills, CA 90210, USA
* Corresponding author.
E-mail address: gracejanegraw@gmail.com

Clin Plastic Surg 49 (2022) 137–148
https://doi.org/10.1016/j.cps.2021.08.003

> **Box 1**
> **Sources for nasal dorsal augmentation**
>
> Autologous
>   Cartilage (septal, auricular, costal)
>   Bone (calvarium, rib, iliac crest)
>   Osseocartilage (rib)
>   Diced cartilage fascia (DC-F)
>   Fascia, perichondrium, dermofat
> Allogeneic
>   Allograft costal cartilage
>   Allograft bone
>   AlloDerm
> Synthetic
>   Silicone
>   Expanded tetrafluoroethylene (ePTFE)

a successful dorsal augmentation, all of which will be discussed in this chapter. Although the authors' general preference in technique for nasal dorsal augmentation is the diced cartilage with fascia (DC-F) graft, the various surgical approaches, including their advantages and disadvantages, will be explored here. Ultimately, a thorough knowledge of these facets will optimize overall success for the treatment of the deficient nasal dorsum.

DISCUSSION
Nasal Analysis

A balanced approach, understanding the contributions and effects of the radix, dorsum, tip, and chin on nasal projection, is necessary for a thorough analysis. The nasion is the deepest portion of the nasofrontal angle and serves as the central point of the radix. It establishes the starting point of the nose, as it transitions from the glabella. Typical nasofrontal angles range from 115° to 145°. The ideal position of the nasion resides between the supratarsal crease and upper lash line. Both the vertical height and projection of the radix effectively create the appearance of a shorter or longer nose.[1] Ideal tip projection should reside at a height two-thirds the length of the nose.[5] Once an evaluation of the radix and tip has been performed, dorsal curvature should be assessed by forming a line from the radix to the nasal tip. In general, the dorsum should lie 2 mm posterior to this line in the female population and directly on this line in the male population. If the dorsum lies significantly posterior to either of these lines, dorsal

augmentation should be considered.[6] However, the importance of maintaining the perspective of the patient's radix and tip positioning, while analyzing the dorsal height, should be emphasized because this key facet helps achieve the overall nasal balance. For example, a patient with a low radix and underprojected tip may not require as large of a dorsal augmentation once these factors are addressed.

Considerations

Other facial features that should be taken into consideration are the patient's midface (ie, malar eminences and premaxilla) and lower face (ie, lips, mandible, and chin) projections to ensure proper nasofacial harmony. For example, in a nose with adequate dorsal height, overprojected malar eminences can create the appearance of an underprojected nose because of an imbalance of proportions. Similarly, a prognathic or macrognathic chin may also give the appearance of an underprojected nose.

In revision rhinoplasty cases, several nasal deformities can be commonly associated with a deficient dorsum, including a saddle nose deformity (**Figs. 1** and **2**), collapsed columella, excess or deficient caudal septum, pollybeak deformity, among others. As with considerations of other facial features, treatment of these deformities concomitantly is pertinent in achieving optimal results by creating the overall facial balance.

Lastly, ethnic variations should be taken into account when considering the extent of dorsal augmentation required. In general, those of Asian, black, and Creole descent present with low dorsal heights, and those of Mexican descent present with low radix heights.[7–9] Please see Chapter 13 for a full discussion in regards to non-Caucasian rhinoplasty. Goals of the rhinoplasty should be discussed in detail with the patient, in regards to the desire for the Westernization of the nose or preservation of ethnic characteristics.

Operative Goals

The patient's goals and surgeon's expertise are combined to achieve desired, conceivable results. Open and closed surgical approaches may be used. However, in most cases, to attain optimal and precise outcomes, the authors' preference is to perform the operation via the open approach. Through transcolumellar and marginal incisions, the surgeon gains direct visualization of, and immediate access to, the underlying, osseocartilaginous framework. This approach purports a thorough assessment of the esthetic, structural, and functional needs of the nose. Additionally,

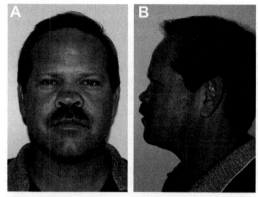

Fig. 1. A patient with congenital dorsal agenesis, resulting in a saddle nose deformity. (*A*: frontal view, *B*: side view).

direct exposure enables the accurate placement of grafts, allowing for precise results (**Fig. 3**).[10] Furthermore, the open approach avoids unnecessary contact of the graft with the nasal cavity, minimizing bacterial contamination.[11,12] Although the open approach for rhinoplasty remains the preferred option for the authors because of the aforementioned advantages, certain special circumstances may deem the closed approach a reasonable choice (**Video 1**). Cases whereby compromised vascularity is a concern and/or a

contracted skin envelope is present because of prior rhinoplasty could benefit from limited dissection and thus the closed approach.[13]

A complete nasal analysis performed preoperatively helps determine the degree of dorsal augmentation required. In turn, the amount of augmentation needed establishes the type of material appropriate for the graft. Smaller augmentations may just require septal or auricular conchal cartilage harvest. However, larger augmentations require a substantial amount of material, which may necessitate a costal cartilage harvest. Similarly, for minimal nasal dorsal augmentations just requiring camouflage of contour irregularities, perichondrial grafts may be used. However, for those requiring significant volume, fascia grafts [ie, rectus fascia or deep temporalis fascia (DTF)] may serve as crucial conduits for diced cartilage, the core bulk providing augmentation, and as camouflage of surface irregularities. As mentioned earlier, the authors' preference is to perform nasal dorsal augmentations with autologous grafts—the authors believe these grafts to be the gold standard for reasons that will be discussed later in discussion.

However, at times, the following may call for the usage of nonautologous grafts: patient preference, the desire to limit donor-site morbidity, and insufficient cartilage due to prior harvest or

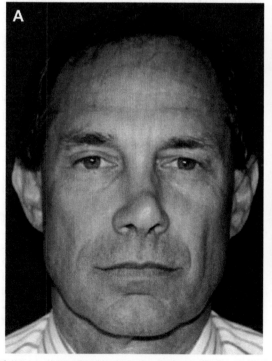

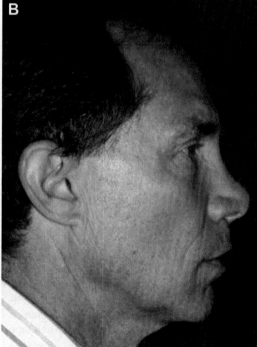

Fig. 2. A patient with a history of boxer trauma to the nose, followed by subsequent repeat nasal fractures, resulting in a saddle nose deformity. (*A*: frontal view, *B*: side view).

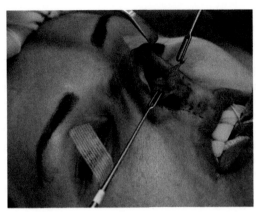

Fig. 3. Exposure gained through transcolumellar and marginal incisions in a quaternary revision rhinoplasty case. The open approach allows for direct visualization and immediate access to the osseocartilaginous framework.

calcifications. Although the aforementioned reasons should be taken into consideration, achieving optimal, long-lasting results should preside as the ultimate overarching theme in operative planning.

Surgical Techniques

Autologous grafts

In the authors' opinion, autologous grafts should be the gold standard in rhinoplasty, as they carry many qualities paramount to a successful and reliable nasal dorsal augmentation, such as the following: natural consistency, moldability, durability, biocompatibility, and decreased vulnerability for infection.[1,14,15] These factors are especially advantageous in revision cases.[1] Certainly, aspects of potential donor-site morbidity and resorption should be taken into consideration.[16] However, in the senior author's prior work and breadth of experience, no resorption has been noted with the usage of DC-F grafts for nasal dorsal augmentation. This finding continues to hold true as evidenced by not having the need to overcorrect during the operation to achieve long-lasting results.[2,14] In the following section, the authors discuss the various types of autologous grafts that have been used and purported by rhinoplasty specialists for nasal dorsal augmentation.

Cartilage Several sources for autologous cartilage may be used. The 3 main options are septal cartilage, auricular conchal cartilage, and costal cartilage. As mentioned previously, for smaller augmentations, septal or auricular conchal cartilage may be used. In this instance, septal cartilage is often preferred, as it avoids a secondary donor site. Furthermore, conchal cartilage has been known

to be more susceptible to resorption and thus contour irregularities.[17] Additionally, because of the fragility of conchal cartilage, the graft may at times be less amenable to contouring techniques and therefore offer less structural support.[13,18] However, oftentimes in posttraumatic or revision cases, the septum is frequently deficient.[17] As such, a conchal graft may serve as a viable option with its ease of harvest and minimal donor-site morbidity.[18]

By and large, costal cartilage is an excellent graft source that offers the abundant supply required in a significantly deficient nasal dorsum (**Fig. 4**). However, with the abundant source of graft material comes issues related to donor-site morbidity, such as the potential risk for pneumothorax, increased postoperative pain, scarring, and mild chest contour irregularities. As well, the surgeon should be well versed in the costal cartilage graft harvest to decrease operative times and associated morbidities.[17,19,20] Despite these potential drawbacks, if performed in skilled hands, costal cartilage harvest is an essential tool in nasal dorsal augmentation, especially in revision cases whereby a deficient septum is often present and in those cases whereby a considerable degree of augmentation is required.

Bone Bone grafts may be harvested from the calvarium, rib, and iliac crest. Although a viable option to using cartilage, bone grafts have decreased in popularity over time because of their characteristic rigidity and potential donor-site morbidities.[1,18] Their rigidity lends to several disadvantages, including an inability to contour the grafts optimally, an increased risk of palpability, a possibility for extrusion, and a potential to create an unnatural appearance.[15,19,20] Furthermore, the bone grafts' risk for donor-site morbidity is not insignificant. Although advantages of a calvarial bone harvest include an adjacent operative site, decreased postoperative pain, and ability to camouflage scar, it is associated with an entailed harvest, potential alopecia, and devastating complications such as dural tears, intracranial bleeding, and cerebral injury.[19,20] Risks associated with a costal bone harvest are similar to that as mentioned previously for a costal cartilage harvest.[17,19,20] And, lastly, as with a costal bone harvest, harvest from the iliac crest bone carries the potential for increased postoperative pain and contour irregularities.[15] Overall, the suboptimal characteristics attained from bone grafts are likely not worth the plausible risks associated with their donor-site morbidity.

Osseocartilage A more versatile alternative to the bone graft is the osseocartilaginous graft, which

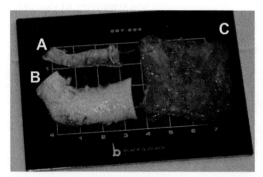

Fig. 4. Various grafts harvested from a single eighth rib harvest site. (*A*: perichondral graft, *B*: rib cartilage graft, *C*: rectus fascia graft).

is typically harvested from the rib. The costal osseocartilaginous graft provides not only structural adaptability conformable to the native nose but also significant structural support and framework.[1] The graft can be used as a composite, using the osseocartilaginous portion to enhance the nasal dorsum and the cartilaginous region to build up on the columella.[1,21] Alternatively, based on the senior author's experience, if a sizable augmentation and structure are needed, the graft can be split into a layered graft, where a bony portion underlies a DC-F portion, to augment a considerably deficient nasal dorsum. These grafts have demonstrated durability and resistance to warping and resorption.[1,21] Dynamic in nature, the costal osseocartilaginous graft is a compelling source for dorsal augmentation cases that require an extensive build-in framework.

Diced cartilage with fascia graft As mentioned previously, the DC-F graft is the authors' main workhorse graft for achieving nasal dorsal augmentation (**Figs. 5** and **6**). Constant issues of warping, visibility (specifically when wrapped with fascia), and resorption, associated with other autologous grafts, have been shown to not exist with diced cartilage.[14,22] Furthermore, this graft offers the benefit of moldability up to 3 weeks postoperatively, allowing the surgeon to shape the graft to the patient and surgeon's esthetic desire.[14,23] The DC-F technique has stemmed as a modification from Erol's technique of the "Turkish delight," which is diced cartilage wrapped in Surgicel (Ethicon, Somerville, NJ, USA). In Erol's study of 2365 patients who underwent the "Turkish delight" technique, only 0.5% experienced resorption.[23] However, in a study performed by Daniel and Calvert of 22 patients, using the same exact technique as described by Erol, 100% experienced resorption. Given the unexpected resorption rate seen in all cases, the technique was immediately aborted.

Thus, these findings led to the modification of Erol's technique, using diced cartilage wrapped in fascia, which was first described by Daniel and Calvert in 2004. In this study, they described the discrepancy of resorption rates seen for the "Turkish delight" technique to be attributed to the indication for using the DC-F graft. Erol seemed to use the graft to camouflage dorsal contour irregularities, whereas Daniel and Calvert used the graft to augment the dorsum. Subsequently, in the study by Daniel and Calvert of 20 patients who underwent DC-F grafting for radix or dorsal augmentation, none experienced resorption; thus, these results were also confirmed histologically. Interestingly, because of initial uncertainty of resorption rates in DC-F grafts, overcorrection was performed in earlier cases, in the anticipation of possible resorption; however, lack of resorption was seen, which led to excessive augmentation, requiring revision surgery for graft reduction in these cases.[14]

In the senior author's experience, the source of diced cartilage (ie, septum, ear, or rib) does not affect the quality and outcome of the graft. This is thought to be likely secondary to the size of the cartilage pieces (0.5 mm to 1 mm) after they have been diced; their miniscule size likely negates any effect from the cartilage source's intrinsic properties. A reliable, robust source of fascia is the DTF, which can be accessed through a variety of incisions. In patients with long hair, a linear incision can be placed 1 cm above and 0.5 to 1 cm posterior to the root of the helix and remain hidden within the hair-bearing scalp. Otherwise, the DTF may be accessed through a temporal brow lift incision, an incision along the hairline just above the helical root for those with short hair, or a posterior helical incision with the assistance of an endoscope. Regardless of the type of access, crucial to the success of this graft is the size harvested. Adequate size of DTF should be at least 4 cm in length and width to sufficiently wrap the diced cartilage (Video 2).[2] Another reasonable option for fascia is the rectus fascia. One should consider harvesting the rectus fascia if already harvesting a costal graft to limit donor sites.

Possible complications with the DC-F graft include low-grade infection and graft migration. Typically, infections will resolve with antibiotic therapy. However, infection can lead to resorption because of the progressive destruction of diced cartilage.[2] At times, if the DC-F graft does not incorporate well into its recipient site, graft migration can occur.[24] In cases such as these, the surgeon may reactivate and mobilize the graft with a hyaluronidase injection and place the graft in its proper position again.[2]

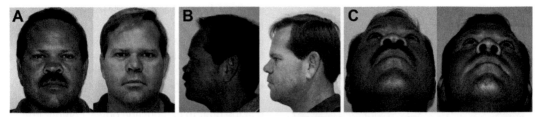

Fig. 5. A patient with congenital dorsal agenesis, resulting in a saddle nose deformity, who underwent dorsal augmentation with diced rib cartilage wrapped in rectus fascia graft. Follow-up time on this patient is 1 year. (*A*: frontal view, *B*: side view, *C*: basilar view; left, before; right, after).

Fascia, perichondrium, and dermofat In patients who require minimal nasal dorsal soft-tissue augmentation, especially to create a smoother surface contour and camouflage irregularities, fascia grafts may be considered. These grafts may be taken from sources such as the DTF, superficial musculoaponeurotic system, mastoid fascia, and rectus fascia.[1,3,25] Alternatively, to limit donor-site morbidity, and if the surgeon is already harvesting a costal graft, a perichondrial graft may also be harvested for the same purpose (see **Fig. 4**). For additional bulk, these grafts may be folded to create a layered, or stacked, graft. For a comprehensive overview

of autologous soft-tissue grafts, dermofat, a technique popular in East Asian countries, will be briefly mentioned.[26] The dermis and fat layers are harvested from the sacrococcygeal region on either side of the intergluteal crease.[27] Despite their popularity, dermofat grafts have been shown to have an unusually high resorption rate (40% to 70%), likely correlated with increasing amounts of fat taken.[28] As such, surgeons have had to overcorrect by 30% to 40% when using dermofat grafts.[27] Overall, with these autologous soft-tissue grafts, it is important to remember that generally they do not add much for augmentation purposes, but rather, they

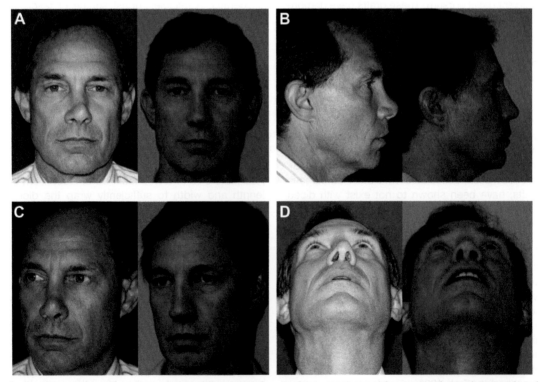

Fig. 6. This patient suffered traumatic saddle nose deformity from repeat nasal fractures, who underwent dorsal augmentation with diced rib cartilage wrapped in rectus fascia graft. Follow-up time on this patient is 3 years. (*A*: frontal view, *B*: side view, *C*: oblique, *D*: basilar view; left, before; right, after).

best serve the purposes of creating a smoother profile and hiding any contour irregularities.

Allogeneic grafts

Although autologous tissue is favored by many surgeons for the purpose of dorsal augmentation, allogeneic (ie, biologic, nonautologous) and synthetic (ie, nonbiologic implant) sources may be considered, or even preferred, in certain settings, especially in Asian countries. Surgeon choice plays a role here because there is controversy and support for each type of graft. In favor of non-autologous graft includes patient preference to limit donor-site morbidity, insufficiency of autologous graft, ready availability, ease of use, and lower perioperative morbidity.[3] Some debate that allogeneic grafts have less tendency for warping than autologous sources. As there is much in the literature that supports the usage of autologous grafts in nasal dorsal augmentation, there is also much to support the use of nonautologous grafts.[4,29–32] The next 2 sections will review and compare a range of sources to include allograft costal cartilage, allograft bone, AlloDerm (LifeCell Corporation, Branchburg, NJ, USA), silicone implant, ePTFE, among others.

Allograft costal cartilage The success of autologous costal cartilage has led to allograft costal cartilage as an obvious extension. One known source is irradiated homologous costal cartilage (IHCC), which has a track record of safe use in a variety of plastic surgical reconstructions.[3,15] IHCC is taken from human cadaveric specimens, readily available, relatively malleable, and, therefore, easy to contour.[33] Other benefits include minimal tissue immunoreactivity and near-zero risk of disease transmission, which can be attributed to current preparation methods that include robust donor testing and gamma radiation treatment at a level of 60,000 Gy before distribution.[14,18,19] Concerns of warping and resorption exist; however, a range of rates have been reported from minimal to 100%.[3,33] To decrease the risk for warping, certain techniques have been applied as follows: delaying graft insertion by 30 minutes from the end of thawing, eliminating perichondrium from the graft, contouring the graft uniformly, and securing the graft with K-wire fixation.[18,19,34] The results of IHCC augmentation have been favorable without the evidence of significant or extrusion.[34]

Next, related to IHCC, Tutoplast (RTI Surgical Holdings Inc, Alachua, FL, USA), a proprietary allograft cartilage alternative with a unique preparation, will be discussed. The allograft costal cartilage is dehydrated with peroxide and acetone and then irradiated up to 25,000 Gy. Initial studies have shown concerns of complication rates reaching approximately 30%; these complications included warping and resorption. As a result, Tutoplast was thought to be deficient for the purposes of nasal dorsal augmentation.[35] However, these poor results did not bear out in a later study performed by Vila and colleagues. In fact, the rates of complication were statistically equivalent to those of autologous costal cartilage and IHCC grafts.[31]

The meta-analysis of Vila and colleagues demonstrated no difference in outcomes between autologous and allograft, including IHCC and Tutoplast, costal cartilage grafts. Published in 2020, their study analyzed 28 studies, which provided a total of 1041 patients in their final analysis. Of these 1041 patients, 72% underwent autologous costal cartilage grafting and 28% underwent allograft costal cartilage grafting (both IHCC and Tutoplast) for nasal dorsal augmentation. There was no statistical difference in warping (5%), resorption (2%), contour irregularity (1%), infection (2%), or revision surgery (5%). Limitations to this analysis included lack of patient-reported outcomes, difficulty in assessing true revision rates, and differentiating the use of all graft types for structural or nonstructural use.[31] Overall, allograft costal cartilage grafts have the benefit of decreased surgical morbidity and the potential for both durable and favorable esthetic outcomes.[3,31]

Allograft bone Allograft bone can also be considered for nasal dorsal augmentation, although because of its rigidity, it has a tendency toward being more difficult to shape and handle, in addition to creating an unnatural, stiff appearance of the nose.[3] Graft sources include cortical bone of the tibia and femur and can be obtained from DCI Donor Services in Nashville, TN. After extensive processing to minimize immunoreactivity, the product is freeze-dried at DCI Donor Services. Once ready for usage in a dorsal augmentation case, the product is rehydrated in a combined saline and antibiotic solution 4 hours before graft placement.[36]

Advantages of allograft bone are its ready availability, no donor-site morbidity, and decreased risks of warping, as compared with autografts.[37] However, disadvantages include difficulty with contouring and unpredictable rates of resorption. Oftentimes, as with autograft bone, high-speed saws and burrs are required for contouring. Potentially, partial demineralization of the allograft bone could improve ease of carving; however, further studies need to be performed to verify this hypothesis. As mentioned earlier, resorption in allograft bone can be an issue because it is difficult to antic-ipate, likely secondary to multiple components, which include donor factors, time to processing, irradiation amount, and host immune response.[30]

Recently, Clark and colleagues published a 10-year follow-up study on the use of freeze-dried cortical allograft bone in nasal dorsal augmenta-tion. Of 19 grafts, 84% had objective evidence of neovascularization with volume persistence. And, of 43 grafts, 86% demonstrated subjective evi-dence of volume persistence. Overall, the study by Clark and colleagues recommended freeze-dried allograft bone as a safe and comparable source for nasal dorsal augmentation without hav-ing any donor-site morbidity.[30]

AlloDerm AlloDerm is an acellular, human cadav-eric dermis sometimes used for the augmentation of the nasal dorsum, in a similar manner to autolo-gous fascial and perichondral grafts. After the product undergoes decellularization and process-ing to minimize immunoreactivity, it is freeze-dried into a collagen matrix sheet that allows for recip-ient tissue ingrowth.[38] AlloDerm may be inserted as a single layer, multiple layers, or as a composite with other components.[18] Although the material may lend to a smooth and natural appearance, studies have reported rates of resorption as high as 45%. For this reason, overcorrection is recom-mended when using AlloDerm.[39] Of note, when stacked, the acellular dermal substitute has been found to achieve, at most, an augmentation of 3 mm[39] As such, similar to autologous fascial and perichondral grafts, AlloDerm should not be the main source for substantial dorsal augmentations but should rather be considered when there is a need to camouflage contour deformities.

Synthetic implants
Silicone Globally, silicone, made of polymerized silica (SiO_2), is the most frequently used synthetic material for nasal implants, especially in Asian countries.[16] Cross-linking and extension of this material allow it to form a variety of lengths, shapes, and thickness. In the setting of dorsal nasal augmentation, silicone rubber is used for a variety of reasons, including its chemical inertness and high resilience against compression, deforma-tion, and temperature. Several prefabricated shapes exist in regards to thickness (ranging from 2 to 10 mm) and design, with L-shaped and I-shaped implants being the most common.[4] To some surgeons, mostly in Asia, silicone implants are ideal, given the following characteristics: little tissue reactivity due to its inert property, ready availability, ease of use and customization for each patient, no need for a donor site, thereby

simplifying the operation, and resistance to resorption and distortion.[3,4] Much support for sili-cone implants stems from the treatment of the Asian rhinoplasty population, which often comes with the desire for significant dorsal augmentation (in some cases, greater than 5 mm). Some sur-geons believe silicone implants to be a superior choice over autologous costal cartilage grafts because of their strong preference to limit donor-site morbidity and prevent postoperative nasal rigidity.[4]

Silicone implants cannot be mentioned without a discussion of their complications, including the significant issue of implant extrusion through the skin and soft-tissue envelope. Extrusion rates have been reported to range from 0.5% to 50%.[40–42] Two main culprits exist as main causes of extrusion: redundancy and infection. Redun-dancy can cause undue tension on the nasal tip or membranous septum, placing the implant at high risk for extrusion. As well, not securing the implant to the nasofrontal angle or within the sub-periosteal pocket may place the implant at risk for migration distally, with the potential for subse-quent extrusion (Video 3). Lastly, infection may create a deeply inflamed and macerated environ-ment, leading to fragile soft tissue overlying the implant, which could be a nidus for implant expo-sure.[4,16,17] Other complications include chronic inflammation, infection, migration, resorption of the underlying native bone, skin discoloration, and capsular contracture.[3,4] Complication rates have ranged from 4% to 36%, and thus, silicone implants have largely fell out of favor in Western countries. However, significantly lower complica-tion rates have been noted in Asian countries, which have been thought to be due to the thicker nasal soft-tissue envelope of Asian patients.[43] For this reason, in addition to the flexibility and size variety of these implants, silicone implants still see widespread use for dorsal augmentation in Asia. Kim and colleagues share a comprehensive review of the surgical technique including graft sculpting, placement, and tip extension.[4]

Although the authors strongly discourage the use of silicone implants, because of significant is-sues of extrusion and infection, among others, un-derstanding their role and usage in nasal dorsal augmentation is crucial to best manage these cases when they present for revision rhinoplasty in the setting of a complication (**Figs. 7** and **8**).

Expanded tetrafluoroethylene (Gore-Tex) ePTFE, a polymer of carbon bound to fluorine, laid out in a fine grid pattern, has been a solid, consistent implant material used for dorsal nasal augmenta-tion.[11,12] Despite discontinuation by its

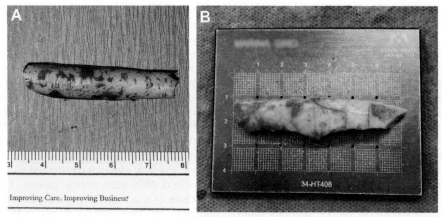

Fig. 7. (*A*) Extruded implant completely removed. (*B*) Rib cartilage graft harvest in preparation for diced cartilage + fascia graft for nasal dorsal augmentation in the same patient.

manufacturer for applications in plastic surgery, medical-grade ePTFE, or Gore-Tex, sheets are still in production for applications in general and vascular surgery and can be acquired as such. ePTFE is a favorable implant because of its inert nature, excellent biocompatibility, cost, and good track record of use.[11,25] Furthermore, it has the ability to incorporate well into the surrounding soft-tissue envelope, yet can still be removed without difficulty, if retrieval is necessary.[11,12,18]

As with silicone implants, complications of ePTFE can include infection and extrusion. Infection and tissue reactivity can lead to short-term extrusion with a reported rate of 3%.[25]

Joo and colleagues evaluated 244 patients who underwent dorsal augmentation rhinoplasty using either autologous costal cartilage or ePTFE. Comparable esthetic outcomes were seen in both the autologous costal cartilage and ePTFE groups. However, the autologous costal cartilage group

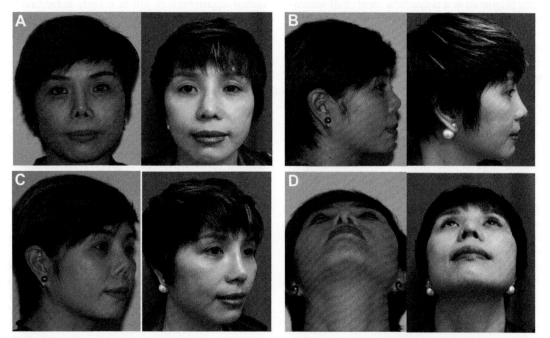

Fig. 8. This patient previously underwent nasal dorsal augmentation with a silicone implant and subsequently suffered an implant extrusion. She then underwent removal of the implant and complex nasal reconstruction, which included dorsal augmentation with diced rib cartilage wrapped in rectus fascia graft. Follow-up time on this patient is 1 year. (*A*: frontal view, *B*: side view, *C*: oblique, *D*: basilar view; left, before; right, after).

demonstrated a significant increase in dorsal and radix heights after augmentation over the PTFE group. As well, complication rates, related to resorption and warping, were found to be significantly higher in the autologous costal cartilage group (11.8% vs 4.0% in the ePTFE group). In general, their study was in favor of ePTFE for dorsal augmentation, given its ease of use, lack of donor-site morbidity, equivalent esthetic outcome, and lower complication rates. Of note, the study did mention a potential for selection bias because of the use of autologous costal cartilage in cases with a more deficient framework and lower dorsal height.[32]

In regards to technique, ePTFE patches often come in 2-mm thickness and can be cut into strips or designed into a "boat shape" to layer onto the nasal dorsum. Up to 2 to 3 layers can be used, depending on the degree of augmentation required, and are sutured into place with 5-0 polydioxanone.[32] Important to note is that the sheet form of Gore-Tex is too thin to serve any structural function but rather should be used to smoothen contours and/or hide irregularities.[44]

Other synthetic implants (ie, supramid, mersilene, proplast, medpor, hydroxyapatite) There are a series of other synthetic implants worth mentioning, although they are not as prevalent as silicone or ePTFE, and thus with a less satisfactory track record. Supramid is a polyamide mesh that resembles Mersilene and has a high resorption rate, likely caused by a modest foreign body tissue reaction.[18,45,46] However, this tissue reaction, in a positive light, could prevent implant migration.[18,46] Another synthetic implant is Mersilene, which is a polyethylene terephthalate mesh that is durable and easily contoured. Infection rates, thought to be secondary to bacterial colonization of the material, have been reported at about 4%, with resultant need for removal in half of these cases. A disadvantage of this product is its difficulty in removal because of excessive fibroblast ingrowth.[12,18] Despite decreased resorption rates compared with Supramid, Mersilene has often been surpassed by ePTFE, as the ePTFE has shown less propensity to infection and more accessible removal when required.[45] Another comparable synthetic option, Proplast, also has similarities to Gore-Tex, in that is a PTFE polymer combined with carbon fiber. Although compared with Supramid, Proplast is more susceptible to infection and extrusion and it offers more structural support and versatility in contouring ability.[3,47] A recent formulation, named Proplast II, combines PTFE with aluminum oxide fibers and hydroxyapatite, which improves bony compatibility and integration.[17] Proplast II may be shaped in a similar fashion to silicone implants, providing versatility in use.[47] However, the material's durability is limited given its increased porosity, lending it toward the susceptibility for fragmentation and collapse.[17,18] As such, Proplast II should not be used in cases requiring significant structural support.

Medpor is a different category of synthetic implants in that it is made of high-density pure polyethylene with a framework of interconnecting pores. The final material consists of 54% polyethylene and 46% pore space volume. The microstructure of the material enables the expeditious ingrowth of vascularized tissue and collagen, creating a robust and stable construct. Given that Medpor is easy to contour, biocompatible, and generally resistant to infection, resorption, and distortion, the implant has shown favorable use in nasal dorsal augmentation.[17,48] Some disadvantages found with this porous polyethylene implant have been its rigidity, lending toward an unnatural appearance, as well as the difficulty of insertion due to its irregular surface.[18] As in the literature surrounding silicone implants, much of the use of Medpor has been in the Asian population, whereby significant degrees of dorsal augmentation are required.[48]

Lastly, hydroxyapatite (HA) should be mentioned as another synthetic source for nasal dorsal augmentation. HA is a bony substitute in composition and can lead to bony ingrowth given its microscopic structure.[44] The material comes in both block and granular forms. The block form can be difficult to handle given its brittle nature and requirement for rigid fixation to the nasal bone.[17,44] The granular form is more pliable; however, because of this property, it does not provide much structural support and serves best to fill or hide contour irregularities. Although fixation to the nasal bone is not required for the granular form, a splint would be required postoperatively until adequate fibrovascular ingrowth has occurred. Because of HA's porosity, vascularization from tissue ingrowth occurs, rendering the implant less susceptible to infection. Furthermore, no resorption and distortion has been found with usage of HA in nasal dorsal augmentation.[44]

The aforementioned review shows the range of synthetic implants applicable to nasal dorsal augmentation. Although Silicone and ePTFE are the most common, other materials have been tried with limited success. Variables such as patient and surgeon preference, implant incorporation, resorption, ease of use, and risks of infection and extrusion should be considered before choosing an implant type for a specific patient.[29]

SUMMARY

Achieving optimal outcomes in nasal dorsal augmentation involves a multifaceted approach. Pertinent to the initial analysis is the evaluation of the entire face, including the frontonasal region, nasal dorsum, malar eminences, premaxilla, lips, chin, and mandible, to best attain nasofacial harmony. As well, in determining the degree of augmentation required, proper diagnosis of the source of deficiency is key to planning out the type of graft needed. For example, if only a minor soft-tissue deficiency is noted, then one can plan for harvesting just a fascia graft. However, if both soft-tissue and structural deficiencies are noted, then one can plan for harvesting a DC-F and osseocartilaginous graft. In general, the authors believe that autologous tissue is the gold standard for grafts in dorsal augmentation because of its biocompatibility, natural appearance, decreased susceptibility to infection, reliability, and long-lasting outcomes. However, some surgeons may choose a nonautologous source because of its ready availability, ease of use, and ability to avoid a complex autologous tissue harvest with associated donor-site morbidity. Overall, a customized, comprehensive plan needs to be agreed upon by both the patient and surgeon to ultimately achieve optimal, long-lasting outcomes.

CLINICS CARE POINTS

- A comprehensive approach in nasal analysis, noting the importance of maintaining overall nasofacial balance and accurate diagnosis of the degree of dorsal augmentation required (ie, soft tissue only, soft tissue and structural support, and so forth), is essential to achieving desired outcomes.

- A breadth of autologous and nonautologous (ie, allogeneic and synthetic) graft sources exist and therefore require a rhinoplasty specialist, well versed in these techniques, to select the best option for dorsal augmentation in his/her patient.

- Owing to their biocompatibility, reliability, natural semblance, and durable outcomes, the authors believe autologous grafts to be the optimal sources for nasal dorsal augmentation.

- Although autologous sources are favorable, nonautologous sources may be preferred by some surgeons because of their accessibility, ease of use, and avoidance of donor-site morbidity.

DISCLOSURE

The authors report no commercial or financial conflicts of interest and any funding sources for all authors.

SUPPLEMENTARY DATA

Supplementary data related to this article can be found online at https://doi.org/10.1016/j.cps.2021.08.003.

REFERENCES

1. Daniel RK. Radix and dorsum. In: Mastering rhinoplasty. Berlin: Springer; 2010. p. 67–100.
2. Calvert J, Kwon E. Techniques for diced cartilage with deep temporalis fascia graft. Facial Plast Surg Clin N Am 2015;23:73–80.
3. Dresner HS, Hilger PA. An overview of nasal dorsal augmentation. Semin Plast Surg 2008;22:65–73.
4. Kim IS. Augmentation rhinoplasty using silicone implants. Facial Plast Surg Clin N Am 2018;26:285–93.
5. Byrd HS, Hobar PC. Rhinoplasty: a practical guide for surgical planning. Plast Reconstr Surg 1993;91:642.
6. Orten SS, Hilger PA. Facial analysis of the rhinoplasty patient. In: Papel ID, editor. Facial plastic and reconstructive surgery. New York, NY: Thieme Medical Publishers; 2002. p. 361–8.
7. Toriumi DM, Pero CD. Asian rhinoplasty. Clin Plast Surg 2010;37:335.
8. Rohrich RJ, Muzaffar AR. Rhinoplasty in the African-American patient. Plast Reconstr Surg 2013;111:1322–40.
9. Daniel RK. Hispanic rhinoplasty in the United States, with emphasis on the Mexican American nose. Plast Reconstr Surg 2003;112:244–57.
10. Adamson PA, Doud Galli SK. Rhinoplasty approaches. Arch Facial Plast Surg 2005;7:32–7.
11. Godin MS, Waldman R, Johnson CM. The use of polytetrafluoroethylene (Gore-Tex) in rhinoplasty. A 6-year experience. Arch Otolaryngol Head Neck Surg 1995;121:1131–6.
12. Lohuis PJFM, Watts SJ, Vuyk HD. Augmentation of the nasal dorsum using Gore-Tex: intermediate results of a retrospective analysis of experience in 66 patients. Clin Otolaryngol 2001;26:214–7.
13. Murrell GL. Auricular cartilage grafts and nasal surgery. Laryngoscope 2004;114:2092–102.
14. Daniel RK, Calvert JW. Diced cartilage grafts in rhinoplasty surgery. Plast Reconstr Surg 2004;113:2156–71.
15. Gurley JM, Pilgram T, Perlyn CA, et al. Long-term outcome of autogenous rib graft nasal reconstruction. Plast Reconstr Surg 2001;108:1895–905.

16. Deva AK, Merten S, Chang L. Silicone in nasal augmentation rhinoplasty: a decade of clinical experience. Plast Reconstr Surg 1998;102:1230–7.

17. Niechajev I. Porous polyethylene implants for nasal reconstruction: clinical and histologic studies. Aesthet Plast Surg 1999;23:395–402.

18. Lovice DB, Mingrone MD, Toriumi DM. Rhinoplasty and septoplasty. Grafts and implants in rhinoplasty and nasal reconstruction. Otolaryngol Clin North Am 1999;32:113–41.

19. Clark JM, Cook TA. Immediate reconstruction of extruded alloplastic nasal implants with irradiated homograft costal cartilage. Laryngoscope 2002; 112:968–74.

20. Sherris DA, Kern EB. The versatile autogenous rib graft in septorhinoplasty. Am J Rhinol 1998;12: 221–7.

21. Ciolek PJ, Hanick AL, Roskies M, et al. Osseocartilaginous rib graft L-strut for nasal framework reconstruction. Aesthet Surg J 2020;40(4):NP133–40.

22. Daniel RK. Rhinoplasty: an atlas of surgical techniques. New York: Springer; 2002. p. 11–2.

23. Erol OO. The Turkish delight: a pliable graft for rhinoplasty. Plast Reconstr Surg 2000;105:2229.

24. Celik M, Haliloglu T, Baycin N. Bone chips and diced cartilage: an anatomically adopted graft for the nasal dorsum. Aesthet Plast Surg 2004;28:8–12.

25. Davis RE, Wayne I. Rhinoplasty and the nasal SMAS augmentation graft. Arch Facial Plast Surg 2004;6: 124–32.

26. Na DS, Jung SW, Kook KS, et al. Augmentation rhinoplasty with dermofat graft and fat injection. J Korean Soc Plast Reconstr Surg 2011;38(1):53–6.

27. Suh MK. Dorsal augmentation using autogenous tissues. Facial Plast Surg Clin N Am 2018;26:295–310.

28. Conley JJ, Clairmont AA. Dermal-fat-fascia grafts. Otolaryngology 1978;86:641–9.

29. Barrett DM, Wang TD. Dorsal augmentation—choosing the right material for the right patient. JAMA Facial Plast Surg 2016;18(5):333–4.

30. Clark RP, Pham PM, Ciminello FS, et al. Nasal dorsal augmentation with freeze-dried allograft bone: 10-year comprehensive review. Plast Reconstr Surg 2019;143:49e–61e.

31. Vila PM, Jeanpierre LM, Rizzi CJ, et al. Comparison of autologous vs homologous costal cartilage grafts in dorsal augmentation rhinoplasty. JAMA Otolaryngol Head Neck Surg 2020;146(5):347–54.

32. Joo YH, Jang YJ. Comparison of the surgical outcomes of dorsal augmentation using expanded polytetrafluoroethylene or autologous costal cartilage. JAMA Facial Plast Surg 2016;18(5):327–32.

33. Murakami CS, Cook TA, Guida RA. Nasal reconstruction with articulated irradiated rib cartilage. Arch Otolaryngol Head Neck Surg 1991;117: 327–30.

34. Adams WP, Rohrich RJ, Gunter JP, et al. The rate of warping in irradiated and nonirradiated homograft rib cartilage: a controlled comparison and clinical implications. Plast Reconstr Surg 1999;103:265–70.

35. Song HM, Lee BJ, Jang YJ. Processed costal cartilage homograft in rhinoplasty. Arch Otolaryngol Head Neck Surg 2008;134(5):485–9.

36. Wong G, Johnson LM, Hagge RJ, et al. Nasal dorsal augmentation with freeze-dried allograft bone. Plast Reconstr Surg 2009;124:1312–25.

37. Christophel JJ, Hilger PA. Osseocartilaginous rib graft rhinoplasty: a stable, predictable technique for major dorsal reconstruction. Arch Facial Plast Surg 2011;13:78–83.

38. Gryskiewicz JM, Rohrich RJ, Reagan BJ. The use of alloderm for the correction of nasal contour deformities. Plast Reconstr Surg 2001;107:561–70.

39. Gryskiewicz JM. Waste not, want not: the use of AlloDerm in secondary rhinoplasty. Plast Reconstr Surg 2005;116:1999–2004.

40. Peled ZM, Warren AG, Johnston P, et al. The use of alloplastic materials in rhinoplasty surgery: a meta-analysis. Plast Reconstr Surg 2008;121(3):85e–92e.

41. Lee MR, Unger JG, Rohrich RJ. Management of the nasal dorsum in rhinoplasty: a systemic review of the literature regarding technique, outcomes, and complications. Plast Reconstr Surg 2011;128:538e–50e.

42. Loyo M, Ishii LE. Safety of alloplastic materials in rhinoplasty. JAMA Facial Plast Surg 2013;15:162–3.

43. Ahn J, Honrado C, Horn C. Combined silicone and cartilage implants. Augmentation rhinoplasty in Asian patients. Arch Facial Plast Surg 2004;6:120–3.

44. Byrd HS, Hobar PC. Alloplastic nasal and perialar augmentation. Clin Plast Surg 1996;23:315–26.

45. Adamson PA. Grafts in rhinoplasty. Arch Otolaryngol Head Neck Surg 2000;126:561–2.

46. Adams JS. Grafts and implants in nasal and chin augmentation. Otolaryngol Clin North Am 1987;20: 913–30.

47. Baran CN, Tiftikcioglu YO, Baran NK. The use of alloplastic materials in secondary rhinoplasties: 32 years of clinical experience. Plast Reconstr Surg 2005;116:1502–16.

48. Pham RTH, Hunter PD. Use of porous polyethylene as nasal dorsal implants in Asians. J Cosmet Laser Ther 2006;8:102–6.

Non-Caucasian Rhinoplasty

Roxana Cobo, MD

KEYWORDS

- Rhinoplasty • Non-Caucasian rhinoplasty • Ethnic rhinoplasty • Thick-skin rhinoplasty
- Latino/mestizo rhinoplasty • African American Rhinoplasty • Asian rhinoplasty

KEY POINTS

- Non-Caucasian rhinoplasty patients are patients of ethnic origin or patients coming from different ethnic groups.
- Surgeons need to be able to understand the interplay of culture, race, and ethnicity when trying to define and understand patients' specific desires with their rhinoplasty operation.
- Performing an adequate anatomic diagnosis of the patient's particular features will help aid in planning the adequate procedure to be able to obtain the surgical goals patients want to achieve.
- A preservation and structural approach is presented in which minimal resection and structuring of existing anatomic structures is performed to obtain the best surgical result.

INTRODUCTION

"Non-Caucasian" is a term that is often used when mentioning patients who are not "white" or who are not considered "Caucasian." In facial plastic surgery the term "non-Caucasian" has been used interchangeably to speak about patients of ethnic origin or patients coming from different ethnic groups. Standards of beauty during many years were based on findings described for the "white Caucasian" individuals, and most surgeries were targeted to obtain these ideals. Today this has changed completely. With globalization, most of the world today has mixed racial patterns and although beauty patterns are still dictated by what is found in the magazines and in social media, these images have also changed, and what is frequently seen are models and actresses of mixed backgrounds, thus changing patterns for beauty.

The term "non-Caucasian" includes all groups that are not considered from white Caucasian origin. This includes patients from Asia, African descent, and Latino/mestizo background. There are thousands of ethnic groups and within ethnic groups there can be important racial differences.

Ethnicity is defined as groups of people that share religious, linguistic, cultural, and tribal origins or backgrounds.[1] Race is more oriented toward physical characteristics and phenotype and frequently is used interchangeably with the term "ethnic" but has also been used for political purposes, making its use less frequent. Trying to classify patients according to race or ethnicity makes it extremely difficult and impractical, as there are no set values or fixed characteristics related to the different groups or classifications.[2] For this reason, instead of trying to classify rhinoplasty patients depending on where they come from, it becomes important to be able to focus on the individual nasal characteristics of the patient when they are examined.[3–5]

GENERAL CLASSIFICATION FOR NON-CAUCASIAN PATIENTS BASED ON ANATOMIC FINDINGS

As mentioned previously, "mixed race" patients are impossible to fit into specific anatomic categories. We need to remember that the final shape of the nose will depend on the interaction of the underlying bony and cartilaginous framework and

Private Practice Facial Plastic Surgery, Department of Otolaryngology, Clinica Imbanaco, Grupo Quiron Salud, Carrera 38A #5A-100, Consultorio 222A, Cali 760044, Colombia
E-mail address: rcobo@imbanaco.com.co

Clin Plastic Surg 49 (2022) 149–160
https://doi.org/10.1016/j.cps.2021.07.008
0094-1298/22/© 2021 Elsevier Inc. All rights reserved.

the external covering that is the skin soft tissue envelope (S-STE). If we use general anatomic findings to classify noses, they can be grouped into 3 main types depending on the size and general characteristic of the bony and cartilaginous framework: leptorrhine, platyrrhine, and mesorrhine. The leptorrhine noses are usually characteristics reserved for patients of Caucasian origin and are out of the scope of this article. In this article, we focus more on noses with mesorrhine or platyrrhine characteristics (**Table 1**).

Mesorrhine Nose

This type of nose is usually found in the mestizo patients of Latin America but also patients from East Asia (China, Korea, Japan, and southeast Asia). This type of nose is situated in the middle between the flat noses seen in patients with platyrrhine characteristics and the big, strong noses seen in patients with leptorrhine features. The bony vault tends to be small and wide with short nasal bones, tips tend to have poor rotation and projection, and nostrils tend to be round. This translates in a weak osseocartilaginous skeleton. The S-STE can be thicker and more sebaceous. The septal cartilage in these patients is not big, it is not thick, and the caudal septum is frequently retrusive (**Fig. 1**).

Platyrrhine Nose

This type of nose is the flatter nose with small osseocartilaginous skeletons that result in a low radix, small bones, and relatively flat nasal tips with poor projection and rotation. The platyrrhine nose is commonly found in patients of African descent. The S-STE is usually thicker than in the mesorrhine patients. Availability of septal cartilage for grafting can be limited, with retrusive caudal septums and small nasal spines (**Fig. 2**).

Leptorrhine Nose

Although out of the scope of this article, it is worth mentioning that leptorrhine characteristics are commonly found in Caucasian patients and has the opposite characteristics of the platyrrhine nose. Dorsums are high, strong with high osseo-cartilaginous frameworks. The S-STE tends to be thinner than in the other 2 nasal categories. Septal cartilage tends to be thicker and more developed, and caudal septums more prominent. Nasal spines tend to be bigger (**Fig. 3**).

Today we know most patients will be a mixture of these nasal types and it will become our responsibility as specialists to make the proper diagnosis and try to define our patients' needs depending on what they want from their surgery.

THE CONSULTATION

The consultation is the most important part when dealing with non-Caucasian rhinoplasty patients and listening to our patients becomes particularly important. We need to be able to understand what our patients want and what bothers them the most about their nose. Knowing our patients' background is important in helping us define and understand their cosmetic desires. Even though it is constantly stated that patients want to retain their ethnic features, it really becomes important to define if this is particularly true. As surgeons,

Table 1
Nasal characteristics in ethnic patients

Characteristics	Platyrrhine (African Descent)	Mesorrhine (Latin American/Asian Descent)	Leptorrhine (Caucasian)
Nasal dorsum	Very low radix/flattened nasal bridge	Normal to low radix/wide nasal bridge	Normal to high radix/high nasal bridge
Nasal bones	Short	Normal to short	Normal to long
Cartilaginous nasal vault	Flattened	Weak/wide	Normal trapezoidal shape/narrow
Nasal tip	Flimsy unsupportive/lack of projection and rotation	Flimsy unsupportive/poor projection and rotation	Strong/defined/adequate projection and rotation
Nasolabial angle	Acute	Normal to acute	Normal to obtuse
Nasal spine	Very short	Short	Normal to long
Nostril shape	Horizontal shape/flaring	Normal to horizontal shape	Oval shape
Alar base	Wide	Normal to wide	Normal to narrow

Adapted from Cobo R. Ethnic rhinoplasty. HNO. 2018 Jan;66(1):6-14.

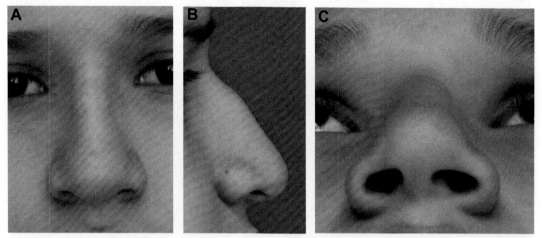

Fig. 1. Mesorrhine nasal characteristics. (*A*) Frontal view where skin tends to be thicker, nasal bones are short and have a tendency to be slightly wide, upper lateral cartilages are weak. Nasal tips are bulbous with poor definition. (*B*) On the lateral view, dorsums tend to be low and sometimes small humps or pseudohumps can be present. (*C*) Base view shows short columellas, with a relatively wide nasal base. Tips show poor support.

we need to be able to identify if what we have to offer will give our patients what they are looking for.

A complete assessment of the nose and face is performed, including a dynamic and static internal and external nasal valve evaluation. All information is recorded in our standard nasal evaluation chart (**Fig. 4**). Systematic standard rhinoplasty photographs are taken, and patients' images are evaluated and modified using computer imaging programs. All patients are asked to point out specifically what they do not like about their nose and what are the areas they want modified or repaired. This is recorded in the patients' charts.

At the end of the consultation, the surgeon should be able to answer the following questions:

1. Type of skin: is it thin, thick or normal? In patients with thick skin, the skin is additionally classified in type I, II, or III depending on the skin's specific characteristics and the presence or absence of oiliness, sebum production, and acne[6] The thick skin classification used by the author is as follows:

   Type I: Thick skin with elasticity. Oiliness is absent, no acne or redness. Pinch test positive over rhinion and supratip (ability to elevate skin when pinched with thumb and finger).

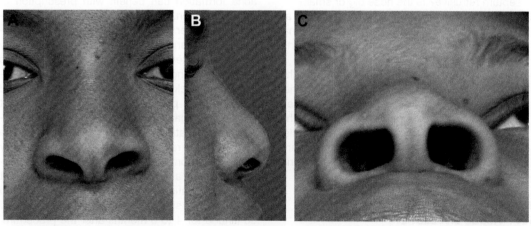

Fig. 2. Platyrrhine nasal characteristics. (*A*) Frontal view shows short, flat, and wide nasal bones with poor osseocartilaginous framework. Tips are bulbous with poor definition. (*B*) Lateral view shows a low osseocartilaginous dorsum with tips with poor projection and rotation. (*C*) Base view can show a short columella with a base that shows wide flaring horizontally shaped nostrils.

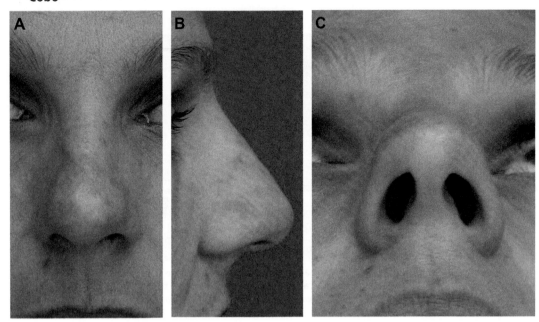

Fig. 3. Leptorrhine nasal characteristics. (*A*) Frontal view shows a strong osseocartilaginous framework with strong nasal tips. (*B*) Lateral views show high dorsums with tips that have important projection. (*C*) Base view shows a longer columella, more defined nasal tip structures, a bigger nasal spine, and a thinner S-STE.

Type II: Thick skin with little elasticity. Oiliness is present. Mild-to-moderate acne/acne-prone skin. Open pores are present.

Type III: Thick skin with no elasticity. Oiliness is present. Moderate-to-severe acne is present. Moderate-to-severe/redness can be present. Open pores are present. Pinch test negative (skin will not elevate when pinched with thumb and finger).

2. Type of underlying bony and cartilaginous framework: is it strong, normal or weak? Is the dorsum low or is there a hump? Are bones big or small? How is the cartilage? Is the caudal septum retrusive? Is the nose big or small?

3. Grafting options: Will septal cartilage fulfill all my grafting requirements? Will I need additional cartilage? If so, from where? Conchal cartilage? Rib cartilage?

4. Surgical Plan: What surgical options does the patient have? It is interesting to note that most surgical techniques today are focused on strengthening support structures of the nose and preserving as much as possible. Most surgical techniques are geared toward improving symmetry, creating balance, and improving definition and refinement.

INTEGRATED MANAGEMENT OF THE SKIN SOFT TISSUE ENVELOPE

Many of our non-Caucasian patients are patients with thick skin. Establishing an integrated management of the skin in rhinoplasty patients can enhance results and reduce postsurgical swelling and inflammation.

When patients have thick skin, this is classified into types I, II, or III and management prescribed according to patients' individual needs. All rhinoplasty patients receive skin conditioning promoting skin exfoliation and controlling sebum and oil production. If possible, topical treatment is begun before surgery and continued at least for 4 to 6 months after surgery. This will help control swelling and inflammation.[6]

It has been shown that patients with overly thick skin, increased sebum production, and acne formation can benefit with prescription of oral isotretinoin. Today low dose schemes (0.25–0.40 mg/kg per day) are just as effective as standard dosing and have fewer side effects. Every time more, intermittent dosing (20 mg 2–3 times a week) is being used with positive results in patients with thick skin, sebaceous hyperplasia and increased oil production.[7–9] Surgery does not have to be delayed if patients are taking oral isotretinoin.[6] Treatment is stopped the week before surgery and restarted 2 weeks post surgery when tapes come off. In patients who have undergone surgery, and have not started treatment but have an indication for oral isotretinoin, it is started 2 weeks after surgery (when tapes come off) and continued for 4 to 6 months after the procedure. All patients are monitored with hepatic function tests and in women pregnancy must be avoided rigorously.[6,7,9]

Fig. 4. Nasal evaluation chart.

NASAL EVALUATION

1. SKIN TYPE:

   Normal ☐ Thick ☐ Thin ☐ Sebaceous ☐ Dry ☐ Acne ☐

   Thick Skin Classification: I ☐ II ☐ III ☐

2. NASAL VALVE: N:normal C:compromised

   Internal Nasal Valve: Right☐   Left ☐

   External Nasal Valve: Right☐   Left ☐

3. NASAL SEPTUM

   Straight ☐

   Deviated: Right ☐   Left ☐

   Area of Cottle (1-4):

   Caudal ☐ Basal _____ Cephalic _____

4. INFERIOR TURBINATES

   Normal ☐ Augmented ☐ Other_____

5. NASAL BONY DORSUM

Height of Radix in mm:_____

Normal ☐   Low ☐   High ☐   Hump ☐ Narrow ☐ Wide ☐

Deviated: Right ☐ Left ☐

Depression: Right ☐   Left ☐

6. UPPER LATERAL CARTILAGES

Normal ☐   Wide ☐   Narrow ☐

 Collapse: Right ☐ Left ☐

 Deformity:_____

7. NASAL TIP

Alar Cartilages: Normal ☐ Thin ☐ Wide ☐ Strong ☐ Flimsy☐ Scar Tissue☐

Pinched: Right ☐   Left ☐

Other: _____

8. NASOLABIAL ANGLE

    Degrees:_____   Acute☐   Obtuse☐

9. NASAL BASE

   Normal ☐   Narrow ☐   Wide ☐ Asymmetric ☐

10. NOSTRIL ORIENTATION

  Oval ☐   Vertical ☐   Horizontal ☐

  Flaring ☐   Non-Flaring ☐

11. NASAL TIP RECOIL

  Weak ☐Strong ☐

   Nasal Spine: Normal ☐ Prominent ☐ Small ☐ Deviated: ☐ _____

12. DONOR SITES FOR CARTILAGE GRAFTS

     Nasal Septum ☐ Auricle: Right ☐   Left ☐   Rib ☐

13: NASAL DEVIATION

     Straight: ☐

     Deviated: ☐

          Upper Third: Right ☐   Left ☐

          Middle Third: Right ☐   Left ☐

              Lower Third (Nasal Tip): Right ☐ Left: ☐

14. MEASUREMENTS (mm)

  N-T : _____

  A-T: _____

  Height of Radix_____

  Height of Rhinion_____

  Intercanthal Distance_____

  Nasal Base Distance_____

SURGICAL TECHNIQUES

The objective of this article was not to concentrate on surgical techniques. This would be impossible. The philosophic surgical approach for managing non-Caucasian patients is presented with emphasis on African, Asian, and Latino/mestizo patients. All of these are ethnic groups that have a predominance of mesorrhine and platyrrhine anatomic characteristics. These surgeries are procedures oriented toward structuring, strengthening, augmenting, and refining. A structural and preservation approach has been used by the author for more than 10 years, with some variations and includes the following:

- Adequate anatomic diagnosis
- Definition of available cartilage for grafting purposes
- Preservation and reinforcement or reconstruction of support nasal structures using structural grafting techniques
- Definition of the different nasal structures with sutures and grafts
- Refinement techniques
- Management of the S-STE

The most important question that must be answered before surgery is: will the available septal cartilage I have be enough for the possible techniques I will be using in this patient? In patients of Asian, African, and sometimes mestizo descent, it is not uncommon to have to perform dorsal augmentation techniques. In these cases, additional cartilage will be necessary. A similar scenario can be seen when important support is needed to reinforce the pedestal and nasal tip lobule.

The first choice for cartilage is always the nasal septum. In cases in which we know this will not supply our needs, conchal cartilage or rib cartilage are good harvesting options. These additional options need to be explained to our patients. Rib cartilage is a preferred option if structural grafts will be needed. Conchal cartilage, although a good and easy source of cartilage, will not make the ideal structural graft. In these cases, rib cartilage is the preferred choice. Surgical options are endless. It becomes useful to plan surgery using a "problem-solving approach" (**Table 2**).

Dorsal Augmentation

Dorsal augmentation is frequently needed in patients of Asian and African origin and sometimes in Mestizo patients. Many surgical techniques have been described, including use of solid rib cartilage grafts and nasal implants.[4,10–12]

Table 2
Problem-solving approach in non-Caucasian rhinoplasty

Anatomic Problem	Surgical Solution
Low dorsum	Dorsal augmentation • Solid cartilage grafts • Finely diced cartilage + fibrin glue covered with fascia or perichondrium
Weak Pedestal/retrusive caudal septum	Overlapping septal extension graft
Flaring nostrils/retracted ala/ weak lateral sidewall	• Free-floating alar rim graft • Articulated alar rim grafts • Lateral crura repositioning
Nasal tips with poor projection and rotation	• Lateral crural steal • Lateral crural tensioning • Angulated tip defining sutures
Nasal tips with poor definition	• Shield graft • Cap graft
Camouflaging techniques	• Superiorly pediculated superficial musculoaponeurotic system (SMAS) flap • Finely diced cartilage • Cartilage paste
S.STE thinning techniques	• SMAS ligament resection

All techniques can have complications. Implants are commonly used in Asia for dorsal augmentation. Materials commonly used today are mainly silicone and expanded polytetrafluoroethylene.[11] The big drawback to these techniques is the risk of infection requiring meticulous planning and execution of the operation.

The author prefers autologous materials, such as cartilage, for dorsal augmentation. Cartilage can be harvested from septum, auricular concha, or rib. Solid cartilage grafts have successfully been used for dorsal augmentation with excellent long-term results.[13] Other very popular options include finely diced cartilage grafts either wrapped in fascia (also known as DC-F) or mixed with fibrin glue (the Tasman technique).[12,14] Cartilage used for dicing can be harvested from septum, concha, or rib. The choice of the cartilage will really depend on the specific grafting needs of the patient. Temporalis fascia or rectus abdominis fascia can be used to wrap the DC-F graft. When using finely diced cartilage with fibrin glue, the author covers the dorsal portion of the graft that will be against the S-STE with perichondrium or fascia to avoid any long-term visibility of any of the cartilage pieces (**Fig. 5**).

Reinforcing the Pedestal

The shape of the nasal tip is given by the alar cartilages and their relationship to the base of the nose or pedestal, which is formed by the caudal end of the septum and the nasal spine and its S-STE covering. It is not uncommon to find retrusive caudal septums and short nasal spines in patients with mesorrhine and platyrrhine characteristics. This translates into bulbous tips with poor projection and rotation. The S-STE is thicker and more inelastic and their septal cartilage is thinner and more flimsy than that found in Caucasian patients. The main goal in nasal tip surgery for this group of patients is focusing on surgical techniques that will improve projection, rotation, and definition.[15,16] If the foundation is not strong enough, the weight of a heavy S-STE over a flimsy graft will tend to push the nasal tip backward, increasing rotation excessively. It becomes particularly important to have a sturdy foundation on which the lower lateral cartilages can be repositioned and kept in place.[17]

A structural approach is frequently needed and is the first step to establish a solid foundation over which tip grafting techniques can be performed. This stabilization is frequently obtained

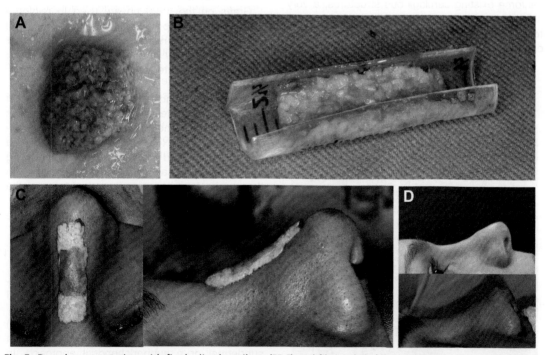

Fig. 5. Dorsal augmentation with finely diced cartilage (FDC) and fibrin glue. (*A*) Cartilage can be harvested from septum, ear concha, or rib, and should be finely diced. (*B*) FDC is placed in a template fashioned from a 3-mL syringe cut lengthwise and mixed with fibrin glue. (*C*) Dorsal portion of graft is covered with temporalis fascia or rectus abdominis fascia. (*D*) Preoperative and immediately postoperative images of patient after dorsal augmentation graft with FDC and fibrin glue.

with a strong septal extension graft (SEG) that can be placed end to end or overlapping the existing natural caudal septum.

The first question that needs to be answered is from where the cartilage is going to be harvested. In patients undergoing primary rhinoplasty, the ideal choice is septal cartilage. Alternative choices are conchal and rib cartilage. Conchal cartilage is not the best choice for a structural graft, and rib cartilage is probably the best choice for its strength but many times is not accepted, especially in patients undergoing primary rhinoplasty.

The shape and position of the SEG will define the degree of rotation and projection. Today the author prefers an overlapping septal extension graft (OSEG) that has a more triangular shape. This gives more stability to the pedestal. Frequently a small bolster graft is placed on the contralateral side to stabilize the graft, especially when important projection is needed. This helps keep the graft in the midline (**Fig. 6**). Once the graft is stabilized, the feet of the medial crura are sutured to the OSEG using a tongue-in-groove technique. Work on the nasal tip is performed when stabilization of the base has been completed. It is important to note that to be able to execute important changes in the nasal tip that include use of sutures to reorient cartilages and grafts to reinforce existing cartilaginous structures, a very solid and stable foundation is required to be able to support all the contracting forces that will be created over time.

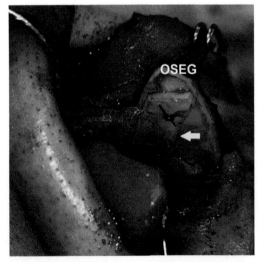

Fig. 6. OSEG. OSEG in place with bolster graft fixed on contralateral side. Angulated bolster graft (*yellow arrow*) helps give additional stability to OSEG.

Managing the Nasal Tip in Non-Caucasian Patients

Nasal tip techniques have changed dramatically over the past years independent of what ethnic group the patient belongs to. Most of the changes obtained in the nasal tip are done reorienting and structuring the existing nasal tip structures and resecting very little, if any tissue in the nasal tip area. Today emphasis is placed on the lateral crura and the lateral sidewall trying to create a smooth transition between the nasal tip and alar lobule. The main objectives are as follows: decreasing the bulk in the supratip area and supraalar groove, creating a smooth transition between the nasal tip and the alar lobule, and defining extent of tip projection, rotation, and definition.[17] Multiple techniques are used today to flatten the lateral crura and create a smooth transition in the lateral crura. This is done with sutures and grafts. Sutures used are angulated dome-defining sutures where the objective is to define the existing dome or create a new dome where the caudal edge is placed angulated and slightly higher than the cephalic edge of the alar cartilage. These types of sutures help reorient the alar cartilages in a more favorable position.[17,18] Tensioning of the lateral crura using the SEG is also another extremely useful way to reorient and structure the nasal tip.[19]

Grafts on the nasal tip are used to reinforce structures and help improve definition. The lateral sidewall can be reinforced using alar contour grafts, articulated alar rim grafts, alar strut grafts, or performing lateral crural repositioning[20–22] (**Fig. 7**).

It is not uncommon to find in the non-Caucasian population that after all "possible" tip techniques have been performed, additional refining procedures need to be executed. Onlay tip grafts like a cap graft or a shield graft can be important grafting techniques that can help improve definition. In these patients, it becomes important to cover the leading edge of these grafts with either perichondrium or fascia to help camouflage any visible edges of the graft.

Surgical Management of the Skin Soft Tissue Envelope

In patients with ultra-thick inelastic skin (type III thick skin), it becomes necessary to perform superficial musculoaponeurotic system (SMAS) debulking. Debulking can be performed using a subdermal or a subperichondrial approach. In both approaches, the SMAS is resected "en block" respecting the dermis and the vascular supply of the nose. This means avoiding use of cautery and avoiding extending dissection laterally

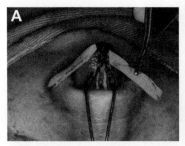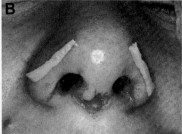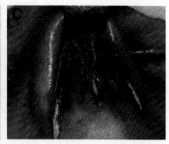

Fig. 7. Grafts used to support the lateral sidewall and smooth out the transition from the nasal tip to the alar lobule. (*A*) Articulated alar rim grafts (*B*) Alar contour grafts. (*C*) Lateral crura repositioning.

in the alar groove to avoid vascular compromise of the flap (**Fig. 8**).

Eliminating dead space over the supratip and scroll area is an important maneuver that should be performed at the end of surgery before closing the skin flap, especially in patients with thick skin. An absorbable suture is placed approximating the supratip area to the anterior septal angle. This will help in flap redraping, will reduce blood accumulation in this area, and will decrease the swelling and possibility of secondary scar formation.

Surgery of the Nasal Base

Surgery of the nasal base is performed at the end of the surgery after all incisions have been closed. Alar base resection is more frequent in patients of African descent and Asian descent because they have more prominent platyrrhine characteristics. In Mestizo patients (Latino patients) it is not infrequent to find that after appropriate projection, rotation, and definition have been achieved, alar base resection is not as important.[16,23,24] Planning and execution of procedures on the nasal base should be meticulous, and closure of incisions should be performed precisely to avoid asymmetries and unnecessary scars.

Management of Swelling and Postsurgical Edema

Preventing swelling and managing postsurgical edema is important in non-Caucasian patients, especially if they have thick skin. A good surgical technique can result in a poor surgical outcome if proper postsurgical recommendations are not followed.

Immediate postsurgical management

All measures are geared toward diminishing postsurgical swelling. The nose should be taped properly, and a thermoplastic or metallic splint should routinely be used over the taped nasal dorsum. This will reduce edema, dead space formation, and bleeding. Patients should remain with their

head elevated 45 to 60° the first weeks after surgery and use ice packs or cold compresses over eyes and cheeks, especially in the first 72 hours after the procedure. This will help reduce chemosis and edema.

Tapes and cast are removed on day 7 and additional tapes are used for a second week. Two weeks postoperative, all tapes are removed, and patients are restarted on their skin regimens. These skin-cleansing protocols will aid in reducing swelling and controlling sebum, oil, and acne formation, and should be used at least during the first 6 months after the procedure.

Late postsurgical management

Long-term prevention and management of edema formation is critical. Patients should prevent sun

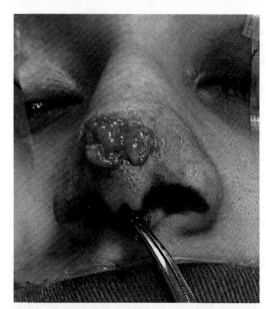

Fig. 8. SMAS resected en bloc to thin out the S-STE. This SMAS can be used as a graft to fill in depressions in the radix, at the nasal spine to help push out the nasolabial angle, or over the dome area as camouflage.

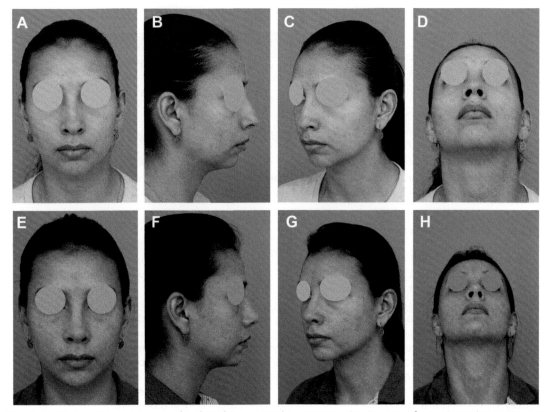

Fig. 9. (*A–D*) Preoperative images. (*E–H*) Eighteen months postoperative images of non-Caucasian patient. A structural and preservation procedure was performed with conservative remodeling of dorsum, spreader flaps of upper lateral cartilages, placement of an OSEG, lateral crural tensioning of alar cartilages, and placement of articulated alar rim grafts. Domes were defined using angulated dome-defining sutures.

exposure, strenuous exercise, and spalike activities like saunas and Turkish baths. If patients feel their nose is swollen, they should use ice packs and, if possible, elevate the head of the bed when sleeping.

Additional treatments include use of intranasal topical steroid sprays (fluticasone, mometasone) to reduce intranasal swelling. When indicated, oral isotretinoin is started 2 weeks after surgery and used for 4 to 6 months to control sebum production and acne formation and decrease inflammation of the nasal tip area (see integrated management of S-STE, earlier in this article).

Patients should be followed routinely. All should understand that swelling will be more prominent and that real results will be seen between 12 and 18 months postsurgery.

Minimally invasive procedures have also been described to treat postsurgical swelling and prevent fibrosis and scar formation in the supratip and tip area. Some surgeons routinely inject triamcinolone acetonide (Kenalog) 10 mg/mL at a dose of 0.05 to 0.1 mL starting as early as 2 weeks postsurgery and repeating injection every 4 to 6 weeks. It has been reported that corticosteroids reduce fibroblast proliferation and the inflammatory response,

reducing fibrosis and scar formation. Possible side effects are subcutaneous atrophy, telangiectasia, skin necrosis, and possible ulcerations.[25,26] Other investigators have advocated the use of 5-fluorouracil injected in the subdermis, starting injections as early as 1 week postoperatively, and repeating every 4 weeks, totaling 4 to 6 injections. These injections can be very painful, so they can be combined with triamcinolone to reduce the pain.[27]

SUMMARY

Non-Caucasian patients are also known as ethnic patients. The world's population today is multiracial, and every time we are treating more non-Caucasian patients in our offices. The rhinoplasty surgeon needs to be able to understand the interplay that culture, race, and ethnicity play in patients' self-image and their particular desires when seeking surgery. Rhinoplasty today is not a one-size-fits-all surgery. It is important to be able to make the proper anatomic diagnosis, understand the different possible surgical options, and be able to offer our patients an individualized integrated approach to their rhinoplasty procedure (**Fig. 9**).

CLINICS CARE POINTS

- Non-Caucasian patient evaluation should include nasal characteristics based on the 3 anatomic groups mentioned: platyrrhine, mesorrhine, and leptorrhine. This will give the surgeon important information that will help plan surgery in a proper fashion.

- The 5 key points that should be answered during consultation are as follows:
  - What does the patient want of his or her surgical procedure
  - What type of skin does the patient have
  - What are the characteristic of his or her cartilaginous dorsum
  - What are the grafting options for that specific patient
  - What is the possible surgical plan for this patient

- All patients are offered an integrated management of the S-STE to reduce and control swelling and inflammation and, in this way, achieve improved surgical outcomes.

- Surgical approaches include a preservation and structural approach. This means the following:
  - Very limited if any tissue resection
  - Preservation and reinforcement or reconstruction of support nasal structures using structural grafting techniques
  - Definition of the different nasal structures with sutures and grafts
  - Refinement techniques
  - Surgical management of the S-STE when necessary

DISCLOSURE

The author has nothing to disclose.

AUTHOR DISCLOSURE STATEMENT

No financial interests exist.
  No funding was received for this article.

REFERENCES

1. "ethnic." Merriam-Webster.com. Available at: https://www.merriam-webster.com/dictionary/ethnic. Accessed March 1 2021

2. Leong SC, Eccles R. Race and ethnicity in nasal plastic surgery: a need for science. Facial Plast Surg 2010;26(02):63–8.

3. ÓConnor K, Brissett A. The changing face of America. Otolaryngol Clin North Am 2020;53:299–308.

4. Cobo R. Ethnic rhinoplasty. HNO 2018;66(01):6–14.

5. Cobo R. Ethnic rhinoplasty. Facial Plast Surg 2019; 35:313–21.

6. Cobo R, Camacho JG, Orrego J. Integrated management of the thick-skinned rhinoplasty patient. Facial Plast Surg 2018;34(1):3–8.

7. Cobo R, Vitery L. Isotretinoin use in thick-skinned rhinoplasty patients. Facial Plast Surg 2016;32(6): 656–61.

8. Zaenglein AL, Pathy AL, Schlosser BJ, et al. Guidelines of care for the management of acne vulgaris. J Am Acad Dermatol 2016;74(05):945–73.e33.

9. Spring LK, Krakowski AC, Alam M, et al. Isotretinoin and timing of procedural interventions: a systematic review with consensus recommendations. JAMA Dermatol 2017;153(08):802–9.

10. Peng GL, Nassif PS. Rhinoplasty in the African American patient. Anatomic considerations and technical pearls. Clin Plast Surg 2016;43:255–64.

11. Na Hg, Jang YJ. Use of nasal implants and dorsal modification when treating the east Asian nose. Otolaryngol Clin North Am 2020;53:255–66.

12. Tasman AJ, Diener PA, Litschel R. The diced cartilage glue graft for nasal augmentation morphometric evidence of longevity. Facial Plast Surg 2013;15(2):86–94.

13. Toriumi D. Dorsal augmentation using autologous costal cartilage or microfat-infused soft tissue augmentation. Facial Plast Surg 2017;33(2): 162–78.

14. Calvert J, Brenner K. Autogenous dorsal reconstruction: maximizing the utility of diced cartilage and fascia. Semin Plast Surg 2008;22(2):110–9.

15. Jin HR, Won TB. Rhinoplasty in the Asian patient. Clin Plast Surg 2016;43:265–79.

16. Cobo R. Management of the mestizo nose. Otolaryngol Clin North Am 2020;53:267–82.

17. Toriumi D. Nasal tip contouring: anatomic basis for management. Facial Plast Surg Aesthet Med 2020; 22(1):10–24.

18. Kovacevic M, Wurm J. Cranial tip suture in nasal tip contouring. Facial Plast Surg 2014;30(6):681–7.

19. Davis R. Lateral crural tensioning for refinement of the wide and underprojected nasal tip rethinking the lateral crural steal. Facial Plast Clin North Am 2015;23(1):23–53.

20. Rohrich RJ, Raniere J Jr, Ha RY. The alar contour graft: correction and prevention of alar rim deformities in rhinoplasty. Plast Reconstr Surg 2002; 109(7):2495–505.

21. Goodrich J, Wong BJF. Optimizing the soft tissue triangle, alar margin furrow, and alar ridge aesthetics:

analysis and use of the articulate alar rim graft facial. Plast Surg 2016;32:646–55.

22. Toriumi DM, Asher SA. Lateral crural repositioning for treatment of cephalic malposition. Facial Plast Surg Clin North Am 2015;23(1):55–71.

23. Kim JH, Park JP, Jang YJ. Aesthetic outcomes of alar base resection in Asian patients undergoing rhinoplasty. JAMA Facial Plast Surg 2016;18(6):462–6.

24. Boahene K. Management of the nasal tip, nasal base, and soft tissue envelope in patients of African descent. Otolaryngol Clin North Am 2020;53: 309–17.

25. Hanasono MM, Kridel RW, Pastorek NJ, et al. Correction of the soft tissue pollybeak using triamcinolone injection. Arch Facial Plast Surg 2002; 4(1):26–30.

26. Hussein W, Foda H. Pollybeak deformity in Middle Eastern rhinoplasty: prevention and treatment facial. Plast Surg 2016;32:398–401.

27. Irvine LE, Nassif PS. Use of 5-fluorouracil for management of the thick-skinned nose. Facial Plast Surg 2018;34(1):9–13.

Alar Base Reduction
Nuances and Techniques

Nazim Cerkes, MD

KEYWORDS

- Nasal tip • Alar base • Nasal base • Alar lobule • Nostril sill • Alar base reduction • Alar flare

KEY POINTS

- The alar base should be proportional with the upper part of the nose and other facial structures for a harmoniously balanced appearance. The width of the nasal base is an important guide in surgical planning and treatment of the appropriate width of the upper parts of the nose.
- Several anatomic variations are seen on the nasal base. The common alar base deformities are horizontal excess or deficiency, vertical excess or deficiency, and cephalic malposition or caudal malposition of alar base.
- There are 3 basic types of excision on alar base surgery. Alar wedge excision, nostril sill excision, and combined alar wedge and nostril sill excision.
- The alar wedge excision is an elliptical excision that is placed in the alar crease and it is used to reduce the size and shorten the vertical length of alar lobule and correct the excessive flaring on the frontal view.
- Nostril sill excision is used to decrease the interalar distance and nostril sill length. It is performed in patients with a wide nasal base without alar flare.
- Combined alar wedge and nostril sill excision is used in cases with a wide alar base and additionally, there is excessive flaring and large alar lobule.

INTRODUCTION

The alar base plays an important role in the appearance of the nose. The alar base should be proportional with the upper part of the nose and other facial structures for a harmoniously balanced appearance.[1–4] Overly wide or flared alar base will lead to a bottom-heavy appearance of the nose. Although alar base surgery is considered in patients with wide alar bases, dynamic changes during rhinoplasty operation may affect the width of the alar base and alar flaring.[3] Decreasing tip projection will result in widening of the alar base and alar flaring, and increasing tip projection will do an opposite effect. After a significant dorsum reduction, lower part of nose may become proportionally larger and an alar base reduction may require for the harmoniously balanced nose. The width of the nasal base is also an important guide in surgical planning and treatment of the appropriate width of the upper parts of the nose.[3,5]

Alar base surgery is typically performed at the end of the operation and the final decision-making process should be after all other steps of the surgery have been completed and the incisions closed as changes in tip projection and dorsal height will affect the shape of the alar base.

ANATOMIC CONSIDERATIONS

Nasal base consists of 3 components, the columellar base, nostril sills, and alar lobules. Columellar base is the medial subunit of the nasal base, nostril sills, and alar lobules are lateral subunits (**Fig. 1**). The columellar base is composed of medial crural footplates and soft tissues between the footplates and caudal septum/anterior nasal spine. Alar lobules form the lateral walls of nostrils and nasal base. They are composed of fibrofatty soft tissue and some amount of muscle and may assume a variety of shapes and sizes. Nostril sill is the area between the columellar

Private Practice, Hakki Yeten Cad. No:17/6, Fulya, Besiktas, Istanbul 34365, Turkey
E-mail address: ncerkes@hotmail.com

Clin Plastic Surg 49 (2022) 161–178
https://doi.org/10.1016/j.cps.2021.08.007

plasticsurgery.theclinics.com

base and alar lobule which forms the part of the nostril base. The alar crease (alar fascial groove) is the junction between the cheek and nose and is an important landmark in the planning of alar base surgery.

Interalar width is the distance from lateral alar projection to the opposite lateral alar projection point. Nasal base width (alar base width) is the distance from the alar base insertion point to the opposite alar base insertion point. Alar flare is the distance from lateral alar projection point to alar base insertion point (**Fig. 2**).

The ideal nostril has a teardrop shape. Lateral alar rim should be straight and smooth in contour, whereas the medial aspect of the nostril should be concave creating a smooth curvature of the lateral nostrils (**Fig. 3**).

PREOPERATIVE ASSESSMENT

During preoperative nasal analysis, the analysis of the nasal base with the other features of the face is crucial for a successful outcome. Evaluating the shape, dimensions, position, and symmetry of the alar base from frontal and basal views are necessary Alar base width is best evaluated from the frontal view. Basal view is essential in the evaluation of the anatomy of the nasal base, alar flaring, nostril circumference, and asymmetries. In Caucasians, the interalar width (distance between the lateral alar projection points) should not be wider than intercanthal distance as long as the intercanthal distance is optimal.[6–8] (**Fig. 4**) When considering African American rhinoplasty, the normal index for African American patients is to actually have the nostril attachment lateral to the medial canthus. Alar flare refers to the maximum degree of convex bowing of the alar base above the alar crease. Excessive alar flare, in which the alar edge extends more than 2 mm lateral to the alar base attachment, may commonly be seen in the African American nose.[9,10]

The nostril shape and size are the important considerations to be taken into account in planning the alar base surgery. If the nostril size of the patient is within normal limits, the alar base modification should only involve the resection of a skin ellipse along the most lateral portion of the ala, creating a scar to hide in the groove without resection from nostril sills.

Diagnosis of nasal base deformities is critical for success. During the examination, all units of the nasal base should be evaluated in detail. Several anatomic variations are seen on the nasal base. Alar base deformities can be horizontal excess or deficiency, vertical excess or deficiency, cephalic malposition, or caudal malposition of alar base.[3]

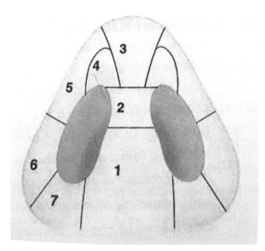

Fig. 1. Subunits of nasal base and nasal tip: (1) Columellar base, (2) columellar body, (3) infratip lobule, (4) soft triangle, (5) lateral nasal wall, (6) alar lobule, and (7) nostril sill.

Nostril sills can be wide or narrow. Soft tissue deformities of columellar base or deviation of caudal septum compromise nostril aperture resulting in external nasal valve dysfunction and airway obstruction.

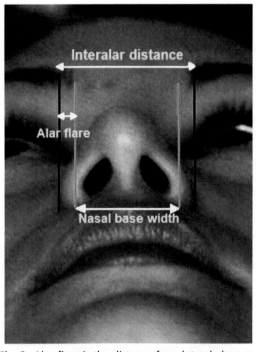

Fig. 2. Alar flare is the distance from lateral alar projection point to the alar base insertion point.

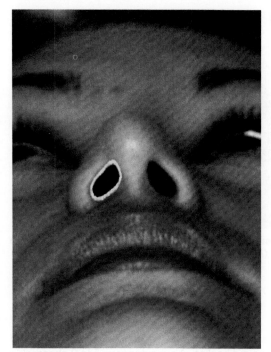

Fig. 3. Ideal nostril has a teardrop shape. (The yellow *line* indicates the nostril circumference).

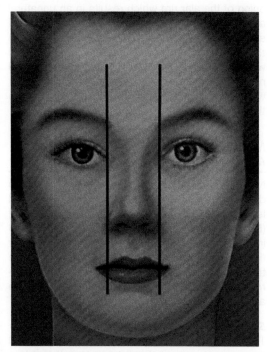

Fig. 4. Interalar width is the distance between the lateral alar projection points. Ideally, it is equal to intercanthal distance.

Columellar base deviations, malposition, or flaring of medial crural footplates are fairly common deformities that lead to functional and aesthetic problems.[8] In patients with flaring footplates or hypertrophic ANS, the orientation of the nostrils may change and diagnosing nostril sill deformities can be difficult.

MANAGEMENT OF NASAL BASE DEFORMITIES

Alar base management is one of the integral parts of rhinoplasty operation which has to be planned carefully and executed conservatively. Aggressive excisions may cause irreparable deformities.[11]

Columellar base should be addressed before alar base resections. Correction of columellar base deformities and positioning of medial crural footplates should be the primary step of nasal base surgery to attain aesthetic ideals of the columellar base and improve external nasal valve function.[7,8] These maneuvers also alter the shape of the nostrils and position of the other elements of the nasal base. If caudal septum is deviated, it must be repositioned to the midline. If the anterior nasal spine is not on the midline, it can be osteotomized and repositioned. A hypertrophic ANS may distort the columellar base and widen the columellar-labial angle. In this case, it should be reduced to improve the columellar base. If exists, medial crural deformities and asymmetries are corrected.

Flaring medial crural footplates presented with a wide columellar base may compromise the airway. In such cases, the resection of soft tissues from in between the medial crura, extending down to the ANS area should be performed to be able to properly approximate the medial crura with sutures to narrow the columellar base (**Fig. 5**). The suturing of the opposing faces of the footplates has the effect of increased tip projection and enlarge the external nasal valve (**Fig. 6**).

Alar Base Surgery

Deformities requiring alar base modification include wide nasal base, alar flaring, large nostril size, and asymmetries of nostrils or alae. The actual design of alar base excisions should be made once all incisions are closed. The location and amount of excision are performed depending on the site of excess. It is crucial to meticulously plan the incisions, to make the scars inconspicuous, remove tissue precisely to achieve adequate reduction and symmetry while avoiding overresection.

There are 3 basic types of excision on alar base surgery.

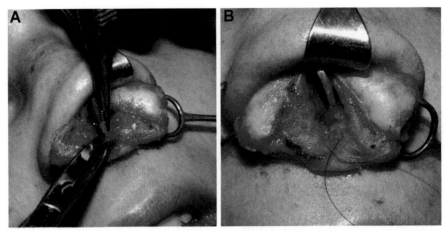

Fig. 5. (*A*) Removal of soft tissues from in between the medial crura to be able to properly approximate the medial crura with sutures to narrow the columellar base. (*B*) Approximation of medial crural footplates with a suture passing through both footplates.

1. Alar wedge excision
2. Nostril sill excision
3. Combined alar wedge and nostril sill excision

The axis of alar base excisions can be horizontal or vertical. When a horizontal axis excision is performed, the nasal base will narrow and alar lobule will move medially. Nasal sill excision is an excision from the horizontal axis. A wedge resection from the alar lobule is an excision on the vertical axis which shortens the alar rim and decreases the alar flare.[3,5–8,10]

Correction of Alar Flaring (Alar Wedge Excision)

The alar wedge excision is an elliptical excision that is, placed in the alar crease (**Fig. 7**). It is used to reduce the size and shorten the vertical length of the alar lobule and correct the excessive flaring on the frontal view.[3,5–9,12–14] Reduction of alar flare also orients the nostrils toward a more vertical axis. Alar wedge excision does not decrease a wide nasal base. To avoid reducing nostril size and shape, the incision is not extended into the vestibule.

Surgical technique
Markings should be conducted meticulously with measuring accurately with calipers before injection of local anesthetic solution. Incision is placed in the alar crease or just 0.1 to 0.2 mm above the alar crease and performed with a No: 15 blade. The excised wedge includes the skin and deeper tissue including alar musculature and fibrofatty tissue (**Fig. 8**). Excessive hemostasis with cautery

should be avoided which can lead to impaired wound healing. A subcutaneous 5 to 0 absorbable stitch is used to approximate edges. Skin is closed meticulously with 6 to 0 nylon sutures. The sutures are removed 6 to 7 days after the surgery.

Alar wedge excisions should be planned meticulously and executed conservatively. Excessive reduction of alar flare may lead to over straightening of the alar rim which results in an unnatural and imbalanced appearance. In the planning of alar wedge resection, it is imperative to preserve the 1:1 ratio between the infratip lateral nasal wall and alar lobule (**Fig. 9**). If the infratip lateral nasal wall is large, it is better not to do an alar wedge excision to preserve proportion between these units (**Fig.10**).

Narrowing Wide Alar Base (Nostril Sill Reduction)

Nostril sill excision is the technique that is used to decrease the interalar distance and nostril sill length, and reduce the size of the nostril (**Fig. 11**).[7,8,10,13] Nostril sill excision is performed in patients with a wide nasal base without alar flare. However, care must be taken to preserve the external nasal valve aperture. Excessive narrowing of nostrils causes unnatural appearance and functional problems.

Surgical technique
The midcolumella is marked and calipers are used to measure and mark the distance from the midcolumellar point to the alar crease which is usually 10 to 12 mm from the midcolumellar point. The area

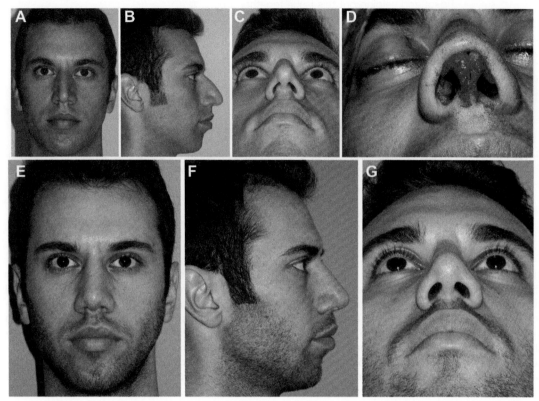

Fig. 6. (*A–C*) This 20-year-old man was seeking aesthetic and functional improvement. He had a dorsal hump, concave lateral crura and alar pinching, and excessive flaring of medial crural footplates. No septal deviation causing airway obstruction was observed at the internal examination. (*D*) Using the open technique, bony and cartilaginous dorsum was reduced. Lateral crural strut grafts were used for the correction of concave lateral crura. To widen the external nasal valve, the soft tissue between the medial crural footplates was resected and medial crural footplates were approximated with a 5 to 0 PDS suture. (*E–G*) Two-year postoperative pictures show that dorsal hump is reduced, alar pinching is corrected, and excessive flaring of medial crural footplates is corrected with the widening of the external nasal valve. The patient states that his airway improved significantly after the surgery.

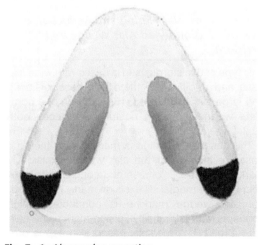

Fig. 7. *1- Alar wedge resection.*

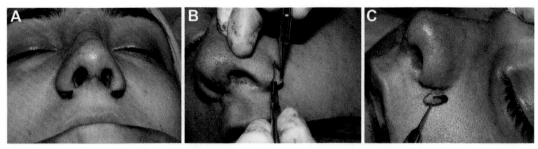

Fig. 8. (*A*) The alar wedge excision is an elliptical excision that is placed in the alar crease. (*B, C*) The excision includes the skin and deeper tissue including alar musculature and fibrofatty tissue.

that will be excised is marked. The excess nostril sill to be excised is marked by 2 lines almost parallel to each other and connected by a horizontal line along the alar fascial crease to avoid dog-ear formation. The lateral mark of the sill resection should be medial enough to preserve the lateral curve of the alar rim. The width of the excised wedge can vary between 1 and 4 mm. If a minimal sill excision is required the incision can be planned as a trapezoid shape that tapers inside toward the nostril floor and externally over the sill without doing a horizontal cut along the alar crease (**Fig. 12**). In larger resections, it is useful to create an alar flap with an incision in the alar crease to rotate the ala medially, narrow the nasal base, and make the nostril smaller (**Fig. 13**). 6-0 nylon sutures are placed at the sill border externally and 5-

0 absorbable sutures are placed internally for closure. Closure of incision advances the lateral flap medially, thereby decreases the interalar distance. Incisions made in the nostril sill are at high risk of visible scarring and require meticulous excision and suturing.

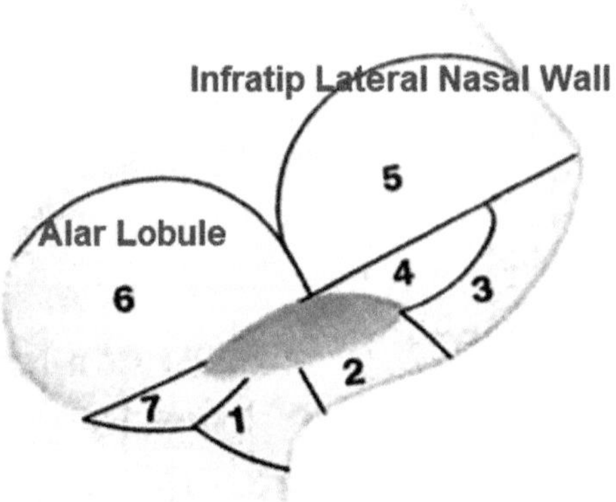

Nostril sill excision can have 2 effects on the nasal base. The sill has an inner or vestibular circumference. An excision in the internal circumference reduces the nostril size. A reduction of the outer circumference will narrow the nasal base.[7] Sill excision does not improve alar flaring because the tissue is removed in a horizontal axis. Nostril sill excision alters the shape of the nostril. Because the base of the nostril is narrowed, initially round shape of the nostril becomes oval (**Fig. 14**).

In patients with cephalic malposition of the alar base if nostril sill is wide, sill resection results in caudal transposition of alar lobule and corrects the deformity.[7] (**Fig. 15**)

Correction of Alar Flaring and Reduction of Nostril Sill (Combined Alar Wedge and Sill Excision)

This type of excision is used in cases with wide alar base and additionally, there is excessive flaring and large alar lobule (**Fig. 16**). Excision of a complete wedge including nostrill sill reduces both nostril size and alar flaring.[3,5–8,10,13]

The nasal sill excision is marked first, then the posterior incision of the alar wedge excision is marked on the alar crease and continued to connect with the medial sill excision mark. Then superior alar wedge marking is conducted which connects with lateral sill excision mark using calipers (**Fig. 17**). A medially based skin flap is preserved at the nostril sill to prevent notching of

Fig. 9. Ideally infratip lateral nasal wall/alar lobule ratio is 1:1. This ratio has to be considered in planning alar wedge resections.

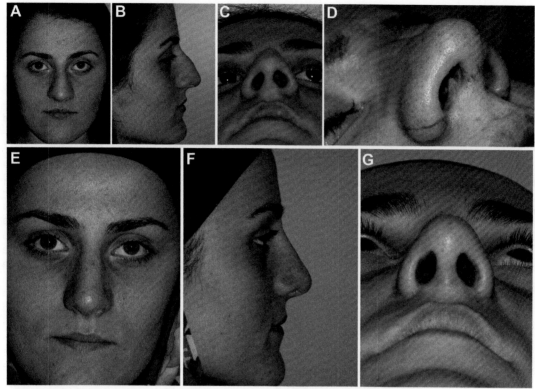

Fig. 10. (*A–C*) This 19-year-old patient had bony and cartilaginous hump with a deviation of nasal septum and bony pyramid, and alar flaring with optimal size nostrils. (*D*) Using open approach bony and cartilaginous dorsum reduction, septoplasty, and septal reconstruction using septal grafts, and 4 mm ala wedge resection bilaterally were performed. (*E–G*) 12 months postoperative pictures reveal that dorsal hump is reduced, a smooth dorsum is achieved, septum deviation and airway obstruction are corrected and alar flaring is decreased.

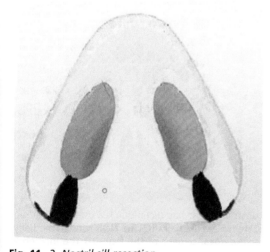

Fig. 11. *2- Nostril sill resection.*

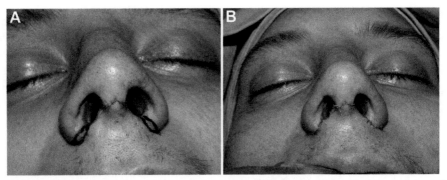

Fig. 12. (*A*) For minimal alar base narrowing, a trapezoid shape excision is planned without doing a horizontal cut along the alar crease. (*B*) After the closure of incisions, the alar base is narrowed, nostril shape is improved, and nostril size is reduced.

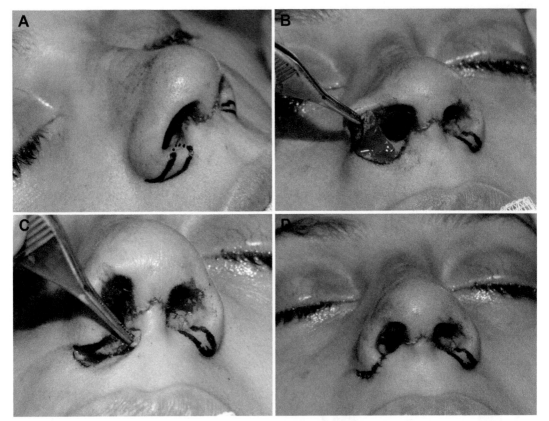

Fig. 13. (*A*) In patients who require large resection from the nostril, sill alar flap technique is a useful technique. (*B*) Alar flap is created with an incision in the alar crease to rotate the ala medially. (*C*) The ala is rotated medially. The amount of resection from the nostril sill is decided after the advancement of the flap. (*D*) The incision is closed with 6/0 nonabsorbable sutures.

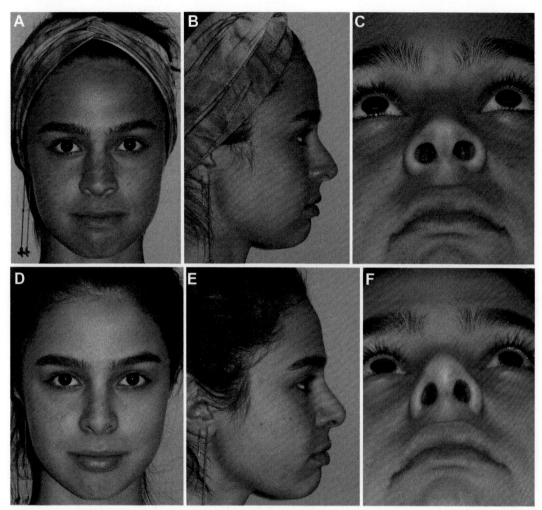

Fig. 14. (*A–C*) This 19-year-old woman presented with broad dorsum, wide alar bases, and large nostrils. Her nostrils are round rather than teardrop shape. (*D–F*) Dorsal aesthetic lines were narrowed with paramedian, transverse, and low to low osteotomies and modified spreader flap technique. 3 mm resection was performed from the nostril sill bilaterally. The patient is shown 18 months postoperatively with the refinement of the broad nasal dorsum, narrowing of alar bases, and reduction of the size of nostrils with improved shape.

the nostril. At first vertical sill incisions are performed, and then the lower alar wedge incision and the superior wedge incision are conducted using No 15 blade. The full-thickness wedge that includes fibrofatty tissue and alar musculature is resected. The sill incision is closed first followed by the alar wedge incision using 6-0 nylon suture (**Figs. 18** and **19**).

Unusual Deformities

Thick alar lobule
In patients with thick alar lobule, an elliptical excision along the vestibular aspect of the alar lobule can be used (**Fig. 20**).

Hanging ala
Caudal malposition of alar lobule presented with hooding of the base and decreased columellar show. An elliptical excision from the vestibular lining of the alar lobule is performed to remove the caudal excess of alar lobule. If necessary, a strip of alar the lining from the alar base can be removed and an alar rim graft to the anterior part of alar rim can be placed to straighten the alar rim (**Fig. 21**).

Reduction of excessively large alar lobule
In patients with excessively large lobule, a crescentic resection including the cephalic portion of the lobule can be performed. Possible visibility of

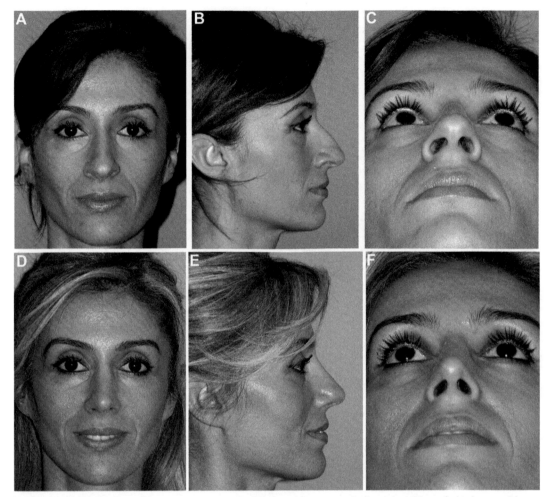

Fig. 15. (*A–C*) This 38-year-old woman presented with dorsal hump, cephalic malposition of alar base, wide nostril sills with large nostrils, and large interalar distance. (*D–F*) Bony and cartilaginous dorsum reduction and 2 mm upward rotation of the nasal tip were carried out. Alar flap was raised with an extended alar crease incision for the medial rotation and caudal transposition of the alar lobule and 3 mm resection from the nostril sill was performed. 36-months postoperative pictures reveal that alar lobules are transposed caudally and nostril size is reduced.

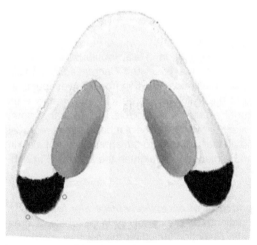

Fig. 16. *3- Combined resection.*

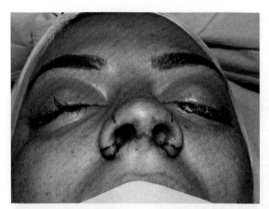

Fig. 17. Marking of a combined alar wedge and sill excision in a patient with large alar lobules and wide alar base.

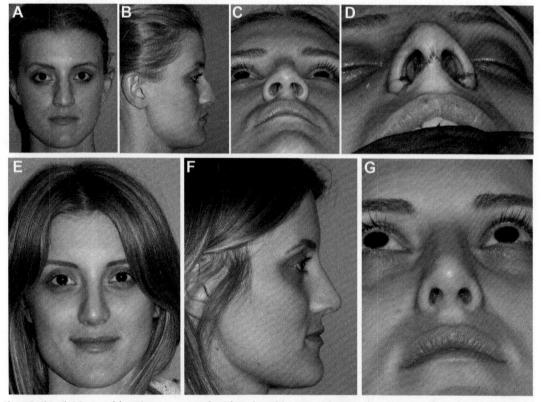

Fig. 18. (*A–C*) 26year-old patient presented with a dorsal hump with irregular dorsal aesthetic lines, broad tip,- wide interalar distance, large alar lobules, and large nostrils. (*D*) Bony and cartilaginous hump reduction, osteotomies, and modified spreader flaps were performed to restore nasal dorsum and dorsal aesthetic lines. Cephalic resection of the lateral crura and tip sutures were used to refine the tip. A combined alar wedge and nostril sill resection were performed to narrow the nasal base and reduce large nostril circumference. (*E–G*) One-year postoperative pictures reveal that a smooth dorsum is achieved with the refinement of dorsal aesthetic lines and nasal tip is refined. The nasal base is narrowed, nostril size is reduced, and a balance between the parts of the nose is achieved.

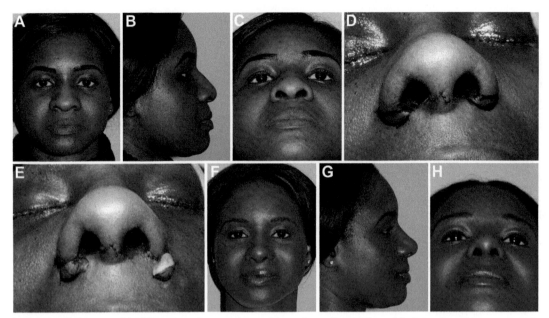

Fig. 19. (*A–C*) 29-year-old African American patient with underprojected tip, wide interalar distance, and alar flaring. (*D, E*) To increase tip projection, lateral crural steal, columellar strut, and onlay tip grafts were performed. A combined excision from the alar lobule and nostril sill was conducted to decrease the alar flare and narrow the alar base. (*F–H*) Two-years postoperative pictures show that tip projection is increased and alar flare is decreased with a reduced nostril size.

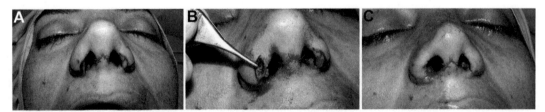

Fig. 20. (*A*) In a patient with thick ala an elliptical excision along the vestibular aspect of the alar lobule is planned. (*B*) Elliptical excision is performed on the right ala. (*C*) After the closure of the incision, there is a noticeable improvement on the right ala and in the shape of the right nostril.

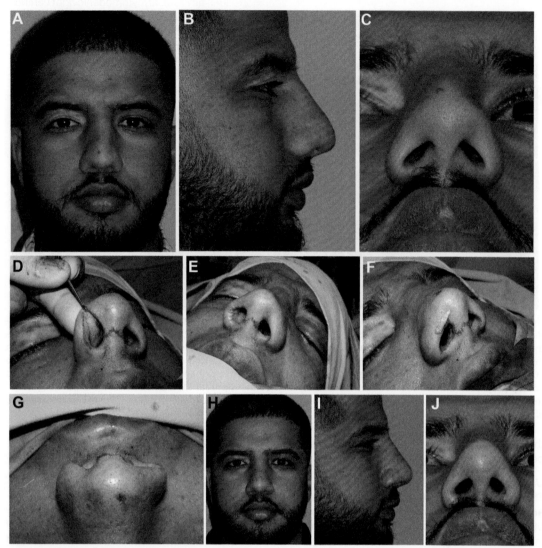

Fig. 21. (*A–C*) This 25-year-old man presented with hanging ala with thick nasal tip skin. He has medial footplate flaring with narrow external nasal valves. (*D, E*) Using the open approach, the medial crural footplates were approximated. An elliptical excision from the vestibular aspect of the alar lobule was performed. Notice that after elliptical excision, the right nostril is wider comparing the other side. (*F*) An alar rim graft to the anterior part of the alar rim was placed to straighten the alar rim and augment the soft triangle. (*G*) Intraoperative picture shows the straightened of the alar rim on the right side after elliptical excision and alar rim graft. (*H–J*) 18-months postoperative pictures of the patient show that Caudal malposition of the ala is corrected, alar rim is straightened, and nostril circumference is enlarged.

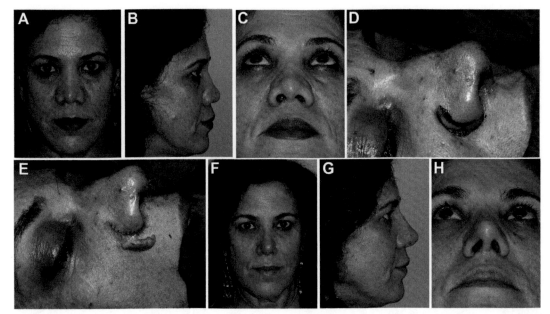

Fig. 22. (*A–C*) This 48-year-old woman was seeking aesthetic improvement of her nose. She has retracted columella, low nasal dorsum, excessively large alar lobule, and alar flaring. (*D, E*) With the open approach, a columellar strut was placed to increase the tip projection and augment the columellar base. A crescentic excision including the cephalic part of the alar lobule was performed. A diced cartilage fascia graft was placed to augment the low dorsum. (*F–H*) The patient is shown 16-months postoperatively. Nasal dorsum is augmented and tip projection is increased with the refinement of the nasal tip. Alar lobules are reduced, alar flaring is corrected, and a better ratio between alar lobule and infratip lateral nasal wall is created. The excision scar in the alar crease is not noticeable.

the scar should be discussed with the patient before the surgery (**Fig. 22**A–H).

Underdeveloped alar lobule

This is a very difficult problem to correct. To augment the alar lobule, a cartilage graft can be placed into the alar lobule. A pocket is prepared in the lobule using delicate scissors through an incision in the alar crease and the cartilage graft is placed into the pocket (**Fig. 23**).

Secondary Deformities

Treatment of secondary deformities of alar base surgery is a challenge.[7,11] In an overly narrowed alar base placement of lateral crural, strut graft can increase nostril flare. Lateral repositioning of alar lobule is the method of treatment in severe deformities. There is no very effective method to augment the overresected alar lobule (**Fig. 24**).

Widenining of Narrow Alar Base and Enlargement of Constricted Nostrils

Constricted nostrils are usually iatrogenic problem that causes severe nasal obstruction. V-Y advancement technique can be used to reposition of alar lobule laterally to widen the nostrils and alar base (**Fig. 25**). Another method to widen the small

nostril is the transpositioning of a flap from the lateral side of the alar lobule (**Fig. 26**).

DISCUSSION

The goal of alar base surgery is obtaining an alar base that is in harmony with the other units of the nose and the other features of the face and symmetric nostrils in proper size and shape. Patients requiring alar base resection may have a variety of alar base configurations. Before alar resection is undertaken, it is important to identify the components of the alar base which should be altered and planning of the resection should be conducted accordingly. The location and amount of excision should be performed depending on the site of excess. If the circumference of the nostril is the optimal size, care should be taken to avoid making the nostril smaller. Nostril shape is another important consideration in the planning of resection. If the nostril shape is ideal, the incision should not be extended into the vestibule of the nostril sill to avoid the distortion of the nostril. When performing an alar wedge resection to correct alar flaring, it is essential to preserve the curvature of the nostril. If the normal curvature of the alar lobule is lost due to excessive excision, this will cause an unnatural appearance of the nose.

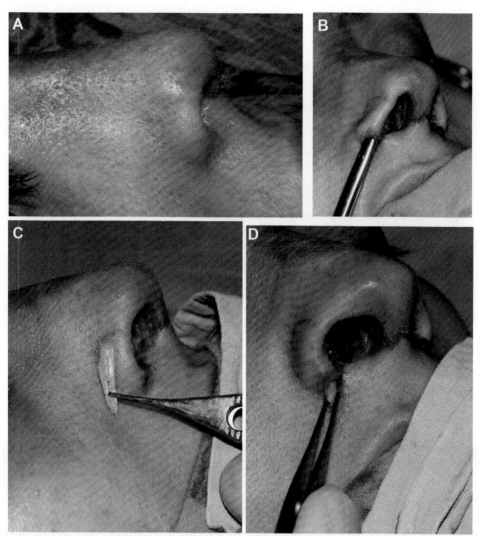

Fig. 23. (*A*) Underdeveloped alar lobule is one of the most difficult deformities to treat. (*B*) An incision in the alar crease was performed, and then a pocket was prepared in the lobule using delicate scissors. (*C*) To augment the alar lobule, a septal cartilage graft was fabricated. (*D*) The cartilage graft was placed into the pocket to augment the alar lobule.

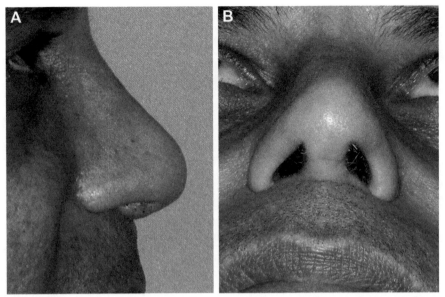

Fig. 24. (*A*, *B*) In this patient, excessive reduction of alar lobule resulted in an unnatural and imbalanced appearance with over straightening of the alar rim.

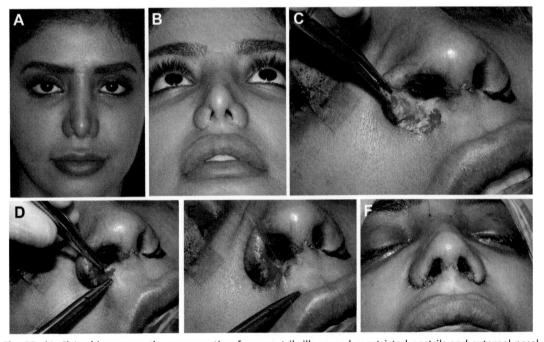

Fig. 25. (*A*, *B*) In this woman, the overresection from nostril sills caused constricted nostrils and external nasal valve obstruction. (*C*) Alar lobule was elevated as a flap with incisions in alar crease and vestibule. (*D*, *E*) The vestibular skin was released and sutured to the skin external side of the nostril sill and the alar lobule was moved laterally with V–Y advancement suture technique. (*F*) The V–Y advancement technique recreated nostril sills and enlarged the nostrils.

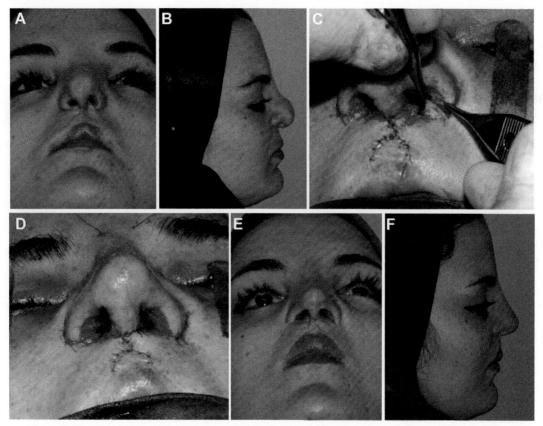

Fig. 26. (*A, B*) Bilateral cleft lip patient who had 4 previous rhinoplasties presented with constricted nostrils. (*C, D*) After structural reconstruction of the nasal tip, a flap from the lateral side of the alar lobule was transposed to the nostril sill. (*E, F*) 2-years postoperative picture shows that a symmetric tip tripod is achieved with enlarged nostrils.

Alar base resections should be executed conservatively because there is no going back after excision is performed and the procedure is irreversible. For a beginner surgeon, it is advisable to do slightly less resection than planned to avoid overresection. If inadequate reduction is performed, further resection can be performed easily under local anesthesia easily in another stage.

SUMMARY

Alar base surgery is one of the integral parts of rhinoplasty operation which is performed to obtain an alar base that is, in harmony with the other units of the nose and the other features of the face and optimize the size and shape of nostrils. Deformities requiring alar base modification include wide nasal base, alar flaring, large nostril size, and asymmetries of nostrils or alae. The location and amount of excision are performed depending on the deformity.

CLINICS CARE POINTS

- Careful analysis of the nasal base and masterful execution of the surgical plan is crucial for a successful outcome.
- Columellar base should be addressed before alar base resections.
- Before alar resection is undertaken, it is important to identify the components of the alar base which should be altered and planning of the resection should be conducted accordingly.
- Alar base resections should be designed meticulously and executed conservatively because there is no going back after excision is performed and the procedure is irreversible.

DISCLOSURE

Adviser, Marina Medical Company, Florida,USA.
Cerkes Video Series, Quality Medical Publishing-
St.Louis-Missouri-USA.

REFERENCES

1. Crumley RL. Aesthetics and surgery of the nasal base. Facial Plast Surg 1988;5:135–42.
2. Constantian MB. An alternate strategy for reducing the large nasal base. Plast Reconstr Surg 1989;83: 41–52.
3. Guyuron B. Alar base abnormalities: classification and correction. Clin Plast Surg 1995;23:263–70.
4. Sheen JH, Sheen AP. Aesthetic rhinoplasty. 2nd edition. St Louis: Quality Medical Publishing; 1998.
5. Adamson PA. Alar base reduction. Arch Facial Plast Surg 2005;7:98.
6. Kridel RW, Castellano RD. A simplified approach to alar base reduction: a review of 124 patients over 20 years. Arch Facial Plast Surg 2005;7:81–93.
7. Guyuron B. Alar base surgery. In: Gunter JP, Rohrich RJ, Adams WP, editors. Dallas rhinoplasty: nasal surgery by the masters. 2nd edition. St Louis: Quality Medical Publishing; 2007.
8. Ahmad J, Rohrich RJ, Lee MR. Aesthetics and surgical refinement of the nasal base. In: Rohrich RJ, Adams WP, Ahmad J, editors. Dallas rhinoplasty :nasal surgery by the masters. 3rd edition. St Louis, Missouri/Boca Raton, Florida: QMP/CRC Press; 2014.
9. Rohrich RJ, Muzaffar AR. Rhinoplasty in African-American patient. Plast Reconstr Surg 2003;111: 1322–39.
10. Toriumi DM. Structure Rhinoplasty: lessons learned in 30 years. Chicago: DMT Solutions; 2019.
11. Sheen JH. Alar resection and grafting. In: Gunter JP, Rohrich RJ, Adams WP, editors. Dallas rhinoplasty: nasal surgery by the masters. 2nd edition. St Louis: Quality Medical Publishing; 2007.
12. Oneal RM. Managing the alar base. In: Gunter JP, Rohrich RJ, Adams WP, editors. Dallas rhinoplasty: nasal surgery by the masters. 2nd edition. St Louis: Quality Medical Publishing; 2007.
13. Foda HM. Nasal base narrowing: the combined alar base excision technique. Arch Facial Plast Surg 2007;9:30–44.
14. Tellioglu AT, Vargel I, Cavusoglu T, et al. Simultaneous open rhinoplasty and alar base excision for secondary cases. Aesthet Plast Surg 2005;29: 151–5.

Complications in Rhinoplasty

Danielle F. Eytan, MD[a],*, Tom D. Wang, MD[b]

KEYWORDS

- Rhinoplasty • Complications • Risks • Challenges • Deformity

KEY POINTS

- Consider individual patient factors to determine the need for antibiotics or topical antimicrobials.
- Treat all hematomas and infections immediately with drainage and antibiotics to avoid and minimize untoward outcomes.
- Overresection of a dorsal hump and inadequate tip support can lead to a variety of deformities that can often be prevented with appropriate surgical techniques.
- Patient counseling around possible complications and expectations is critical in the preoperative discussion and consent process.

INTRODUCTION

Although many complications of rhinoplasty are preventable with good surgical planning and technique, the competent surgeon must be prepared to deal with the range of complications that can result from this complex procedure. Understanding the diagnosis and management of the most frequently encountered complications in rhinoplasty is critical to excellent care.

Complications from rhinoplasty are fortunately relatively rare. A recent database study looking at nearly 5000 rhinoplasties found major complications, defined as those occurring within 30 days of surgery that require an emergency room visit, admission, or surgery, were at an overall rate of 0.7%.[1] Although rare, complications and suboptimal outcomes can be a source for postoperative litigation. In fact, rhinoplasties are among the most litigated procedures in facial plastic surgery.[2] One study found that 80% of lawsuits after rhinoplasty were due to suboptimal esthetic outcomes, whereas 40% were attributed to poor functional outcomes.[3] A thorough and honest informed consent process has been critically identified as key to

minimizing litigation should complications occur and highlights the importance of open communication between surgeons and patients about the possible risks inherent in this complex procedure.[4]

DISCUSSION

Although not a comprehensive list, this discussion delves into further detail on some of the more commonly encountered or notable complications of rhinoplasty. These complications are divided into early, late, and technical complications.

Early Complications

These complications tend to present within the first week after surgery.

Postoperative hemorrhage/hematoma

Bleeding-related complications such as epistaxis or hematoma are the most common complications encountered following rhinoplasty, with incidence reported to be 0.2% to 6.7%.[1,4,5] Bleeding is most commonly from traumatized nasal mucosa and incision sites and typically responds well to head elevation, topical decongestants such as oxymetazoline, and nasal pressure to the anterior septum as

The authors have no conflicts of interest to disclose.
[a] Division of Facial Plastic & Reconstructive Surgery, Department of Otolaryngology-Head and Neck Surgery, New York University School of Medicine, 222 E 41st Street, 8th. Floor, New York, NY 10017, USA; [b] Division of Facial Plastic & Reconstructive Surgery, Department of Otolaryngology-Head and Neck Surgery, Oregon Health and Science University, 3181 Southwest Sam Jackson Park Road, SJH01, Portland, OR 97239, USA
* Corresponding author.
E-mail address: danielle.eytan@gmail.com

Clin Plastic Surg 49 (2022) 179–189
https://doi.org/10.1016/j.cps.2021.07.009
0094-1298/22/© 2021 Elsevier Inc. All rights reserved.

needed. Packing with absorbable (Surgicel, Gel-foam, NasoPore) or nonabsorbable (Rhinorocket, Merocel) options can be used and removed in 2 to 4 days if necessary. If bleeding persists despite this, trauma to a branch of the sphenopalatine artery must be considered. Such serious bleeding is uncommon and occurs in less than 1% of patients.[6]

In recent years, there has been growing interest in the use of tranexamic acid, an antifibrinolytic agent, to reduce bleeding in a variety of surgical procedures. Evidence for its role in rhinoplasty has emerged as well, with studies showing a decrease in intraoperative bleeding, as well as improvement in postoperative periorbital ecchymoses and edema with administration of a preoperative dose.[7–9] Some studies have also introduced the idea of using desmopressin (DDAVP) in low doses for routine bleeding in rhinoplasty, although this is not common practice.[10,11]

Hematomas of the nasal soft tissues or the septum following rhinoplasty must be drained, which can typically be done in the office. If untreated, soft tissue hematomas can lead to fibrosis and risk causing contour irregularities.[12] If located in the septal mucosal pocket, hematomas can lead to cartilage necrosis, loss of dorsal support, and a saddle nose deformity.

Infection

The overall rate of infection following rhinoplasty is reported to be 0% to 4% in the literature.[1,4,5] Infection following rhinoplasty can range from a mild soft tissue cellulitis to an abscess, or ultimately to a severe complication such as brain abscess or meningitis, although exceedingly rare (**Fig. 1**). Cellulitis can be adequately treated with oral antibiotics and observation, whereas suspected abscesses of the soft tissue envelope or septum require drainage and potentially intravenous antibiotics. Although rare, an untreated septal abscess can lead to cavernous sinus thrombosis and additional sequelae, such as meningitis and brain abscess.

The use of perioperative antibiotics in rhinoplasty has continued to be a source of variability among surgeons. Although many rhinoplasty surgeons use antibiotics in the perioperative setting, the details of duration and benefits are not clearly known. Some advocate for prophylactic antibiotics with a single preoperative dose or for 3 perioperative doses as opposed to a postoperative antibiotic course, noting that no significant difference in postoperative infection rates has been shown in prospective studies.[13,14] The current guidelines for rhinoplasty from the American Academy of Otolaryngology–Head and Neck Surgery do recommend against routinely prescribing postoperative antibiotics for greater than 24 hours.[15] However,

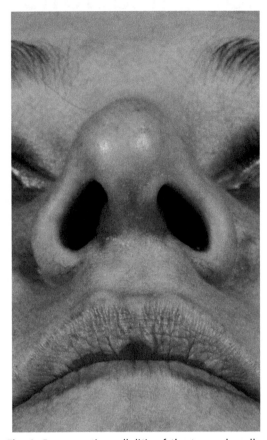

Fig. 1. Postoperative cellulitis of the transcolumellar incision; this was successfully treated with a course of oral antibiotics with full resolution.

they do note exceptions to this guideline, including revision or complicated surgery, patients with baseline colonization of methicillin-resistant *Staphylococcus aureus* (MRSA), extensive cartilage grafting, immunocompromised patients, concurrent medical conditions requiring antibiotics (such as rhinosinusitis), or nasal packing.

Nasal packing is used by some surgeons to aid in postsurgical hemostasis and assist with septal healing. Although limited to rare case reports, the use of nasal packing has been rarely linked to toxic shock syndrome.[16–21] In these reports, onset of toxic shock syndrome after surgery was rapid with symptoms including nausea, fever, tachycardia, hypotension, and need for intensive care. Treatment has included systemic antibiotics and supportive care. Given these reports, there has been ongoing controversy on the need and benefit of prophylactic antibiotics in the setting of nasal packing. A recent meta-analysis with 990 patients showed no significant difference in infection rate in patients treated with or without antibiotics.[22] Without an obvious benefit to treatment, the surgeon must carefully weigh the associated risks of prophylactic antibiotics if nasal packing is used.

MRSA, however, is a unique exception that requires special consideration. Many patients are colonized by methicillin-sensitive *S aureus* (MSSA), whereas a certain percentage of healthy patients harbor the more virulent MRSA and are at risk for more aggressive infection following rhinoplasty. The incidence of colonization of MSSA and of MRSA in the US population has been reported at approximately 28.6% and 1.5%, respectively.[23] This rate is known to be higher in health care workers or those who have been recently admitted to a hospital or residential care facility, reaching as high as 15% in some studies.[24–26] Meanwhile, data have shown that patients who are colonized with MRSA do indeed have a 4-fold higher incidence of clinical infection.[27] Mupirocin ointment has been shown to be 97% effective in reducing nasal carriage of both MSSA and MRSA, and preoperative treatment with mupirocin was shown to reduce infection rates by 50% in general surgery procedures.[28] Given these findings, a preoperative 5-day course of topical treatment with mupirocin ointment to the nasal vestibules and perioperative antibiotics has been suggested for patients undergoing rhinoplasty who are deemed at high risk for MRSA colonization.[28,29]

Complications associated with rib cartilage use

Rib cartilage is a valuable asset to rhinoplasty surgery but brings additional potential for complications that must be discussed with patients and considered in surgical planning and management. Both homogeneous irradiated rib cartilage and autologous rib cartilage carry risk. Complications with autologous rib cartilage use are related to both donor site issues and, more often, recipient site issues. In a systematic review including 21 studies evaluating rates of complications with autologous costal cartilage done in 2015, pooled donor site complications were identified at a rate of 3.2%, whereas recipient site complications were 11.4%.[30]

The most serious complication at the donor site is pneumothorax (0.1%), whereas pleural tears and breeches without pneumothorax are more frequently reported (0.6%). The most common long-term donor site complication was scarring, reported in 2.9%. Techniques to address and minimize donor site complications have been described. To improve safety and prevent pneumothorax or pleural breech, conservative harvest techniques in which only a central segment of costal cartilage is removed have been described.[31,32] To minimize the impact of any scarring, using a limited incision length or selecting an inframammary incision can be beneficial, particularly in female patients.

Recipient site complications tend to be more common yet less severe, although they can affect long-term functional and cosmetic outcomes of the rhinoplasty itself. The most frequently reported recipient site complications in the literature were warping (5.2%), infection (2.5%), graft resorption (0.9%), displacement or extrusion (0.6%), and graft fracture (0.2%).[30]

Warping refers to distortion of the cartilage, which can ultimately lead to changes in the nasal structure requiring revision surgery. This complication is seen both in autologous rib cartilage grafts and donated irradiated rib grafting and thus has been frequently studied. Some studies suggest a decrease in warp rates with increasing patient age, related to an increase in calcification of the cartilage.[33] The carving plane, level of costal cartilage harvest, and oppositional suturing techniques have all failed to show any effect on warping.[34] There are several suggested approaches to minimize this complication, with the primary method involving immersing the grafts in saline for delayed use to evaluate for warping. This method has a varied range of reported warp rates in the literature, with the mean rate found to be 3.08% in a meta-analysis of 10 studies done by Wee and colleagues.[35] Differential approaches to carving of the cartilage have also been described, with primary methods including concentric carving[36] and oblique carving.[37–39] In 2013 Tastan and colleagues[38] first described this technique of oblique carving of grafts at a 30° to 45° angle from the long axis of the rib and had no incidences of warping in his 43 patients initially studied using this approach. Later studies comparing the concentric and oblique split carving techniques have demonstrated equivalent rates of warp.[39]

Soft tissue complications

Soft tissue complications after rhinoplasty are typically minor, consisting of localized and temporary issues such as acne or dermatitis. Contact dermatitis related to adhesives used for nasal taping and dressing applications can be observed, and all patients should be queried for any known adhesive allergies before surgery.[40,41] If encountered, this can typically be managed with topical cortisone and gentle cleansing (**Fig. 2**).

In rare occasions, however, the devastating complication of skin necrosis can occur, with reported incidence of 1.7%.[4] Skin necrosis can result from an improper plane of dissection, overly aggressive thinning of the subcutaneous layer,

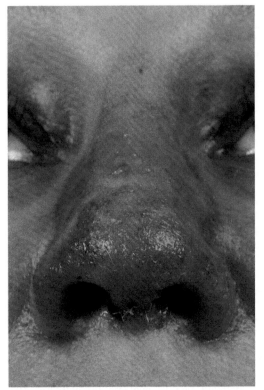

Fig. 2. Contact dermatitis in a patient due to Mastisol liquid adhesive. This condition resolved with topical cortisone cream and gentle cleaning.

excessively tight closure or dressing application, inadequately treated postoperative infection, or patient smoking (**Fig. 3**A–D). Treatment may require a range of approaches, from local wound care to major reconstruction, depending on the severity and extent.

Understanding the nasal anatomy is critical to maintaining a safe tissue dissection plane. There are 5 layers above the bony and cartilaginous framework of the nose, including the skin, superficial areolar layer, fibromuscular layer, deep areolar layer, and perichondrial/periosteal layer.[42] The blood supply is found in the deep fat layer above the nasal superficial musculoaponeurotic system, and thus dissection must occur below this layer to maintain safe perfusion of the soft tissue.[42,43] In patients with thick nasal skin, defatting or thinning of the soft tissue envelope is often used to help achieve a more desirable and defined outcome. However, this must be done conservatively to maintain adequate blood supply. Vascular compromise can also occur without sacrifice of the vessels directly, but by either excessive internal or external compression. Internal compression can be seen with significant dorsal augmentation approaches, with rare cases reported.[44] Alternatively, external

compression from tight nasal taping and splinting, most frequently with metal splints, has been associated with nasal skin necrosis as well.[45,46] It has thus been suggested that the more malleable thermoplastic splints with pores in it can better accommodate postoperative edema and prevent excessive compression.

Finally, patient factors can contribute to soft tissue complications. Most notably, heavy smoking is a known factor in impaired wound healing.[47] A thorough social history must be taken in the preoperative evaluation, and if the surgeon is to offer rhinoplasty to a smoking patient, the possibility of wound healing complications must be adequately addressed in the patient's preoperative counseling. The rhinoplasty surgeon must thus be acutely aware of patients' smoking history and factor this into their surgical decision making when considering use of the higher-risk techniques of soft tissue debulking or significant dorsal augmentation.

Late Complications

Late complications tend to occur in the weeks to months following surgery, and oftentimes even years later. These complications are often more gradual in onset and present in continued follow-up with patients. Rhinoplasty must always be performed with care and thought given to the long-term success of the procedure both for functional and esthetic outcomes.

Unfavorable scarring

There are limited data regarding unfavorable scarring in rhinoplasty, but available data report incidence rates of 0% to 7%.[5,48,49] Unfavorable scarring includes hypertrophic scarring and keloids, hyperpigmentation, or notching irregularities. As in other areas of the body, certain patients are predisposed to hypertrophic scarring, especially those with darker skin pigmentation or a personal or family history of scarring. Closure must be meticulous and tension free to minimize this complication. If keloids do occur, they can be treated as they would at other locations with intralesional steroid and/or 5-fluorouracil injections.

Patient dissatisfaction

As with any operative procedure, appropriate patient selection and preoperative counseling is critical to set patient expectations appropriately. Full discussion of the risks, benefits, and potential complications of rhinoplasty is necessary. Thorough discussion and understanding of the possible need for additional procedures to achieve the patient's desired outcome is important. Expected changes over long-term course should be addressed. **Fig. 4**A,B demonstrates a patient who

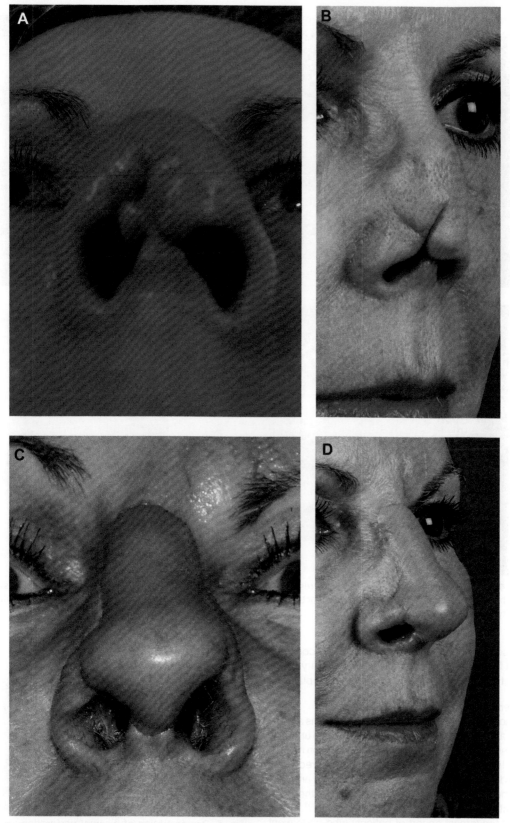

Fig. 3. Patient presented with skin necrosis due to inadequately treated postoperative infection after primary rhinoplasty (*A,B*). Postoperative photographs after undergoing paramedian forehead flap reconstruction of the defect (*C,D*).

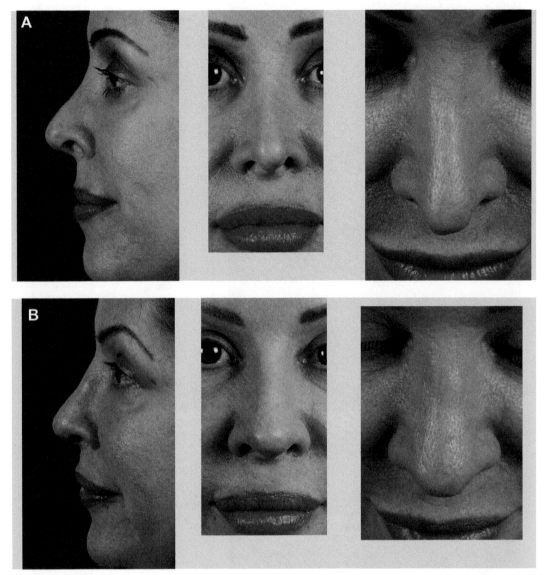

Fig. 4. Patient dissatisfaction related to overresection with pinched tip, alar retraction, nostril asymmetry, loss of the brow-tip esthetic lines, and bilateral functional airway obstruction (*A*). Two years following revision rhinoplasty to address her concerns (*B*).

presented with dissatisfaction with both cosmetic and functional outcomes following a primary rhinoplasty and 2 years following revision rhinoplasty.

Need for revision

Although many postoperative complications are minor and transient, some do lead patients to undergo revision, or, secondary rhinoplasty. Revision rates in the literature vary widely, but are most frequently cited at 0% to 10%.[5,50] Most revisions are performed to address cosmetic concerns rather than functional ones.[5] Spataro and colleagues[51] evaluated the largest cohort of patients who underwent primary rhinoplasty, 172,324 in total from 3 large

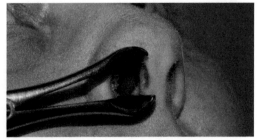

Fig. 5. Demonstration of a septal perforation visible on anterior rhinoscopy.

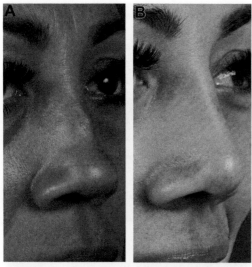

Fig. 6. Saddle nose deformity from prior septorhinoplasty (*A*). Postoperative photograph following reconstruction using autologous costal cartilage grafting (*B*).

state databases, and found a 3.1% rate of revision at 3 years follow-up. The investigators identified independent risk factors to be female sex, younger age, history of anxiety or autoimmune disease, and

surgery for cosmetic or congenital deformities. There is evidence that approximately 30% of patients who undergo revision rhinoplasty within 5 years of their primary procedure change their surgeons, thus suggesting that surgeon-reported revision rates may be underestimating the true value.[52] Understanding these factors may help the surgeons in their own self-assessment in efforts to improve patient satisfaction.

Technical complications

Septal perforation

As septoplasty is commonly performed with rhinoplasty, septal perforation is a known possible complication (**Fig. 5**). The reported incidence rates of septal perforation in the literature vary from 0% to 2.9%.[4,5] This complication typically results from opposing mucosal tears obtained during cartilage harvest. Prudent dissection of the mucoperichondrial flap to avoid unnecessary tears, as well as closure of at least one side in the case of any opposing tears, will help to prevent this complication.

Saddle nose deformity

The saddle nose deformity is a known manifestation of middle vault collapse (**Fig. 6**A,B). This

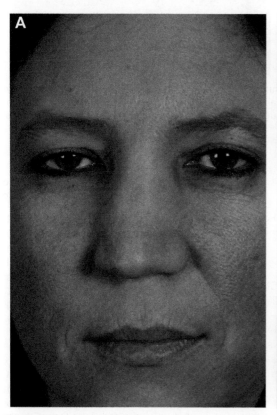

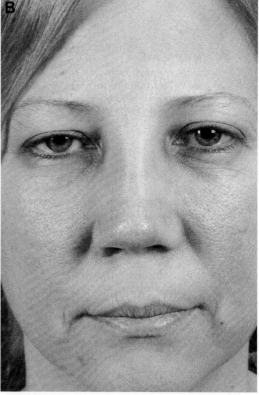

Fig. 7. Wide open roof deformity following previous septorhinoplasty with inadequate medialization of the nasal bones (*A*). Postoperative photograph following bilateral lateral osteotomies to close the open roof (*B*).

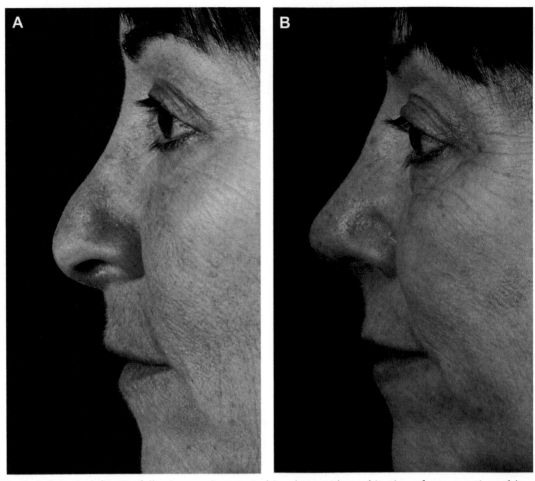

Fig. 8. Pollybeak deformity following previous septorhinoplasty with combination of overresection of bony dorsum, inadequate reduction of cartilaginous dorsum, and loss of tip projection (*A*). Postoperative photograph demonstrating correction of deformity including slight augmentation of bony dorsum, reduction of cartilaginous dorsum, and increased tip projection (*B*).

deformity is commonly due to loss of middle vault support following overly aggressive septorhinoplasty, or septal perforation resulting from iatrogenic, neoplastic, infectious, or granulomatous etiologies.[53,54] Careful consideration of remaining middle vault support is required during septoplasty to prevent iatrogenic collapse. Correction and prevention require restoration of the dorsal-caudal support using grafting materials, frequently from costal cartilage or other sources.[55]

Open roof deformity
As one of the most common aims for rhinoplasty, removal of a dorsal hump can seem a simple task to both patients and surgeons alike. However, care must be taken to prevent postoperative functional and esthetic deformities in the process. The open roof deformity is a well-known deformity that

can result after dorsal hump reduction (**Fig. 7**A,B). In an open roof deformity, following resection of the bony dorsum, the nasal bridge appears flat and wide, in a trapezoidal shape. This appearance is a result of gaps remaining between the septum and each nasal bone. To correct this, lateral osteotomies must be performed and adequate medialization of the nasal bones must be ensured. Incomplete osteotomies that do not allow for full mobilization of the bones will lead to persistent open roof and unsatisfactory outcomes.

Inverted V deformity
The inverted V deformity is another complication that can result from dorsal hump resection and osteotomies. Aggressive resection can lead to dissociation of the upper lateral cartilages from the caudal margin of the nasal bones, which then

creates the shadow effect for which the deformity is named. To maintain the natural brow-tip esthetic line, spreader grafts and suture resuspension of the upper lateral cartilages to the septum are important; this will help prevent the inferomedial migration of the upper lateral cartilages and avoid development of the inverted V. Patients with decreased middle vault support due to short nasal bones and long upper lateral cartilages tend to be predisposed to development of this deformity, and additional care must be taken with these cases.

Pollybeak deformity

The pollybeak deformity is a frequently encountered technical complication and accounts for up to 40% to 64% of revision rhinoplasties in some series.[56–58] This deformity is caused by the relative underprojection of the nasal tip compared with the projection of the dorsum and can thus result from multiple causes (**Fig. 8**A,B). Most frequently, insufficient lowering of the cartilaginous dorsum, particularly at the anterior septal angle, is the culprit. Alternatively, failure to restore adequate tip support can lead to eventual tip ptosis and the appearance of pollybeak. It is thus critical to adequately assess the dorsal height following resection and redraping of the soft tissue in rhinoplasty, as well as to restore the disrupted tip support mechanisms. Alternatively, postoperative pollybeak deformity can also result from development of scar tissue in the supratip region following dorsal reduction; this can often be addressed with localized steroid injections in the office, thereby avoiding the need for revision rhinoplasty.[59]

Rocker deformity

The rocker deformity is a complication following osteotomies in which the nasal bone inferior to the osteotomy sinks relative to the bone superior to the cut. This deformity may occur when osteotomies are carried out superior to the medial canthus. In these cases, steps must be taken to camouflage the often visible bony step off or replace the bone and wait until the bone heals before attempting further osteotomy.

SUMMARY

Fortunately, complications following rhinoplasty are fairly uncommon and can often be avoided. Appropriate patient selection, counseling, and preoperative planning, meticulous technique, and close postoperative management are the keys to successful outcomes. Surgeons must be aware of the range of possible complications to provide adequate patient counseling and be competent in their identification and prompt management should they arise.

CLINICS CARE POINTS

- When preparing patients for rhinoplasty, possible early and late complications should be thoroughly reviewed as part of the consent process.
- Patients with a history of MRSA should be treated with a preoperative course of topical mupirocin and/or systemic antibiotics.
- Routine antibiotics do not need to be given to all patients undergoing uncomplicated rhinoplasty, but should be reserved for complex or revision cases under surgeon discretion.
- When harvesting costal cartilage for grafting, the perichondrium on the deep surface of the cartilage should be carefully dissected and preserved to maintain adequate pleural coverage.
- Any pleural breech during costal cartilage harvest should be repaired immediately, with postoperative imaging to confirm that pneumothorax is not present.

REFERENCES

1. Layliev J, Gupta V, Kaoutzanis C, et al. Incidence and preoperative risk factors for major complications in aesthetic rhinoplasty: analysis of 4978 patients. Aesthet Surg J 2017;37(7):757–67.
2. Svider PF, Keeley BR, Zumba O, et al. From the operating room to the courtroom: a comprehensive characterization of litigation related to facial plastic surgery procedures. Laryngoscope 2013;123(8):1849–53.
3. Razmpa E, Saedi B, Safavi A, et al. Litigation after nasal plastic surgery. Iran J Otorhinolaryngol 2011; 23(65):119–26.
4. Heilbronn C, Cragun D, Wong BJF. Complications in rhinoplasty: a literature review and comparison with a survey of consent forms. Facial Plast Surg Aesthet Med 2020;22(1):50–6.
5. Sharif-Askary B, Carlson AR, Van Noord MG, et al. Incidence of postoperative adverse events after rhinoplasty: a systematic review. Plast Reconstr Surg 2020;145(3):669–84.
6. Cochran CS, Landecker A. Prevention and management of rhinoplasty complications. Plast Reconstr Surg 2008;122(2):60e–7e.
7. McGuire C, Nurmsoo S, Samargandi OA, et al. Role of tranexamic acid in reducing intraoperative blood loss and postoperative edema and ecchymosis in primary elective rhinoplasty: a systematic review and meta-analysis. JAMA Facial Plast Surg 2019; 21(3):191–8.

8. Ghavimi MA, Taheri Talesh K, Ghoreishizadeh A, et al. Efficacy of tranexamic acid on side effects of rhinoplasty: a randomized double-blind study. J Craniomaxillofac Surg 2017;45(6):897–902.

9. De Vasconcellos SJDA, Do Nascimento-Júnior EM, De Aguiar Menezes MV, et al. Preoperative tranexamic acid for treatment of bleeding, edema, and ecchymosis in patients undergoing rhinoplasty a systematic review and meta-analysis. JAMA Otolaryngol Head Neck Surg 2018;144(9):816–23.

10. Gruber RP, Zeidler KR, Berkowitz RL. Desmopressin as a hemostatic agent to provide a dry intraoperative field in rhinoplasty. Plast Reconstr Surg 2015; 135(5):1337–40.

11. Haddady-Abianeh S, Rajabpour AA, Sanatkarfar M, et al. The hemostatic effect of desmopressin on bleeding as a nasal spray in open septorhinoplasty. Aesthet Plast Surg 2019;43(6):1603–6.

12. Teichgraeber JF, Russo RC. Treatment of nasal surgery complications. Ann Plast Surg 1993;30(1): 80–8.

13. Andrews PJ, East CA, Jayaraj SM, et al. Prophylactic vs postoperative antibiotic use in complex septorhinoplasty surgery: a prospective, randomized, single-blind trial comparing efficacy. Arch Facial Plast Surg 2006;8(2):84–7.

14. Rajan GP, Fergie N, Fischer U, et al. Antibiotic prophylaxis in septorhinoplasty? A prospective, randomized study. Plast Reconstr Surg 2005;116(7): 1995–8.

15. Ishii LE, Tollefson TT, Basura GJ, et al. Clinical practice guideline: improving nasal form and function after rhinoplasty executive summary. Otolaryngol Head Neck Surg 2017;156(2):205–19.

16. Allen S, Liland J, Glew R. Toxic shock syndrome associated with use of latex nasal packing - PubMed. Arch Intern Med 1990;150(12):2587–8.

17. Toback J, Fayerman JW. Toxic shock syndrome following septorhinoplasty: implications for the head and neck surgeon. Arch Otolaryngol 1983; 109(9):627–9.

18. Barbour S, Shlaes D, Guertin S. Toxic-shock syndrome associated with nasal packing: analogy to tampon-associated illness - PubMed. Pediatrics 1984;73(2):163–5.

19. Mansfield CJ, Peterson MB. Toxic shock syndrome: associated with nasal packing. Clin Pediatr (Phila) 1989;28(10):443–5.

20. Hull HF, Mann JM, Sands CJ, et al. Toxic shock syndrome related to nasal packing. Arch Otolaryngol 1983;109(9):624–6.

21. Jacobson JA, Kasworm EM. Toxic shock syndrome after nasal surgery: case reports and analysis of risk factors. Arch Otolaryngol Neck Surg 1986; 112(3):329–32.

22. Lange JL, Peeden EH, Stringer SP. Are prophylactic systemic antibiotics necessary with nasal packing? A systematic review. Am J Rhinol Allergy 2017; 31(4):240–7.

23. Gorwitz RJ, Kruszon-Moran D, McAllister SK, et al. Changes in the prevalence of nasal colonization with Staphylococcus aureus in the United States, 2001-2004. J Infect Dis 2008;197(9):1226–34.

24. Ibarra M, Flatt T, Van Maele D, et al. Prevalence of methicillin-resistant staphylococcus aureus nasal carriage in healthcare workers. Pediatr Infect Dis J 2008;27(12):1109–11.

25. Lucet J-C, Grenet K, Armand-Lefevre L, et al. High prevalence of carriage of methicillin-resistant staphylococcus aureus at hospital admission in elderly patients: implications for infection control strategies. Infect Control Hosp Epidemiol 2005;26(2):121–6.

26. Eveillard M, Martin Y, Hidri N, et al. Carriage of methicillin-resistant staphylococcus aureus among hospital employees: prevalence, duration, and transmission to households. Infect Control Hosp Epidemiol 2004;25(2):114–20.

27. Safdar N, Bradley EA. The risk of infection after nasal colonization with staphylococcus aureus. Am J Med 2008;121(4):310–5.

28. Angelos PC, Wang TD. Methicillin-resistant staphylococcus aureus infection in septorhinoplasty. Laryngoscope 2010;120(7):1309–11.

29. Abuzeid WM, Brandt MG, Moyer JS, et al. Methicillin-resistant staphylococcus aureus–Associated infections following septorhinoplasty. Facial Plast Surg 2012;28(3):354–7.

30. Varadharajan K, Sethukumar P, Anwar M, et al. Complications associated with the use of autologous costal cartilage in rhinoplasty: a systematic review. Aesthet Surg J 2015;35(6):644–52.

31. Lee M, Inman J, Ducic Y. Central segment harvest of costal cartilage in rhinoplasty. Laryngoscope 2011; 121(10):2155–8.

32. Boyaci Z, Çelik Ö, Ateşpare A, et al. Conservative costal cartilage harvest for revision septorhinoplasty. J Craniofac Surg 2013;24(3):975–7.

33. Balaji S. Costal cartilage nasal augmentation rhinoplasty: study on warping. Ann Maxillofac Surg 2013;3(1):20.

34. Farkas JP, Lee MR, Lakianhi C, et al. Effects of carving plane, level of harvest, and oppositional suturing techniques on costal cartilage warping. Plast Reconstr Surg 2013;132(2):319–25.

35. Wee JH, Park MH, Oh S, et al. Complications associated with autologous rib cartilage use in rhinoplasty: a meta-analysis. JAMA Facial Plast Surg 2015;17(1):49–55.

36. Kim DW, Shah AR, Toriumi DM. Concentric and eccentric carved costal cartilage: a comparison of warping. Arch Facial Plast Surg 2006;8(1):42–6.

37. Loghmani S, Loghmani A, Maraki F. Oblique split rib graft surgery in primary and secondary septorhinoplasty. World J Plast Surg 2019;8(2):237–44.

38. Tastan E, Yucel OT, Aydin E, et al. The oblique split method: a novel technique for carving costal cartilage grafts. JAMA Facial Plast Surg 2013;15(3): 198–203.

39. Wilson GC, Dias L, Faris C. A comparison of costal cartilage warping using oblique split vs concentric carving methods. JAMA Facial Plast Surg 2017; 19(6):484–9.

40. Ezeh UE, Price HN, Belthur MV. Allergic contact dermatitis to mastisol adhesive used for skin closure in orthopedic surgery: a case report. J Am Acad Orthop Surg Glob Res Rev 2018;2(9):e037.

41. Mabrie DC, Papel ID. An unexpected occurrence of acute contact dermatitis during rhinoplasty. Arch Facial Plast Surg 1999;1(4):320–1.

42. Oneal RM, Beil RJ. Surgical anatomy of the nose. Clin Plast Surg 2010;37(2):191–211.

43. Saban Y, Amodeo CA, et al. An anatomical study of the nasal superficial musculoaponeurotic system surgical applications in rhinoplasty, vol. 10, 2008. Available at: www.liebertpub.com. Accessed February 20, 2021.

44. Eskitascioglu T, Kemaloglu AC. Skin necrosis in nasal dorsum following rhinoplasty. Eur J Plast Surg 2010;33(1):49–51.

45. Mrad MA, Almarghoub MA. Skin necrosis following rhinoplasty. Plast Reconstr Surg Glob Open 2019; 7(2):e2077.

46. Bilgen F, Ince B, Ural A, et al. Disastrous complications following rhinoplasty: soft tissue defects. J Craniofac Surg 2020;31(3):809–12.

47. Silverstein P. Smoking and wound healing. Am J Med 1992;93(1A):22S–4S.

48. Foda HMT. External rhinoplasty for the Arabian nose: a columellar scar analysis. Aesthet Plast Surg 2004; 28(5):312–6.

49. Kim HC, Jang YJ. Columellar incision scars in asian patients undergoing open rhinoplasty. JAMA Facial Plast Surg 2016;18(3):188–93.

50. Christophel JJ, Park SS. Complications in rhinoplasty. Facial Plast Surg Clin North Am 2009;17(1): 145–56.

51. Spataro E, Piccirillo JF, Kallogjeri D, et al. Revision rates and risk factors of 175 842 patients undergoing septorhinoplasty. JAMA Facial Plast Surg 2016; 18(3):212–9.

52. Crawford KL, Lee JH, Panuganti BA, et al. Change in surgeon for revision rhinoplasty: the impact of patient demographics and surgical technique on patient retention. Laryngoscope Investig Otolaryngol 2020;5(6):1044–9.

53. Lee JJ, Hong SD, Dhong HJ, et al. Risk factors for intraoperative saddle nose deformity in septoplasty patients. Eur Arch Otorhinolaryngol 2019;276(7): 1981–6.

54. Hamilton GS. Dorsal failures: from saddle deformity to pollybeak. Facial Plast Surg 2018;34(3):261–9.

55. Kim J, Kim CH, Oh JH, et al. Saddle deformity after septoplasty and immediate correction. J Craniofac Surg 2020;31(1):e62–5.

56. Vuyk HD, Watts SJ, Vindayak B. Revision rhinoplasty: review of deformities, aetiology and treatment strategies. Clin Otolaryngol Allied Sci 2000; 25(6):476–81.

57. Kamer FM, McQuown SA. Revision rhinoplasty: analysis and treatment. Arch Otolaryngol Neck Surg 1988;114(3):257–66.

58. Foda HMT. Rhinoplasty for the multiply revised nose. Am J Otolaryngol 2005;26(1):28–34.

59. Hanasono MM, Kridel RWH, Pastorek NJ, et al. Correction of the soft tissue pollybeak using triamcinolone injection. Arch Facial Plast Surg 2002; 4(1):26–30.

Nonsurgical Rhinoplasty

Rod Rohrich, MD[a,b], Brendan Alleyne, MD[c],*, Matthew Novak, MD[a],
Justin Bellamy, MD[a], Edward Chamata, MD[a,b]

KEYWORDS

- Liquid rhinoplasty • Nasal filler • Nonsurgical rhinoplasty

KEY POINTS

- As the center of the facial canvas, the nose is one of the first areas to draw attention at a conversational distance. Particularly in the era of social media, not only is it the frontal view that is important but also the basal and side profiles that draw increased attention. For these reasons, surgical correction of nasal deformity is frequently sought.
- Patients often request nonsurgical rhinoplasty because of lessened cost and downtime, as well as the concept of "try it before you buy it," where patients would like to see what a surgical rhinoplasty may look like before embarking on a costly and irreversible surgery.
- Given the inherent risk of vascular compromise as well as blindness that has been described in nonsurgical rhinoplasty, expert consultation is warranted.
- Knowledge of the nasal vascular anatomy and danger zones is critical to providing safe use of hyaluronic acid fillers to address cosmetic concerns.

 Video content accompanies this article at http://www.plasticsurgery.theclinics.com.

INTRODUCTION/HISTORY/DEFINITIONS/BACKGROUND

Nonsurgical rhinoplasty has been increasingly sought by patients in the last several years (**Figs. 1–7**, Video 1).[1] The use of hyaluronic acid offers a temporary and relatively safe method for addressing minute and specific nasofacial disharmony. Patients should, however, be counseled regarding the limitations of the procedure.[2–4] Filler cannot directly address, for instance, a wide bony dorsum. It also cannot properly address imperfections in a large nose, as, by adding volume, inherently the nose is made even bigger. Patients need to understand limitations such as these in order to make sure they appropriately realize the goal of liquid rhinoplasty.

Currently, hyaluronic acid fillers are the most common products used in liquid rhinoplasty.[5–7] Permanent substances, such as free silicone, are no longer recommended and are known to cause granulomas and distant migration without respect to tissue planes.

More recently, fat augmentation as also been used, typically at the time of surgical facial rejuvenation, but the principles can be completed under local anesthesia as well.[8,9] Even more recently, fat and platelet-rich fibrin have been shown to augment the nasal soft tissue envelope.[10]

DISCUSSION

The indications for nonsurgical rhinoplasty are small, specific nasal deformities that are safely amenable to camouflage by the addition of filler. Patients with large noses baseline or with severe deformity throughout the nose are better addressed with surgical rhinoplasty. Using mirror-feedback during the procedure can guide the use of fillers and allow the goals of the patient to be fully realized by the surgeon. Personnel using hyaluronic acid fillers need to be trained in the use

[a] Dallas Plastic Surgery Institute, 9101 North Central Expressway, Suite 600, Dallas, TX 75231, USA; [b] Division of Plastic Surgery, Baylor College of Medicine, Houston, TX, USA; [c] Renaissance Plastic Surgery, 145 Saint Peters Centre Blvd, Saint Peters, MO 63376, USA
* Corresponding author.
E-mail address: Brendan@RPSplasticsurgery.com

Clin Plastic Surg 49 (2022) 191–195
https://doi.org/10.1016/j.cps.2021.08.005
0094-1298/22/Published by Elsevier Inc.

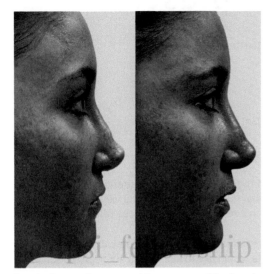

Fig. 1. Twenty-four-year-old woman with 3 prior nasal traumas. (*left*) Preprocedure supratip deformity with partial collapse of caudal mid vault. (*right*) Following nonsurgical rhinoplasty (use of 0.4 cc Juvaderm XC).

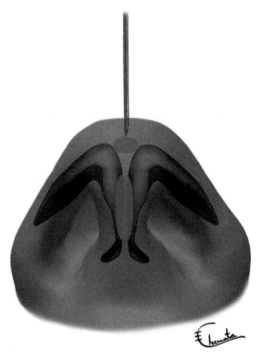

Fig. 3. Basal view of supra-perichondrial depot injection of the tip and columella. (*Courtesy of* Edward Chamata, MD, Houston, TX.)

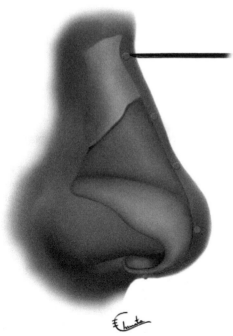

Fig. 2. Five-point technique showing lateral view of supra-perichondrial depot injection of the radix, dorsum, supratip, tip, and columella. (*Courtesy of* Edward Chamata, MD, Houston, TX.)

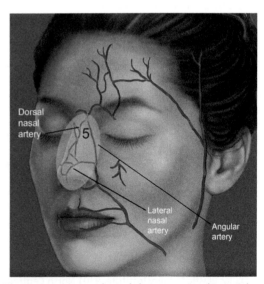

Fig. 4. Anatomy and nasal danger zones. (*From* Scheuer JF 3rd, Sieber DA, Pezeshk RA, Gassman AA, Campbell CF, Rohrich RJ. Facial Danger Zones: Techniques to Maximize Safety during Soft-Tissue Filler Injections. Plast Reconstr Surg. 2017 May;139(5):1103-1108; with permission.)

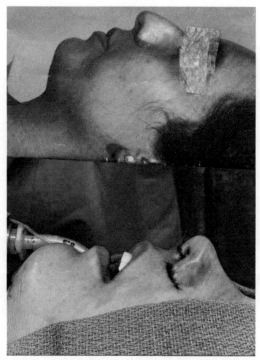

Fig. 5. Preoperative (*top*) and postoperative (*bottom*) view of patient following open rhinoplasty and removal of permanent liquid filler along dorsum and columella, which was an attempt to correct a dorsal hump.

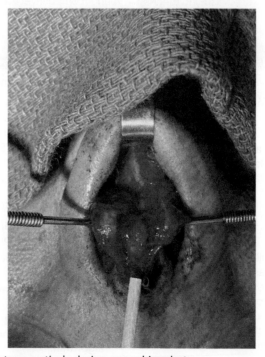

Fig. 6. Bellafill filler found intraoperatively during open rhinoplasty.

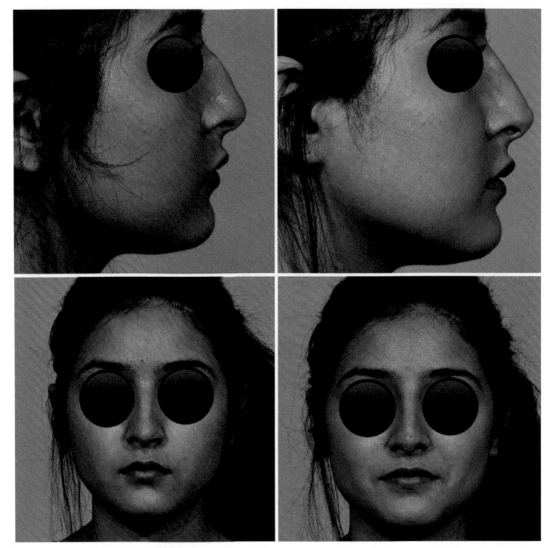

Fig. 7. Patient with bony dorsal convexity (*left*) and after injection of 0.3 cc Restylane (*right*) through Rod J Rohrich 5-Point Liquid Rhinoplasty Technique.

of hyaluronidase protocols and to have a heightened awareness for vascular compromise signs and symptoms, as immediate early intervention is paramount.[11–13]

SUMMARY

In summary, nonsurgical filler-based rhinoplasty can offer patients a less invasive, more affordable, and temporary means of addressing specific nasal deformities. Patients should be counseled regarding the inherent vascular risks. It is pivotal to set realistic patient expectations and to assess these goals several times throughout the procedure.

CLINICS CARE POINTS

- Set realistic patient expectations with what goals can and cannot be attained from nonsurgical injection of filler.
- Stay deep and medial when injecting all fillers in the nasal area.
- Be aware of signs and symptoms of vascular compromise.
- All personnel need training with hyaluronidase as part of an appropriate tissue-rescue algorithm.

DISCLOSURE

Dr R. Rohrich receives instrument royalties from Eriem Surgical, Inc, and book royalties from Thieme Medical Publishing. The remaining authors have no financial interests to declare in relation to the content of this article. No funds were received or used for the research reported in this article.

SUPPLEMENTARY DATA

Supplementary data to this article can be found online at https://doi.org/10.1016/j.cps.2021.08.005.

REFERENCES

1. Moon HJ. Use of fillers in rhinoplasty. Clin Plast Surg 2016;43(1):307–17.

2. Rohrich RJ, Agrawal N, Avashia Y, et al. Safety in the use of fillers in nasal augmentation-the liquid rhinoplasty. Plast Reconstr Surg Glob Open 2020;8(8): e2820.

3. Moon HJ. Injection rhinoplasty using filler. Facial Plast Surg Clin North Am 2018;26(3):323–30.

4. Bertossi D, Lanaro L, Dorelan S, et al. Nonsurgical rhinoplasty: nasal grid analysis and nasal injecting protocol. Plast Reconstr Surg 2019;143(2):428–39. https://doi.org/10.1097/PRS.0000000000005224. Erratum in: Plast Reconstr Surg. 2019 Aug;144(2): 538. PMID: 30531619.

5. Segreto F, Marangi GF, Cerbone V, et al. Nonsurgical rhinoplasty: a graft-based technique. Plast Reconstr Surg Glob Open 2019;7(6):e2241.

6. Rosengaus F, Nikolis A. Cannula versus needle in medical rhinoplasty: the nose knows. J Cosmet Dermatol 2020. https://doi.org/10.1111/jocd.13743.

7. Brito ÍM, Avashia Y, Rohrich RJ. Evidence-based nasal analysis for rhinoplasty: the 10-7-5 method. Plast Reconstr Surg Glob Open 2020;8(2):e2632.

8. Durand PD, Hogan SR, Lamaris GA, et al. Distant migration after clandestine silicone injections: how far is too far? Dermatol Surg 2017;43(7):983–7.

9. Sieber DA, Scheuer JF 3rd, Villanueva NL, et al. Review of 3-dimensional facial anatomy: injecting fillers and neuromodulators. Plast Reconstr Surg Glob Open 2016;4(12 Suppl):e1166.

10. Kovacevic M, Kosins AM, Göksel A, et al. Optimization of the soft tissue envelope of the nose in rhinoplasty utilizing fat transfer combined with platelet-rich fibrin. Facial Plast Surg 2021. https://doi.org/10.1055/s-0041-1723785.

11. Bertossi D, Giampaoli G, Verner I, et al. Complications and management after a nonsurgical rhinoplasty: a literature review. Dermatol Ther 2019; 32(4):e12978.

12. Philipp-Dormston WG, Goodman GJ, De Boulle K, et al. Global approaches to the prevention and management of delayed-onset adverse reactions with hyaluronic acid-based fillers. Plast Reconstr Surg Glob Open 2020;8(4):e2730.

13. Lee W, Oh W, Oh SM, et al. Comparative effectiveness of different interventions of perivascular hyaluronidase. Plast Reconstr Surg 2020;145(4):957–64.

Moving?

Make sure your subscription moves with you!

To notify us of your new address, find your **Clinics Account Number** (located on your mailing label above your name), and contact customer service at:

Email: journalscustomerservice-usa@elsevier.com

800-654-2452 (subscribers in the U.S. & Canada)
314-447-8871 (subscribers outside of the U.S. & Canada)

Fax number: 314-447-8029

Elsevier Health Sciences Division
Subscription Customer Service
3251 Riverport Lane
Maryland Heights, MO 63043

ELSEVIER

Printed and bound by CPI Group (UK) Ltd, Croydon, CR0 4YY

08/05/2025

01864704-0007